Bioethics Yearbook

VOLUME 3
THEOLOGICAL DEVELOPMENTS IN BIOETHICS:
1990-1992

Bioethics Yearbook

VOLUME 3

Bioethics Yearbook

VOLUME 3
THEOLOGICAL DEVELOPMENTS IN BIOETHICS:
1990-1992

THE CENTER FOR ETHICS, MEDICINE AND PUBLIC ISSUES
Baylor College of Medicine
The Institute of Religion
Rice University
Houston, Texas, U.S.A.

Edited by

B. Andrew Lustig, *Senior Editor*
Baruch A. Brody, *Director*
H. Tristram Engelhardt, Jr.
Laurence B. McCullough

SPRINGER SCIENCE+BUSINESS MEDIA, B.V.

ISBN 978-0-7923-2555-0   ISBN 978-94-011-1886-6 (eBook)
DOI 10.1007/978-94-011-1886-6

ISSN 0926-261X

Printed on acid-free paper

TABLE OF CONTENTS

INTRODUCTION

The Center for Ethics, Medicine, and Public Issues, in conjunction with Kluwer Academic Publishers, is pleased to offer this third volume in our series of Bioethics Yearbooks. The Yearbook series alternates between a biennial volume tracing recent theological discussion on topics in bioethics and a biennial volume tracing recent regional discussions in bioethics. Volume One surveyed theological developments from 1988 through 1990. The present volume continues that survey for the period from 1990 through 1992.

In this volume, as in Volume One, we have invited scholars of recognized expertise to chronicle and, if they wish, to interpret recent bioethical discussions in the following religious traditions: Roman Catholicism, the Latter-day Saints, Hinduism, the Anglican Communion, Eastern Orthodoxy, Islam, Lutheranism, Buddhism, Methodism, Baptist-Evangelicalism, Judaism, and the Reformed Tradition. Readers of Volume One will note that we have expanded our coverage in a number of areas. For example, in addition to the authors from Volume One who are again covering Protestant discussions, Drs. Theo Boer and Egbert Schroten have contributed an excellent essay on Protestant developments in continental Europe. For this and subsequent theological volumes, Dr. Kathleen Nolan has assumed duties as commentator on Buddhist developments. Her masterful essay offers both a timely overview of recent Buddhist contributions to bioethics and a broader discussion of Buddhist sources that are generally under-reported to Western readers. In response to suggestions from readers of Volume One, we also invited commentary on Seventh-Day Adventist, Pentecostal, and liberal Jewish developments for this volume. Unfortunately, the scholars we enlisted for those chapters were not able to meet the deadline we must honor to assure the timely publication of each yearbook in the series. However, we hope to include coverage of those traditions, and perhaps others, in Volume Five.

As before, in order to retain a uniformity to the discussions within this volume, as well as among volumes in the series, we have asked our authors to order their remarks, as much as possible, according to the following list of topics: new reproductive technologies, abortion, maternal-fetal conflicts, care of severely disabled newborns, consent to treatment and experimentation, confidentiality, equitable access to health care, ethical concerns raised by cost-containment measures, decisions to withhold or withdraw life-sustaining treatment, assisted suicide and active euthanasia, the definition of death, and organ donation and transplantation. As with Volume One, each author has addressed only those topics on the list that have been recently discussed in his or her tradition. In addition, authors were free to comment on issues not on the list in a final broad category designated "other issues".

Each biennial theological Yearbook is an effort to meet the need for a

B. Andrew Lustig (Sr. Ed.), Bioethics Yearbook: Volume 3, vii-ix.
©1993 Kluwer Academic Publishers.

single volume that provides comprehensive and timely summaries of discussions in a number of religious traditions on specific topics in bioethics. We have commissioned our expert commentators to trace recent trends and developments in their respective traditions – both formal statements by official bodies and study groups, and less formal discussions that reflect currents of thought in the continuing dialogue on particular issues. At the same time, we again left it to the discretion of our authors to place 1990-1992 developments in broader context by including those background documents and discussions they deemed necessary to clarify recent concerns.

Besides offering up-to-date summaries of recent developments, our authors have also provided useful bibliographical references to a wide array of documents, many of which would otherwise prove difficult for individuals to know about, much less to assemble. As always, we invite our readers to contact us with advice on ways to improve and expand the range of resources upon which our authors may draw in subsequent theological volumes.

Both similarities and differences in theological method and in conclusions on particular topics will be noted between and among the religious traditions our authors cover. The interested reader may therefore be tempted to muse about larger matters of fundamental theology or ecclesiology to account for such agreement and divergence. But an immediate word of caution is clearly in order. A yearbook, if successful, achieves the important but limited purpose its name implies. This volume is offered primarily as a summary and analysis of recent theological discussion on specific topics. For scholars and others interested in seeing how more fundamental theological themes and approaches may play themselves out on particular issues, this volume may serve to exemplify those tendencies in concrete fashion. But it should not be misinterpreted as an effort to discuss issues of foundational theology or ecclesiology in other than incidental fashion.

Two other substantive points about Volume Three are in order. First, certain authors, in their respective assignments, sometimes report on the same documents and discussion on particular issues. For example, Drs. Boer and Schroten, in their summary of European Protestant developments, discuss a number of Lutheran documents that Paul Nelson also analyzes in his essay on the Lutheran tradition. In such cases, the different vantages of our commentators may lead to subtle differences in perspective that we trust will make such overlap instructive rather than redundant.

Second, although some commentators have a great deal that is new to report on, official discussion in other traditions has been relatively modest. In the latter cases, we have encouraged our commentators to reflect more broadly, according to their own lights, on the possible implications of fundamental themes for particular bioethical issues. For example, Dr. Courtney Campbell, in a very creative essay, discusses the theology of embodiment set forth in the Latter-day Saint tradition and its relevance to a number of disputed issues. As a second example, Dr. Prakash Dasai, the principal author of the essay on

Hindu developments, emphasizes the need to safeguard human dignity as a central value, both in political efforts to end the religious strife between Hindus and Muslims in India and in the more focused discussions of bioethics. As both these examples attest, the slower pace of recent official discussion in some traditions has not prevented those commentators from making important contributions to Volume Three.

As is always true with a volume of this kind, the overall quality of the yearbook depends primarily on the quality of the individual efforts of its contributors. We trust that the scholarship of our authors will be evident. But in less obvious ways, the professional courtesy and responsibility of our authors has made the editing of Volume Three relatively easy. As with preceding volumes, we owe special thanks to Delores D. Smith for her tireless commitment to the daily chores involved in preparing Volume Three for publication.

B. Andrew Lustig, Senior Editor
Baruch A. Brody, Editor, Director of the Center for Ethics
H. Tristram Engelhardt, Jr., Editor
Laurence B. McCullough, Editor

FOREWORD

It is a commonplace to recognize the pluralism of our societies and of many of our institutions. In cities like Houston, people with different cultural and religious traditions are forced to live together – and they are sometimes threatened and frequently enriched by their interaction. In medical centers like the Texas Medical Center doctors and nurses and patients often have different religious convictions – and so integrate health care into different accounts of the deepest significance of their lives, their deaths, their giving birth, their suffering, and their caring for others.

To be sure, in a pluralistic society and in pluralistic institutions, one strategy to enable cooperation and to sustain a peaceable coexistence is secularization, the effort to distance members of a society or partners in the project of health care from their religious roots. But, especially when people face the truth of human mortality or cope with the human vulnerability to suffering, it is clear that those roots still tangle into decisions, still nurture a sense of identity, still support and sustain certain stances with respect to sickness and health. Because this is so, the volumes of *Bioethics Yearbook* which attend to theological traditions are particularly important and practical contributions to medical ethics.

This third volume surveys recent developments in bioethics within major theological traditions. The focus is on the years 1990-1992, but some earlier material is included in order to supplement Volume I, which covered the years 1988-1990. It summarizes the major efforts to reflect about issues in medical ethics in ways that are faithful to particular religious convictions. It also provides bibliographical references to the original documents.

In a diverse society, doctors and nurses – and ethics committees – need a reference book that will help them understand the methods and the results of the religious reflection of particular communities of faith with which particular patients identify. Respect for the embodied integrity of a patient would seem to require nothing less. The patient, after all, is never to be reduced to mere organism nor merely to his or her choice-making capacities. The patient as an embodied self is always related to communities. How, after all, do Mormons think of the body, and how does that understanding condition and challenge the medical care judged appropriate by them or for them? What is the Orthodox Jewish community's halakhic position on whole brain criteria for the determination of death? How are contemporary Roman Catholics thinking about the withdrawal of nutrition and hydration? What do Islamic scholars think about different methods of birth control?

This reference work serves not just health care providers, however, but also the particular communities of faith and their members who want to think with integrity about these issues. The reports provide a way to track developments

B. Andrew Lustig (Sr. Ed.), Bioethics Yearbook: Volume 3, xi-xii.
©1993 Kluwer Academic Publishers.

in particular traditions. How, for example, did Greek Orthodoxy respond to the liberalization of abortion law in Greece? Moreover, the reports facilitate information exchange within traditions. The article by Judith Granbois and David Smith is exemplary in this way; they have undertaken to correspond with representatives of Anglican communities in many parts of the world in order to provide their report, and the report itself enables and calls for further communication within their particular tradition on bioethical issues. Paul Nelson's account of the Lutheran tradition is similarly served by and useful for such an information exchange.

The *Yearbook* will, of course, also be useful for ecumenical discussions. It provides the basis for local efforts at interfaith dialogue which deal candidly with differences while attentive to agreements. The dialogue might consider not just particular decisions and positions but also the different styles and strengths represented by the traditions and these reports about them. Joseph Boyle gives an account of recent Roman Catholic developments and exemplifies the philosophical rigor which is typical of the tradition. Paul Nelson provides a report on the Lutheran tradition and a model of that tradition's concern for confessional integrity, appreciation for ambiguity, and fear of legalism. The articles provide interesting examples of different traditions concerning appeals to scripture, whether Quran, Torah, or New Testament, and different traditions concerning the teaching authority of the religious leadership. Different particular communities can understand both themselves and others better because of this project.

Finally, the work serves the discipline of bioethics by attending to the importance of religious traditions and communities when people with religious convictions face hard moral choices. It is worth remembering that more people belong to some such community than to a philosophical society – and generally take their membership in such a community more seriously.

The undertaking is a critically important and eminently practical one. It may be the case that not every report in this volume is fully worthy of the project. It surely is the case that the reports, even taken together, are not a complete account of religious reflection about medical ethics. Even so, the volume is an enormous contribution to religious communities and their members, to ecumenical conversations, to medical and nursing professionals, to ethics committees, and to the discipline of bioethics. Andrew Lustig has done an excellent job as senior editor to see to it that the volume approaches an excellence worthy of the project. I commend him and the authors of these reports for a most serviceable book. I am proud and pleased, as the director of the Institute of Religion, to introduce it by means of this brief foreword.

Allen D. Verhey
Institute of Religion
Houston, Texas, U.S.A.

THEO A. BOER AND EGBERT SCHROTEN[1]

BIOETHICAL ISSUES IN PROTESTANT CONTINENTAL EUROPE

I. INTRODUCTION

In this essay, we will examine the way that reflection on bioethical issues in Protestant denominations in continental Europe takes place. Our contribution is the first one on this subject in this biennial series. Thus, we will not confine our attention to developments during the last two years, but will provide a somewhat broader overview. We will base our discussion primarily on (semi-) official church documents within and between Protestant denominations.

What do we mean by Protestant denominations in continental Europe? We mean primarily the churches in traditionally Protestant Scandinavian countries (Denmark, Norway, Sweden, and to lesser extent Finland) that have a predominantly Lutheran population; Germany, which is a mixture of Roman Catholic and Lutheran populations, as well as smaller Reformed minorities; Switzerland, which has a strong Reformed (Calvinist and Zwinglian) tradition; France, a predominantly Roman Catholic country with a strong Calvinist tradition; and The Netherlands, where Roman Catholicism and Calvinism play roughly equal parts in a largely secularized society.

For several reasons, this essay does not offer complete coverage. First, our knowledge of Middle- and East-European countries is sketchy, because five or more decades of totalitarian regimes have prevented open and regular ecumenical contacts. Despite recent political developments, such communication has been only partially restored. Second, in many Southern European countries, as well as in Belgium and France, Roman Catholicism is predominant, with Protestant churches usually small minorities. As a result, they may lack the resources necessary for structured reflection on bioethical issues. They may also lack the intellectual habits or theological ambitions for such reflection. Moreover, Protestants in some Roman Catholic countries, depending on their attitudes toward the Roman Catholic Church, may often rely on statements issued by the Roman Catholic Church in their country. Thus, official internal or external Protestant documents in these countries are exceptional.

A third reason for our hesitation to claim completeness in describing Protestant bioethics in continental Europe has to do with the history and present diversity of the continent. We will reflect upon that diversity in Section II. In Section III, we will discuss three main issues in Protestant thinking on

B. Andrew Lustig (Sr. Ed.), Bioethics Yearbook: Volume 3, 1-18.
©1993 Kluwer Academic Publishers.

bioethics. Finally, in Section IV, we will provide a detailed examination of two particular documents: *Becoming Human Beings*, a Dutch report written by the two largest Reformed denominations and the Lutheran church in The Netherlands; and *God is a Friend of Life*, a consensus statement of the Lutheran and Roman Catholic bishops in the Federal Republic of Germany. In future contributions to the Yearbook, we hope to examine a larger range of denominational and ecumenical documents.

II. BIOMEDICAL ISSUES IN A DIVIDED CONTINENT

Unlike the situation in the Roman Catholic Church, most Protestant churches in continental Europe are not part of a hierarchic network in which bioethical issues receive structured reflection. Moreover, unlike the situation in English-speaking countries, linguistic borders in Europe pose serious obstacles to international cooperation and ecumenical reflection. Therefore, many nationally organized Christian denominations, of necessity, organize their own debates on bioethical issues. As a result, many discussions take place on a domestic and denominational level, leaving the outsider with a somewhat confused impression.

A. *The Character of Church Documents*

Because there are few (semi-)official Protestant documents with an international character, discussions generally take place on a domestic level. While the Scandinavian Ecumenical Institute issued several reports in the early 1980s, virtually all recent discussions have been national rather than international in character.

In the various countries, denominations differ about whether or not to make official statements on bioethical issues. The Danish Lutheran Church, for example, conceives its primary task to be one of bringing the Gospel to the nation, not of issuing official viewpoints on particular bioethical topics. Consequently, religious contributions to the national debate on these questions come entirely from individuals. By contrast, in Norway the Lutheran Church tends to adopt a more active role in influencing public discussion. The Norway Lutheran synod, in a report concerning the value of environment, biotechnology and abortion, states that "it is the task of the church to supply on the basis of God's word the ethical premises that underlie jurisdiction" ([19], p. 19). The Norwegian Lutheran Bishops have also issued a report on human values at the boundaries of life ([2]) and a report about the positive and negative aspects of prenatal screening methods [30]. Most recently, the Norwegian Ecumenical Council has issued a report on questions concerning genetics [20].

In Sweden, most official ecclesiastical positions on bioethical issues tend to be ecumenical in character. During the last ten years, these reports have been almost exclusively reactions to legislative proposals or to statements of parliamentary advisory boards. Reports have been issued on abortion, the concept of death, transplantation, genetic integrity [28], homosexual relationships, the use of force in psychiatry, the use of fetal tissue, withdrawal of life-sustaining treatment, and prenatal diagnosis [29].

The Netherlands has a large number of Protestant denominations, many of which have issued statements on bioethical issues that are primarily addressed to their own church members. However, the two largest Protestant denominations, the Netherlands Reformed Church and the Reformed Churches in The Netherlands, also attempt to influence the national debate on bioethical issues. Both denominations have actively cooperated in writing a number of reports, including the following: a report on the morality of abortion (taking a "no, unless" position) [21]; a report on the theological, moral and pastoral aspects of euthanasia [22]; a report on embryo research, reproductive techniques, and prenatal diagnosis [23]; and, in preparation, a report on the moral and pastoral aspects of decisions involving severely handicapped newborns [24]. In addition, in 1989, *Remonstrantse Broederschap*, a relatively small Arminian denomination, issued a report on reproductive techniques [26].

The German discussion in the 1980s has been dominated by questions concerning reproductive and genetic techniques, but attention has also been paid to organ transplantation. In 1985, the Protestant Church of Western Germany (the *Evangelische Kirche in Deutschland* or EKD) edited a brochure on reproductive techniques, surrogate motherhood, and genetic counseling entitled *Von der Würde werdenden Lebens* ("On the Value of Incipient Life")[7]. The brochure stressed that human life from the moment of conception must be adequately protected because the embryo, from the first cell division onward, is destined to be a person, implying that it has the same ethical value as a fetus. This brochure was followed, and its position reaffirmed, in the 1987 document *Achtung vor dem Leben* ("Respect for Life"), in which criteria for genetic technology and reproductive technology were formulated [8].

In 1988, the Department for the Study of Theology of the Lutheran Church in the German Democratic Republic (East Germany) issued a report on the possibilities and risks of genetic engineering [1]. After the fall of the Berlin wall and the reunification of the two German states, the Protestant Church, which had been separated since 1968, agreed to reunite. Since that agreement, no separate reports on bioethical issues are being edited on either side of the former borderline.

In 1989, the EKD, in close collaboration with the German Roman Catholic Bishops Conference, published a declaration on fundamental and practical questions concerning human responsibility to protect life [9]. We will discuss that declaration in Section IV-B below. In 1990, the same churches issued a treatise on organ transplantation [10]. In 1991, a study was published by the EKD on ethical questions posed by genetic technology and its applications to microorganisms, plants, and animals [11]. In 1992, the German Evangelical Alliance published recommendations for legislation on genetic analysis and its applications [6] .

In Switzerland, the Protestant churches are working together in the Federation of Swiss Protestant Churches (FSPC). The Institute for Social Ethics of the Federation, through its working committee on bioethics, has published a report on in vitro fertilization [16] and a report on procreative techniques and human genetics [18]. It has also issued a report on certain theological and ethical aspects of prenatal diagnosis [17]. In the autumn of 1992, the FSPC issued a notice on the patenting of organisms [14]. In the notice, the FSPC urged that intellectual property be protected in a way that would uphold the justified claims of developing countries and prevent the exploitation of nature. The FSPC also expressed support for a political initiative which would change the Swiss constitution to facilitate the legal protection of animals, plants, and organisms from misapplied reproductive and genetic technologies.

In 1987, the Protestant Federation of France published a text entitled *Biologie et Ethique: Eléments de Réflection* ("Biology and Ethics: Elements of Reflection")[12]. The text espoused a rather liberal position with regard to fertilization techniques, sexuality, procreation, and prenatal diagnosis. France is a Catholic country, although very secularized. It is interesting, therefore, to note that the Preamble characterizes the text not as an "instruction" (like the Vatican's *Donum Vitae*) but as "elements of reflection". So far as we know, there are no other official Protestant documents from France, although the Federation recently issued a statement supporting legislation on ethical issues in the biomedicine [13].

As we conclude this overview, which has focused on (semi)official documents of the Protestant churches in continental Europe, we should also refer our readers to two larger volumes (in German) that provide further detailed information about Protestant bioethics in Europe ([15] and [27]).

B. *The Character of the Arguments: Religious or Humanistic?*

Generally speaking, the arguments about bioethical issues in the documents can be divided into two categories. First, there are those derived directly from religious sources or convictions, such as Scripture or other authoritative sources in the Christian tradition. Second, there are arguments that make no explicit reference to religious sources. The reasons for the second type of argument may be principled or practical in nature. Some church documents presuppose a congeniality between Christian and humanistic thought in Western culture, and thus are strongly opposed to separating Christian and non-Christian arguments. An example of this may be found in Sweden where, despite secularization, the Swedish Church views society as deeply influenced by Christian standards. The epistemology of right norms and values is not seen as confined to confessing Christians, but is a matter of consensus in which everyone may have his or her say. Many documents allow for specifically

Christian contributions to medical ethics, but the latter serve mainly as additions to a rational-humanistic groundwork. In Norway, by contrast, there has recently been a tendency to make explicit reference to Scriptural arguments in bioethical discussion, even in documents meant as contributions to the public debate.

On the other hand, the omission of explicitly religious arguments may be a matter of practical or strategic choice. Although many would say that the deepest epistemological ground of ethics must be found in Revelation, a number of Protestant churches consider the use of such arguments a serious hindrance to an open and wide-ranging national debate on bioethical issues. The arguments they prefer to make generally take the form of appeals to common sense or common experience. Their arguments may also exhibit a consequentialist or even utilitarian character, as in appeals made to the common interest.

C. *The Character of the Documents*

With regard to the character of the documents issued by Protestant denominations in Europe, one should distinguish documents meant to be official viewpoints of a denomination on a particular issue from those that have the less formal character of a contribution to the ongoing debate. An example of the first can be found in the German declaration, "God is a Friend of Life" [9]. The Dutch report, "Becoming Human Beings", is an example of the second category [23]. It passed the synods of the issuing churches only because of its character as an overview and a general commentary on various issues. Although some positions taken in the document may lack the support of a large number of synod members, the synods have given the document an important status by accrediting it as a "contribution to the discussion".

D. *The Place of the Debate*

In many countries, the discussion of theological perspectives on bioethical issues takes place within or between churches. Political parties and social organizations in these countries make less explicit use of religiously based arguments. Instead, religious arguments tend to be made by individuals, groups, or representatives of denominations within parties and organizations. Generally speaking, such is the case in the Scandinavian countries, and the resemblance with the United Kingdom and the United States is obvious.

In other countries, however, there are denominational influences not only on individual persons and their arguments, but also on the structures of political parties and social organizations. In these countries (roughly speaking, all Western European Countries except Scandinavia, Great Britain, and Ireland), health care institutions and their affiliated research institutes have an explicit confessional basis.[2] Theologically informed discussions of bioethical issues are thus not confined to church denominations but also occur in professional organizations. Such discussions may be advantageous because debates are held "on the spot". In addition, professional organizations with a denominational foundation can contribute in their own right (*i.e.*, not necessarily by means of their churches) to national debates on the ethics of health care.[3]

III. MAIN TOPICS IN THE BIOETHICAL DEBATE

Despite national variations, it is possible to recognize certain patterns of discussion that are common to most countries and denominations. In recent years, challenges have arisen mainly from three major developments in medical care and research.

A. *Issues at the Beginning of Life*

1. *Abortion*

The issue of abortion, which in most European churches seemed to be settled a decade ago, has during the last few years gained renewed prominence. Its higher profile has been caused by increasing capacities to perform "therapeutic" or "selective" abortion based on prenatal diagnostic indications. In debating which prenatal indications might serve to justify selective abortion, broader questions arise regarding the morality of common liberal abortion practice. An example of this may be found in a Swedish report [29] that provides commentary on a parliamentary document discussing prenatal diagnosis. The title of the parliamentary document indicates the tenor of its discussion: *Den gravida kvinnan och fostret: två individer* ("The Pregnant Woman and the Fetus: Two Individuals"). Another example is the Dutch report *Mensen in Wording* ("Becoming Human Beings"), described in Section IV.A below [23].

2. *New Reproductive Technologies*

New fertilization techniques, such as in vitro fertilization, embryo transfer, artificial insemination by husband or donor, and surrogate motherhood, have given rise to discussion about the connections between sexuality and procreation, and, in the case of donated gametes, about the desirability of involving non-marital partners in the process of procreation. Because of the immense consequences that such choices may have on marital relationships (and thus on the broadly held view of the family as the corner stone in society), it is not surprising that almost every major Protestant denomination has issued one or more reports on these issues. Generally, the documents express approval of new fertilization techniques so long as they are used in stable heterosexual relationships. Doubts (if not disapproval) are expressed about the use of donated gametes on a number of grounds: because of the monogamous character of matrimony, because mankind should respect the course of nature, because of concern for the mental well-being of the future child, and because of a particular vision of God's providence. Similarly, surrogate motherhood is generally disapproved of. The documents also express doubts about the morality of benefitting from methods that have been developed as the result of morally suspect experiments with human embryos. Most of the reports, however, appear to take the existence of the techniques now available more or less for granted (or see them as blessings). In some cases, this position is qualified by the belief that the techniques should have been developed by means that would not have involved experimentation on human embryos. Most documents agree one should avoid creating "spare embryos" when employing in vitro fertilization.

3. *Human Genetics*

The discussion of human genetics is in a very tentative phase. Long-term efforts to analyze the human genome have created anthropological questions about human identity and about the relationship between freedom and determinism. The discussion has focused most concretely on the consequences of genetic screening. Questions are raised about the use of genetic knowledge to substantiate criminal records, and the use of knowledge about a person's genetic predispositions in applications for employment and insurance. A number of denominations have tried to reach tentative conclusions. Nonetheless, actual developments and future possibilities remain open to question, leaving most churches with the sense either that they are premature in their judgments or always lagging behind developments that take their own course. Still, documents generally express disapproval of the manipulation or modification of the human germ line. However, opinions vary about the legitimacy of somatic gene therapy.

B. *Terminal Illness and Euthanasia*

1. *Withholding/Withdrawing Treatment*

New techniques have made diagnosis more reliable and treatment often more effective. In the process, the expectations and demands placed upon health care professionals have increased steadily, and faith in medical science may have become exaggerated. Christians, then, are challenged to take a benevolent yet critical view toward medical techniques. Their view should be benevolent, because physicians are seen to contribute positively to human well-being. Thus, in many debates in European churches, doubts about the direction of modern medical science are commonly preceded by an explicit statement of gratitude for its possibilities and blessings, and physicians are not generally suspected of any bad intentions. However, Protestant denominations also urge that a critical view be taken toward medical science. Some speak of exaggerated expectations about the possibilities of medical science, and about an unwarranted faith in "medical" solutions to problems that may be primarily emotional or spiritual in nature.

The debate on the appropriate limits of medical treatment has become especially urgent in the discussion of terminal illness. In such cases, some recommend that medical treatment should be foregone in favor of a more natural process of dying. The longer one is kept alive by "artificial" treatment methods, the stronger grows the conviction that medical science tends to transgress its "natural" or otherwise appropriate means and purposes.

2. Euthanasia

The development of medical science prompts many discussions about the proper way to die in an environment that is more and more characterized by medical technique. In several European Protestant churches, this has resulted in internal church debates about euthanasia, i.e., ending the life of a patient by active means. In the Scandinavian countries, Protestant churches have pleaded against the legalization of euthanasia. In Germany, churches are uncertain about putting the issue on the agenda at all. In Europe, the Dutch Reformed churches have gone the farthest. They view euthanasia as an accepted practice in The Netherlands. Their standpoint recognizes the Biblical notion that life is a gift of God, which should not be at the disposal of men. However, they provide for the possibility that, in some cases and under strict conditions, the choice for active euthanasia may be justifiable. Those conditions include the informed consent of the patient, the second opinion of another physician, the presence of a terminal illness, and irreversible and unbearable suffering [22]. More recently, a committee of the Protestant churches has written a report on severely handicapped newborns, which has not yet passed the synods. In that report, the issue is raised as to whether non-voluntary euthanasia may be morally defensible (involuntary euthanasia is rejected under all circumstances). The answer tends to a careful "no, unless"[24].[4]

C. The Provision of Health Care For All

In most European countries, in contrast to the United States, national governments exert a relatively large influence on the way that their systems of health care function. As a result, most European national health care systems operate on a principle of solidarity. According to this principle, large differences in treatment and treatment options for different income groups are considered unjustifiable. Access to necessary medical care for all groups and individuals, despite differences in finances and/or personal characteristics, is the core commitment of this broadly shared concept of health care.

Nonetheless, in being confronted by sharply increasing costs and by the need to reduce national expenses, many governments have been forced to reassess the structure of their health care systems. The unification of Europe, which may imply long-term adjustments of national health care systems to international standards, has given rise to discussions about which health care system should be considered normative. Moreover, the collapse of world socialism may make a new discussion about the responsibility of national governments for the health and well-being of their citizens appropriate.

As a result, almost every Western and Eastern European country has begun to debate the questions: "What sorts of medical therapy and care should, under normal circumstances, be granted to all citizens? What do we mean by 'basic' medical care?". These questions are closely linked to questions about the best way to finance the desired system. The introduction of competitive elements in health care systems has been recommended, although this does not imply the abolition of the principle of solidarity in health care. In the public debate, attempts have been made to introduce an element of personal accountability: the person who lives healthily should have a stronger claim to have access to scarce resources than, for example, the person who is an addict. Among the churches, however, the notion of personal accountability as a discriminatory criterion has not received a warm welcome. Both denominational and political contributions to the debate emphasize that health care should remain equally accessible to all, no matter what their finances, family situation, personal history, contribution to society or "guilt" may be.

The conviction that basic medical care should be accessible to all is, in many countries, deeply rooted in the theological notion of non-discriminatory mercy. Thus, the introduction of competitive elements in health care systems is to be allowed only on the condition that improvement in the quality of medical care and financial savings can be accomplished without restricting access.[5]

IV. AN EXAMINATION OF SOME RECENT DOCUMENTS

As mentioned above, a full overview of all bioethical developments in Protestant continental Europe is beyond the scope of this essay. As an alternative to providing an ideological cartography of the various debates, we will instead focus in this section on two key documents.

A. *Mensen in Wording*
("Becoming Human Beings")[23]

A special commission of the theological subcommittees of the two largest Reformed Churches in The Netherlands (*i.e.*, the *Nederlandse Hervormde Kerk* and the *Gereformeerde Kerken in Nederland*) was installed on June 15, 1988 and charged with the task of preparing a document concerning new developments in biomedicine. In particular, questions posed by human reproduction, especially by in vitro fertilization, embryo research, and prenatal diagnosis were to be addressed. In the intervening years, the small Dutch Lutheran Church also took part in the deliberations. The commission spent three years on its task, in early 1992, issued a document to be discussed and eventually authorized by the united synods of the three churches.

The epistemological basis of the document is a mixture of explicit religious arguments derived from Scripture and arguments from the analytical tradition. Chapter One provides a brief account of the confessional foundation for discussing bioethical issues: the ideas that God is the Creator of every individual human being and that the human being is fully a human person only when she lives in community with her Creator and her fellow men. Chapter Two provides general medical-technical information about the new reproductive techniques and practices. Especially important here is the use of the term "pre-embryo" for an embryo up to 20 days. This choice is based upon contemporary medical terminology and does not imply any necessary conclusions about the dignity or value of the pre-embryo and embryo. Chapter Three, the main body of the report, presents ethical positions as concretely as possible within a theological framework. Chapter Four integrates the reflections of Chapter Three and directs them toward the church pastorate. The report concludes with several appendices that provide more factual information about the techniques outlined in Chapter Two.

1. *The Most Important Ethical Positions*

The point of departure for human actions in creation is the call found in Genesis 2:15 for humanity to "till" and to "keep" the garden. Tilling means making use of our own creative capabilities to give our own form to creation. However, mankind, as never before, runs the risk of neglecting to keep and preserve creation by misusing nature for its own ends rather than in accord with God's purposes. This misuse compels us to greater reflection upon our obligations, although it does not mean that humanity should not use its creativity in organizing creation.

a. *The status of the human embryo.* The report states that from conception onward, the human being is more than a mere mass of cells. What distinguishes the human being from the rest of creation is the nature of its relationship to others and to God. The report urges that human life be protected from its inception but does not suggest that there is no distinction between a newly conceived embryo and a developed fetus. Rather, the growth of the human person is a process to which we have a duty of "increasing protectiveness". The majority opinion of the commission is that the pre-embryo deserves some measure of protection but, under certain limited conditions, may legitimately be the object of research. In practice, this position means that scientific research with pre-embryo until the fourteenth day after conception is deemed acceptable under strict conditions; *viz.*, that the research will have a probable positive effect upon the well-being of future generations. Several commission members, however, held the opinion that the use of pre-embryos solely for research is morally unacceptable, because it amounts to a purely instrumental use of individual human life. For these members, the concept of increasing protectiveness does not include the freedom to use embryos for research purposes. It means, instead, that there is no obligation to attempt to save embryos from dying, in contrast to the obligation to save newborn children from dying.

b. *Artificial reproductive techniques.* The confession of the church that God gives life does not necessarily mean that humanity may not make use of artificial reproductive techniques. IVF may be a blessing for a childless couple, although we must guard against excessive expectations. The report raises questions about so-called "special fields of application", such as the donation of gametes or the application of reproductive technologies outside an enduring and heterosexual relationship, but it concludes that a definitive judgment on such matters would be premature at the present time.

c. *Prenatal diagnosis and selective abortion.* The duty to try to prevent handicaps and other deformities is a first priority. However, when a pregnancy is already underway, that guideline may conflict with others, including the value of the human conceptus and the value of solidarity with handicapped people and their families. In general, the interest of the child-in-process should prevail. Therefore, the interruption of pregnancy, based on diagnostic indications, is only justifiable in situations of very severe handicap; *i.e.*, those circumstances that might be said to be "in conflict with life itself". The document states explicitly that this standpoint may have implications for the contemporary liberal practice of abortion in The Netherlands.

B. *Gott ist ein Freund des Lebens*

In 1989, as mentioned above, a declaration was published in Germany by the Council of the EKD and the Roman Catholic Bishops Conference. The title of that declaration, derived from Wisdom 11:26, was *Gott ist ein Freund des Lebens. Herausforderungen und Aufgaben beim Schutz des Lebens* ("God is a Friend of Life. Challenges and Tasks concerning the Protection of Life")[9]. The declaration was supported by all churches that are (guest) members of the Community of Christian Churches in Germany. Therefore, its content may be viewed as a position supported by nearly all Christian churches in Germany.

Essentially, the declaration pleads for a commitment by all people to affirm God's gift of life, which is threatened in numerous ways, and to resist the life-threatening tendencies of society. In its central emphases, the declaration echoes the same themes developed in earlier EKD publications (*e.g.*, [7] and [8]).

The first chapters show how this theme is rooted in the Bible: God is the Creator of life and protects it against chaos and destructive powers, which are closely linked with sin. In a sinful world, where "the whole creation groaneth and travaileth in pain" (Romans 8:22), God reveals himself as a "friend of life." From this perspective, the earth, despite the "dark side" of creation, should be seen as living space for all creatures. The declaration suggests that we should learn again an attitude of wonder toward creation in order to be more respectful. Nuclear technology and genetic technology are clear examples of the extension of human dominion over nature. Since human dominion should foster all life on earth, the churches should support legal efforts to protect the environment.

One chapter is dedicated to the "special value of human life". This value is rooted in the biblical idea of man created in the image of God (Genesis 1:26ff.), an expression meant to emphasize man's exceptional status in nature. The phrase "image of God", however, characterizes not only mankind as a whole but also every individual human being. Every person may see himself or herself as created by God and accepted, in Christ, by God. As such, every human being has a special value and vocation: he or she is called to live in communion with God and to take part in His glory. In this context, the Declaration asserts the unconditional right to life of every human being.

Nonetheless, the question arises as to whether these claims also hold true for prenatal human life. Referring to the findings of modern embryology, the declaration stresses that, from the moment of conception, a living being is developing, and that, from the beginning, the process of development is continuous and not the emergence of something different in kind. Because the embryo is deemed a human individual-in-development, the unborn human being is also an imager of God. As such, it is entitled to the same protection as other human beings. Consequently, the human embryo should not be made the object of manipulation. Although an embryo is undeniably dependent on the life of the future mother, this does not imply that it may be seen as "part" of the mother. Neither our language (e.g., the expression "to come into the world") nor our emotions (e.g., a sense that killing unborn life is "easier" than killing a mature person) should deceive us. Human life must be protected regardless of its state or condition. That human beings are "images of God" does not depend on their qualities but only on God's acceptance. Thus, even if prenatal diagnosis reveals significant fetal anomaly, the fetus retains an unconditional right to life and thus to protection. The declaration acknowledges that saying "yes" to life may be very difficult in such situations, but calls for faithful response to God, who is able to transform a burden into a blessing.

After these remarks, the declaration identifies a number of social spheres where responsibilities for the protection of life are especially clear: upbringing and education, the media, law and jurisprudence, research and technology, the economy, and health care.

The major part of the declaration sets forth five areas that challenge the responsibility to protect life. The fundamental theme of this discussion is that the value of human life will be protected only if any possibility of manipulation is excluded. The five challenges are: (1) embryo research, (2) abortion and the protection of unborn life, (3) handicapped human life, (4) organ transplantation, and (5) the end of human life.

1. *Embryo research*. The declaration reiterates that, from conception onward, embryonic life should be seen as individual human life. As such, the embryo has the same right to be protected as postnatal human life. Given those premises, the conclusion of the declaration is not surprising. Embryo research is permitted insofar as it is benefits the individual embryo; research that damages or destroys the embryo is illicit, regardless of its aims. The value of human life makes it unacceptable to use the embryo in a merely instrumental way for other aims.

2. *Abortion*. Embryos *in vitro* and embryos *in vivo* have the same value, the same right to life, and are worthy of the same protection. Abortion, therefore, is never justifiable. Even in a situation of conflict, every effort should be made to save the fetus along with (and not against) the life of the mother. If, on medical grounds, a choice must be made between the life of the mother and that of the fetus, abortion might be the lesser evil. The churches, in this context, commit themselves to helping to prevent abortions in a number of ways: (a) by strengthening attitudes about responsible sexuality; (b) by deepening people's respect for unborn life; (c) by reforming conditions that hinder the acceptance of unborn life; and (d) by persuading men and women to accept problematic pregnancies. The declaration also recommends political measures (e.g., an increase of aid to children) to minimize the appeal of abortion as an option.

3. *The acceptance of the handicapped*. People with mental or physical handicaps have greater protection than in the past. But the evils of the Nazi past should keep us vigilant. The rights of all individuals, especially the weak and vulnerable, must be protected. The declaration therefore rejects any eugenic population policies. In addition, it calls for a critical attitude towards prenatal diagnosis so that this technique will not undermine people's willingness to accept handicapped individuals.

4. *Organ donation*. The declaration supports organ donation and transplantation because the churches view donation as a way to show love for one's neighbor, even after death. Nevertheless, the declaration acknowledges the delicate problems that donation may present in particular situations and therefore offers no blanket recommendation of the practice.

5. *The end of human life.* The principles of sanctity of life and respect for the autonomy of human beings are both fundamental. Thus, helping terminal patients means helping them to live. This may imply that withdrawal of medical treatment is appropriate in cases when treatment does not extend life but only the process of dying. Still, the declaration stresses that an incurable patient, even if burdensome to other people, retains a fundamental right to life.

The declaration concludes with a number of general admonitions. Christian hope is rooted in the resurrection of Christ. Living in a world marked by sin, we are encouraged by the Gospel to establish signs of God's coming Kingdom, to take the side of God, who is the "Friend of life", and to protect, to the best of our abilities, the lives of other human beings and those of our fellow creatures.

V. SUMMARY REMARKS

Linguistic barriers, as well as national and denominational boundaries, pose serious obstacles to efforts toward international and interdenominational communication in Europe. Nevertheless, the different Protestant European churches have a great deal in common, for they all have dealt with three major issues that have provoked national bioethical debates: (1) issues raised by the manipulation of human life in its earliest stages; (2) issues in terminal care; and (3) the provision of health care for all.

The arguments made in documents issued by Protestant denominations may be divided into three categories. In the first category, documents make an explicit and exclusive reference to Scripture as the basis of their moral positions. In the second category, documents offer arguments based primarily on "rational" or "humanistic" grounds. The second category of argument may embody the view that our moral knowledge can be ascertained by rational means or may be motivated by the practical desire to remain "on speaking terms" with non-Christians. In either case, the absence of explicit references to Scripture does not necessarily mean that Biblical material is considered irrelevant. The majority of documents are in a third category, in that they offer both Scriptural and rationalistic arguments.

In Section IV, we focused on two documents of the German and the Dutch churches, respectively, both of which discuss the subject of responsibility for human life. We conclude that the position of the German churches is more stringent than that of the Dutch churches, especially regarding the use of reproductive technologies. Both documents, however, base their moral positions primarily on Biblical themes.

Center for Bioethics and Medical Law
Utrecht, The Netherlands

NOTES

1. Dr. Theo A. Boer is research fellow at the Center for Bio-Ethics and Medical Law at Utrecht University, The Netherlands. Dr. E. Schroten is professor for Christian ethics at the Theological Faculty of Utrecht University, and Director of the Centre for Bio-Ethics and Medical Law. Correspondence address: Heidelberglaan 2, NL-3584 CS, Utrecht, The Netherlands.
2. In a smaller subdivision of these countries, influential political parties have a Christian or Christian-Democratic basic philosophy. [4] and [5] are examples of documents issued by a Christian-Democratic party.
3. A recent example of this sort of contribution is [3].
4. The issue was raised recently by the Dutch Pediatric Association and the Dutch Medical Association.
5. This opinion has been reached in many documents issued by Christian organizations and political parties, but has, according to our knowledge, thus far not been the subject of official church statements.

BIBLIOGRAPHY

1. Bund: 1988, *Gentechnologie: die neue Macht des Menschen* ("Genetic Technology: the New Power of Man"). Theologische Studienabteilung beim Bund der Evangelischen Kirchen in der DDR. Berlin.
2. Bispemoetet: 1982, Sak 16/82 *"Vern om menneskeverdet i levets grens-esituasjoner"* ("Protection of Human Value at the Boundaries of Human Life"), (manuscript).
3. Boer *et al.*: 1992. *Zorgen met visie. Zorgverlening vanuit christelijk perspectief* ("Caring with Vision. Christian Perspectives on Health Care"). A contribution by the Dutch Christian Association of Health Care Institutions. Kampen, The Netherlands: Kok Publishers.
4. CDA: 1988, *Zinvol Leven. Een christen-democratische bijdrage aan de discussie over draagmoederschap, kunstmatige inseminatie, gift en in vitro fertilisatie* ("Meaningful Life. A Christian-Democratic contribution to the discussion about Surrogate Motherhood, Artificial Insemination, GIFT, and In Vitro Fertilization"), Wetenschappelijk instituut voor het CDA. Den Haag.
5. CDA: 1992, *Genen en Grenzen. Een christen-democratische bijdrage aan de discussie over de gentechnologie* ("Genes and Boundaries. A Christian-Democratic Contribution to the Discussion about Gene Technology"). Wetenschappelijk instituut voor het CDA. Den Haag.
6. DEA: 1992, *Darf nur noch der gesunde Mensch überleben? Sieben Empfehlungen des Hauptvorstandes der Deutschen Evangelischen Allianz zur gesetzlichen Regelung der Anwendung der Genanalyse* ("Can Only

Healthy Humans Survive? Seven Recommendations of the Central Board of the German Evangelical Alliance about the Legal Coordination of the Use of Genetic Screening"), Informationsdienst der DEA, Dokumentation, No. 3, Wetzlar.

7. EKD: 1985, *Von der Würde werdenden Lebens. Extrakorporale Befruchtung, Fremdschwangerschaft und genetische Beratung* ("The Worth of Life in Process: In Vitro Fertilization, Surrogate Motherhood, and Genetic Counselling"). Handreichung der Evangelischen Kirche in Deutschland. Trier.

8. EKD: 1987, *Kundgebung der 7. Synode der Evangelischen Kirche in Deutschland auf ihrer 4. Tagung zur Achtung vor dem Leben* ("Declaration of the Seventh Synod of the Protestant Church in Germany about Respecting Human Life"). EPD-Dokumentation 49/87.

9. EKD: 1989, *Gott ist ein Freund des Lebens. Herausforderungen und Aufgaben beim Schutz des Lebens* ("God is a Friend of Life. Challenges and Tasks in Protecting Life"). Gütersloher Verlagshaus Gerd Mohn, Gütersloh.

10. EKD: 1990, *Organtransplantation.* Gemeinsame Texte 1. Edited by the Church Office of the EKD, Herrenhäuser Strasse 12, 3000 Hannover 21 (Germany).

11. EKD: 1991, *Einverständnis mit der Schöpfung. Ein Beitrag zur ethischen Urteilsbildung im Blick auf die Gentechnik und ihre Anwendung bei Mikroorganismen, Pflanzen und Tieren* ("Accepting Creation. A Contribution to Moral Deliberation concerning Genetic Technology in Microorganisms, Plants, and Animals"). Gütersloher Verlagshaus Gerd Mohn, Gütersloh.

12. FPF: 1987, *Biologie et Ethique. Eléments de Réflexion* ("Biology and Ethics. Elements of Reflection"), *Autres Temps* (Les Cahiers du Christianisme Social), No. 14, pp. 42-46.

13. FPF: 1992, *Bioéthique: la FPF exprime sa satisfaction à l'annonce d'une loi cadre* ("Bioethics: The Federation of Swiss Protestant Churches expresses its consent to a law proposal"), *Réforme*, (Nov. 1), p. 11.

14. FSP: 1992, Schweizerischer Evangelischer Kirchenbund (SEK), Herbst-Abgeornetenversammlung 1992, *Antrag und Bericht zu Motion und Postulaten der Evangelisch-reformierten Synodalverbandes Bern-Jura betreffend Bio-, Gen-, und Fortpflanzungstechnologie.* Bern.

15. Hübner, Jürgen and Schubert, Hartwig von: 1992, *Biotechnologie und evangelische Ethik. Die internationale Diskussion* ("Biotechnology and Protestant Ethics: The International Discussion"). Campus, Frankfurt am Main/New York.

16. ISE: 1987, *In-Vitro-Befruchtung. Technische Möglichkeiten und ethische Perspektiven* ("IVF. Technical Possibilities and Moral Perspectives"). Studien und Berichte aus dem Institut für Sozialethik des SEK, Nr. 37. Bern/Lausanne.

17. ISE: 10/88, Helmut Kaiser, *Unberechenbarkeit des Lebens. Theologische und ethische Aspekte zur pränatalen Diagnostik.* Institut für Sozialethik der SEK. Bern.

18. ISE: 1990, *Fortpflanzungsmedizin und Humangenetik. Ein Beitrag zur Diskussion über die Beobachterinitiative* ("Reproductive Medicine. Contribution to the Discussion"). Studien und Berichte aus dem Institut für Sozialethik der SEK, Nr. 40. Bern/Lausanne.

19. Kirkemötet: 1989, *Vem om livet. Uttalelser om miljövern, abortlovgivning og bioteknologi* ("Caring for Life: Utterances about Environment, Abortion and Biotechnology").

20. Kirkerådet: 1989. *Mer en gener - Utredning om bioteknologi og menneskeverd. Av en arbeidsgruppe oppnevnt av Kirkerådet* ("More than Genes - Examining Biotechnology and Human Value").

21. NHK: 1977, *Wat te denken over abortus provocatus* ("What to Think about Abortion"). Pastoraal geschrift voor de gemeente. Uitgegeven in opdracht van de moderamina der Nederlandse Hervormde Kerk en van de Gereformeerde Kerken in Nederland.

22. NHK/GKN: 1987, *Euthanasie en pastoraat* ("Euthanasia and Pastoral Care"). Leusden.

23. NHK/GKN/ELK: 1992, *Mensen in Wording. Theologische, ethische en pastorale overwegingen bij nieuwe voortplantingstechnieken en prenataal onderzoek* ("Becoming Human Beings: Theological, Moral, and Pastoral Reflections on New Fertilization Techniques and Prenatal Research"). Rapport van de commissie "Biomedische Ethiek" van het Deputaatschap en de Raad voor de Zaken van Kerk en Theologie van de Nederlandse Hervormde Kerk en de Gereformeerde Kerken in Nederland. Leidschendam/Leusden.

24. NHK/GKN: 1993, *Keuze op leven en dood* ("Choosing life or Death"). Leusden, Holland (not yet authorized).

25. Niekerk, K. van Kooten: 1992, *"Die Diskussion in Skandinavien"* ("The Scandinavian Debate"), in [14], pp. 289-378.

26. Remonstrants Vlugschrift: 1989, *Welgeschapen. Vragen over voortplantingstechnieken* ("Well-Created. Questions about Fertilization Techniques"). Een bundeling van bijdragen aan de medisch-ethische conferentie "welgeschapen". Remonstrants Vlugschrift 1.

27. Schubert, Hartwig von: 1992, *Evangelische Ethik und Biotechnologie* ("Protestant Ethics and Biotechnology"). The International Discussion. Campus, Frankfurt am Main/New York.

28. Svenska Ekumeniska Nämnden, Sveriges Frikyroråd, Sveriges Kristna Ungsdomsråd, De Fria Kristna Samfundens Råd (SAMRÅD), Katolska Biskopsämbetet: 1985, *Yttrande över betänkandet Genetisk integritet,* SOU 1984: 88 ("Comment on Parliamentary Report about Genetic Integrity"). Uppsala.

29. Svenska Ekumeniska Nämnden, Sveriges Frikyrkoråd, SAMRÅD,

Svenska Kyrkans Biskopsmöte, Svenska Kyrkans Centralstyrelse, Katolska Biskopsämbetet: 1990, *Yttrande över slutbetänkandet av utredningen om det ofödda barnet* (SOU 1989:51): *Den gravida kvinnan och fostret: två individer. Om fosterdiagnostik. Om sena aborter* ("Comment on Parliamentary Report about the Unborn Child").

30. Utvalg oppnevnt av Bispemoetet: 1982, *Etiske synspunkter på genetisk veiledning og prenatal diagnostikk* ("Ethical Viewpoints about Genetic Counselling and Prenatal Diagnosis"). En utredning av ett utvalg oppnevnt av Bispemoetet, hoesten.

JOSEPH BOYLE

THE ROMAN CATHOLIC TRADITION AND BIOETHICS

I. INTRODUCTION

This essay continues into the period from the middle of 1990 to the middle of 1992 the survey of Catholic writings on bioethics that I prepared for the first volume of this *Yearbook*. The Catholic literature bearing on bioethical issues continues to be extensive. I have used the same principles of selection for this survey as for the first ([8], p. 5).

The development of the Catholic discussion of bioethical issues during the last few years results in this survey having a particularly American slant. This development has been provoked by legal decisions and legislative initiatives in the United States that have led to a substantial commentary by American bishops and theologians. On the issues of withholding treatment, health care reform, and active euthanasia, American Catholics have had to face challenges on a scale that other Catholics have not, and so, not surprisingly, have made some progress not to be found elsewhere in the Church.

Another difference between the situation surveyed here and the survey of two years ago is that there is no ecclesiastical document that presently dominates Catholic concerns in the manner that *Donum Vitae*, the Vatican instruction on reproductive ethics issued in 1987 ([8], p. 6), dominated the period from 1987 through 1990. Discussions framed by the teaching of this document continue to be central to Catholic bioethical debates about abortion, the status of embryos, and fetal tissue transplants. But other issues have emerged as equally important, and although episcopal statements abound, none is as extensive or authoritative as *Donum Vitae*.

Finally, a number of bioethical issues which have not been much discussed by Catholics are beginning to get some attention. Moral issues concerning AIDS and the new possibilities for genetic therapy are the most notable [34]. But the discussion is still very preliminary and so I will not consider those issues here.

II. THE STATUS OF THE PRE-EMBRYO AND THE EMBRYO

Catholic statements and analyses concerning abortion and the treatment of zygotes and embryos continue to multiply. With few exceptions ([20]; [25]), these are of little bioethical interest, because they are exhortations, political statements, or moral directives to politicians. But this literature also includes

B. Andrew Lustig (Sr. Ed.), Bioethics Yearbook: Volume 3, 19-41.
©1993 Kluwer Academic Publishers.

an extensive debate on the status of pre-embryos and embryos.

Donum Vitae set the context for this debate by stating a presumption, held to be indefeasible, that personal existence begins at conception. This is a presumption because it is not possible to determine decisively when the human soul is present, but indefeasible because no further philosophical or scientific evidence could establish that the individual that begins at conception is not a person ([8], p. 7). Norman Ford, in effect, challenges the assertion that underlies this presumption. He argues that there is no human individual until the primitive streak appears, about two weeks after conception ([8], p. 7; [23], p. 64; [33], p. 301).

Ford's position allows for the genetic individuality of the pre-embryo, but denies that before the appearance of the primitive streak there can be developmental individuality or singleness. Before that time, the inner cell mass is not committed to the production of a single individual; its cells remain totipotential ([18], pp. 68-74; [23]; [33], p. 301; [52], pp. 606-614). Thus, it is not a developmental individual.

Ford's critics do not dispute his statement of the facts. Indeed, in the entire Catholic discussion of whether the pre-embryo is an individual, there appears to be only one factual disagreement ([32], pp. 77-78; [52], p. 608). The dispute concerns how to interpret those facts. The critics propose alternative explanations compatible with developmental individuality for phenomena such as twinning and argue, in effect, that mere genetic individuality is not sufficient to account for the organized and purposeful behavior of the pre-embryo, which on Ford's account is more like a community of cells than an individual organism ([11], pp. 93-98; [21], pp. 64-68; [22], pp. 39-48).

Nicholas Tonti-Filippini uses this kind of consideration to argue that new life begins when the sperm loses its identity after penetrating the membrane of the ovum, not sixteen hours later at syngamy when the two sets of chromosomes come together on the metaphase plate for the first time. The identity of sperm and ovum as distinct components disappears when the sperm head is released into the ovum cell; the new cell moves purposefully towards syngamy, and does other things that the sperm and the ovum cannot do. Thus, a new individual already exists ([58]).

It is unlikely that we have heard the final word in the debate between Ford and his critics, in particular about the important practical question of precisely when conception or fertilization occurs. Still, the debate seems well-focused. Perhaps what remains is only the time needed to sift through the complicated arguments and to decide whether the level of coordination and organization that exists in the pre-embryo is sufficient for developmental individuality.

There is, however, a distinct issue in this debate, namely, what effect denying the individuality of the pre-embryo has on the presumption that a person comes into being at conception. Obviously, the choice between accepting the sperm's penetration of the ovum or syngamy as the beginning of personal life has impact on the permissibility of experimenting with zygotes conceived in vitro, and perhaps on the permissibility of some conception-blocking treatments after rape.

But concerning the larger choice between fertilization and the appearance of the primitive streak as the beginning of individual existence, Ford himself refuses to accept the idea that locating the beginning of individuality at the primitive streak stage undercuts *Donum Vitae's* presumption that personal life begins at conception. He emphasizes that his conclusions are not certain, and so reasonable doubt must be resolved in favor of treating the pre-embryo as a person. Still, if his thesis is established, it will make some difference regarding how women can be treated after rape. Yet, this is hardly the indefeasible presumption of *Donum Vitae*. Neither is Ford's view that, even if his position about early embryos proves correct, he would reach the same practical judgments because he accepts the Church's teaching on contraception ([23], p. 65).

Richard McCormick thinks that Ford's position is more certain than Ford does; he states that science shows "powerfully, indeed convincingly" that the pre-embryo is not yet a person because it reveals that the pre-embryo is not a developmental individual. Thus, McCormick explicitly rejects the presumption as understood in *Donum Vitae*. However, he wants to retain a kind of presumption in favor of generally treating pre-embryos as persons, not because they are persons but to protect potential persons from abuse ([33], p. 302).

McCormick's version of a presumption in favor of the pre-embryo seems a more reasonable result of accepting Ford's arguments than does Ford's own position. Still, one wonders what kind of presumption it is. We usually decide how to treat things on the basis of what they are, but on McCormick's view, we know that pre-embryos are not persons. Thus, treating them as persons is a fiction, not a presumption. It is hard to see how such a fiction could bear much weight in situations of serious moral conflict (*cf.* [11], pp. 101-107).

Nonetheless, Ford and his critics appear to agree in accepting the central normative component of *Donum Vitae's* presumption, namely, that being a human individual is sufficient for being a person ([11], p. 97: [18], pp. 62-64), or at least sufficient to require us to attribute personhood to that entity. However, many people do not regard individuality as a sufficient condition for being a person. For the idea of a person makes essential reference to such things as reasoning, choosing, and having interests, or at least to having the capacity for such activities, and many do not believe that embryos and fetuses have such capacities. There is a Catholic version of this view. It is based on the medieval idea of mediate animation, that is, on the idea that the rational soul, that which makes something a person, is not present in the new human organism immediately upon conception, but later, when the developing body is capable of being informed by a principle of rational thought, which seems to require at least the beginning of neurological development. The point at which this is judged to occur varies, but a recent version of this position puts it at twenty weeks ([52], p. 620). Those who hold this view do not, of course, accept the medieval biology that underlies its traditional formulations. They do, however, employ the precedents of Aquinas and other medieval theologians to show the possibility and legitimacy within a Catholic view of a notion of mediate animation ([18], pp. 80-96; [52], pp. 614-622).

Critics of mediate animation raise the question of what theologians such as Aquinas would say about mediate animation if their inadequate biology were corrected by modern science ([24]; [32], pp. 81-82; [50], pp. 106-121). They argue that scholastic metaphysics, if applied to the modern understanding of reproductive biology, provides no support for the theory of mediate animation.

Stephen Heaney's close textual study of Aquinas's views on this matter is particularly helpful. His work provides an example of how serious work in the history of philosophy can contribute to bioethical discussions. His account is very briefly as follows: Aquinas's position includes the view that before the rational soul is infused, there is first a vegetative soul and then an animal soul. This picture requires an answer to the question why this succession of distinct souls, and of distinct entities as well, should be so ordered as to develop towards a reality that can be informed by a rational soul.

In fact, Aquinas saw this as a question needing an answer, and provided one in terms of his Aristotelian biology: the sperm, which he viewed as the active element in human generation, continues to exist and act after the entities formed by the vegetative and the animal souls come into being. This action of the sperm moves these transient beings toward the condition, completely extrinsic to them, in which matter is sufficiently developed so as to be informed by a rational soul.

But the biology here is, as we now know, all wrong. Thus, if there were transient beings of a vegetative and animal nature, essential to the development of a human person, we would have to know why they are ordered, the first to the second, the second to the rational creature. Since these transient beings are distinct realities, they do not contain an explanation of the development of one from the other. There is a lawlike development here; human persons do not emerge from conception by accident. The explanation of Aristotelian biology is mistaken, and others are equally far-fetched. The only plausible explanation is that there is continuous development of the same reality. But if there is no substantial change in the development of the embryo, then the thing developing must be a human person from the start, and that means that the rational soul must be present from the start ([24], pp. 24-31).

Heaney's argument does not establish conclusively that the rational soul is present from conception. Unlike other substantial changes, there is no direct evidence of when this occurs ([11], pp. 109-110; [50], pp. 117-121). But his argument does successfully respond to one line of criticism of *Donum Vitae's* presumption that personal life exists when a living human individual comes to be. The argument is not that the notion of mediate animation is incoherent, or that the ontology of human generation necessarily excludes mediate animation. It is rather that the theory of immediate animation provides a better account of this process than the theory of mediate animation, and that support for the theory of mediate animation in the writings of Aquinas does not exist once we reject his Aristotelian biology. This is sufficient to cast doubt on the soundness of arguments, like Michael Coughlan's, which maintain that *Donum Vitae's* presumption is arbitrary and without substantial roots in the Catholic tradition itself ([18], pp. 58-95).

III. EQUITABLE ACCESS TO HEALTH CARE

At least since the encyclical *Pacem in Terris* was issued by Pope John XXIII in 1963, Catholic social teaching has included an explicit affirmation that there is a right to health care ([2], pp. 71-75). This right is one of the entitlements that form a significant part of the Church's teaching on social justice. However, there does not exist a detailed account of the nature and extent of this right either in papal or episcopal teaching or in the theological literature ([61], pp. 53-54). It is clear that such an account is needed if this right is to function as more than a slogan in Catholic discussions of such matters as rationing scarce resources and defining a level of health care to which all are entitled.

Nevertheless, the right to health care forms the basis for a considerable body of episcopal teaching and popular Catholic literature that addresses the problems of the American health care system and various public initiatives to deal with them ([10], [16]; [31]; [40]; [60]). This literature is highly critical of the status quo in American health care, in particular, the lack of access on the part of the uninsured to comprehensive care. It includes pointed moral criticism of the Oregon plan for rationing health care to the poor. The main concern is that the Oregon proposal unfairly singles out the poor to bear the burdens of dealing with the public costs of health care.

There is no question that recent American Catholic statements on health care are compatible with the broad lines of Catholic social teaching and are, as far as they go, the correct applications of Catholic principles ([10], p. 285; [17]). Whatever the right to health care means exactly, it requires access for all to some decent level of health care; and rationing schemes that target the poor cannot be just if such a right is assumed to exist.

Still, the context of these statements is political, and they contain much more social criticism than moral analysis. They also convey a sense of unrealistic moralism because they do not face the costs and moral difficulties that Catholic teaching poses for individuals and the community. For example, these statements all endorse the effort to control health care costs and to introduce economic efficiency into the system. But cost-cutting does not guarantee access for the poor and uninsured. People often have good reason to seek expensive and exotic health care, and trimming the fat is an inherently limited enterprise. The health care system is more like the educational system and less like a factory or an industry. Are middle class people, then, to be told that they should be ready to forgo the expensive care they need so that the poor can receive more basic care? Questions like this are not addressed because the underlying moral analysis has not been carried out.

Kevin Wildes's discussion of these issues is an interesting exception, and provides a start on the needed moral analysis. He recognizes the need to define more fully the right to health care ([61], p. 54) but appears to accept the idea that Catholic social teaching requires a safety net of insured access to health care. His main concern is to establish reasonable limits to this kind of entitlement ([61], p. 56).

His discussion is framed by the assumption that in a democratic society with a market economy, a two-tiered system of health care is inevitable. Making this assumption explicit is useful. For it surely underlies the entire American discussion and the statements discussed above. These statements do not see the moral issue to be the level of health care that the rich and middle class should seek for themselves, but the provision of a decent minimum for others, which is tacitly assumed to be less than what wealthier people can buy.

But this assumption is ambiguous, and both its plausible interpretations are probably false. This assumption can be understood as a normative or as a factual belief. As a normative belief, it is the idea that a two-tiered system is morally justified. On this reading, the normative force is hidden in the notions of democracy and the market economy. Thus, the idea would be that a country which rejects a two-tiered system is either undemocratic or unreasonably constrains the market, both of which are unjustified. But the underlying moral judgments are, on Catholic terms at least, false. The need to constrain markets to guarantee that people's basic needs are met is a basic element within Catholic social teaching, and a limited safety net surely will not meet needs that are basic in the relevant sense. Moreover, unless a persuasive definition of democracy is assumed, there is nothing undemocratic about a social policy that significantly limits the ability of the wealthy to buy luxury health care. The Canadian health care system, for example, is surely rooted in democratic political procedures, but it is very substantially a single-tiered system.

Interpreted as a factual belief, this assumption is also false, as the example of the Canadian system shows. Perhaps the point is that in the United States a Canadian style system is politically unfeasible, and that a two-tiered system is the best Americans can do. But if understood in this way, the moral evaluation of the American system and its problems can develop along much more radical lines. For unless the political and economic culture that frames the possibilities for change is itself morally justifiable, the obligations of Catholics and of Catholic institutions to help the poor and uninsured cannot be exhausted by public policy efforts within that framework. The unpleasant challenge not faced in the current literature arises again: are we obliged to accept less so that the poor and uninsured can have what they need?

Moreover, the framework itself cannot simply be accepted as a given but must be challenged. In short, examination of Wildes's assumption raises the question of whether the right to health care as understood within Catholic social teaching requires far more than a limited safety net. The deepest roots of Catholic social teaching suggest that the answer to this question will be affirmative ([17]).

The most constructive part of Wildes's analysis is his effort to answer the question of how much health care people are entitled to. He develops an analogy from the Catholic teaching about the limits of medical treatment that people must accept for themselves or for their family members. The limit is set by the burdens of the treatment. When burdens become excessive, the treatment may be forgone. Because the burdens include those on others besides the patient, there is reason to extend the moral logic to social decisions about providing health care to the poor: "In following this line of thought, just as a family is not obligated to provide family members treatments that are burdensome to the rest of the family, so, too, our national society should not be held to such a strict standard" ([61], p. 55).

This may look like trying to solve one moral problem by reference to another equally difficult problem, but the underlying analogy seems correct. Still, the result will remain abstract until we know how to determine what burdens are excessive when the burdens fall on others than the person needing health care assistance. The debate about the significance of the costs of providing nutrition and hydration to patients in persistent vegetative state, to be considered below, exhibits the difficulty of this question. It is not clear that the burden of paying for the health care of the poor can be defined in terms of what middle class people find disagreeable, a standard that is compatible with Wildes's overall conclusion ([61], p. 56). For the standard that defines what burdens are excessive makes reference to their impact on a person's other obligations, and that is only contingently related to what they find disagreeable. Thus, some consideration of fairness and the duty to help others, including strangers, must surely be part of the determination of what can be considered excessive.

IV. WITHDRAWING/WITHHOLDING CARE

A. *The Duty to Preserve Life*

The long-standing Catholic concern about the morality of withholding life-sustaining treatments continues to be manifested in ecclesiastical teaching and in theological debate. In recent years, bishops and moralists in the United States have turned their attention to the moral issues surrounding decisions to withhold artificially provided hydration and nutrition from dying and otherwise seriously disabled patients, especially those in persistent vegetative state (PVS). This concern goes back at least to the middle 1980s, and no doubt has been driven by the widespread public concern caused by well known court cases such as *Brophy* and *Cruzan*.

In the period just prior to that being surveyed here, there were a number of statements by bishops and considerable theological debate about the permissibility of withholding artificially provided hydration and nutrition from those in a persistent vegetative state. These statements and this debate were based on received Church teaching on withholding treatment, that is, on the traditional doctrine of proportionate and disproportionate treatments. But this teaching does not directly address the issues of artificial feeding and hydration, particularly of those who can be expected to live for a considerable time if they are provided food and water, but in a permanently unconscious condition. Moreover, the common moral principles that define the Catholic approach to these decisions are open to several interpretations.

As a result, bishops have voiced public disagreement among themselves and with theologians. As of two years ago, there was no theological or ecclesial consensus about whether withholding artificially provided nutrition and hydration from patients in PVS is morally permissible ([9], pp. 14-18; [13], pp. 107-119).

This discussion has continued during the last two years, and while there is as yet no consensus, there has been progress towards clarifying the precise points of controversy among Catholics. The most significant contributions to this discussion have been several carefully articulated statements by the American bishops.

There were several brief comments by bishops around the time of Nancy Cruzan's death ([4], pp. 494, 495; [36], pp. 518-519) and passing reference to the questions about nutrition and hydration in some episcopal statements primarily addressed to other issues ([5], pp. 349-350; [37], pp. 279-280). Much of what is said in these statements concerning nutrition and hydration has been said before ([8], pp. 14-18). However, one common theme is worth noting: the Bishops of Missouri affirm a "presumption in favor of life in controverted cases" ([4], p. 495). The Bishops of Oregon and Washington affirm a "presumption in favor of providing these necessities [food and water] by whatever means are most easily tolerated" ([5], p. 350; cf. [55], pp. 110). Their reasoning emphasizes the potential for abuse of the patient's interest or of the sanctity of all human life.

Bishop Myers provides a general argument for a presumption in favor of treatment whenever it is not clear that it is disproportionately burdensome. His argument is based on a careful exegesis of the 1980 "Declaration on Euthanasia" issued by the Congregation for the Doctrine of the Faith. He emphasizes that the Declaration follows earlier Catholic teaching in holding that there exists a certain duty to preserve life and health. That duty is not absolute, but it is to be overridden only when fulfilling it would be disproportionately burdensome:

Therefore, when it is not immediately clear whether the use of therapeutic means is disproportionately burdensome, it is not an entirely open question whether or not such means are to be employed. The presumption is that the necessary or useful means are to be employed unless there is evidence that the means are optional, according to the terms of the declaration ([37], p.

278).

This simple argument introduces three relatively unnoticed elements into the more specific debate about the nutrition and hydration of PVS patients. First, it poses a question that Catholics who think it permissible to withhold nutrition and hydration from those in PVS can hardly ignore: what are the burdens of this sort of treatment, and how are they disproportionate? This question will be considered in the next section. Second, this argument makes clear that the moral issue posed by withholding nutrition and hydration from patients in PVS cannot be reduced to the question of whether or not withholding constitutes intentional killing by omission. For even if the decision to withhold these measures is not the cause of the patient's death and does not ordinarily involve the intention to end life ([8], p. 16), the duty to preserve life remains morally relevant.

Third, the argument indicates that the duty to preserve life and health, as conceptualized within the Catholic tradition, remains operative even for those who are permanently unconscious. This challenges the reading of the tradition proposed by Kevin O'Rourke and others who believe that withholding nutrition and hydration from patients in PVS is morally permissible. These commentators maintain that the duty to preserve life does not apply to those who are permanently unconscious, because such people are no longer able to pursue spiritual goals ([8], p. 17). As O'Rourke puts it in his most recent statement:

In Catholic teaching the goal of human life is eternal life. In order to strive for eternal life, we must perform human acts, (acts of intellect and will) under the influence of charity. Acts of man (vegetative and animal acts) of themselves do not bespeak the power to strive for the goal of human life. Hence, if medical therapy will not restore a person to a condition where human acts can be performed by the person, then that therapy would be ineffective or extraordinary ([42], p. 14; cf. [12], p. 554; [35], p. 214).

This is hard to understand except as a claim that the duty to preserve life does not apply to permanently unconscious patients. It also appears to deny that preserving such a person's life could be a benefit to that person. Bishop Myers's indication that the tradition teaches otherwise puts in clear focus what is probably the central point of contention among Catholics. His analysis of the "Declaration on Euthanasia" is sufficient to cast doubt on the common argument that the less permissive position on this question is a simple mistake or aberration within the Catholic tradition ([26]; [35]; [44], pp. 204-206).

The difference between O'Rourke's view and Bishop Myers's view of the obligation to preserve life exemplifies the central point of contention within the Catholic debate, because the position one accepts on this matter determines the further questions one must address. If one accepts O'Rourke's view, then one can easily justify a negative answer to the question of whether one is obliged to provide nutrition and hydration to those in PVS. On this view, such treatment cannot be obligatory; it is either futile in relation to the only goal that matters, or it is a positive impediment to realizing that goal, and so evidently a grave burden. Moreover, any further benefits of treatment, such as the communal value of maintaining solidarity with the debilitated person ([36], p. 519; [59], p. 707) could hardly be real benefits if keeping the person alive were futile or harmful. But if one accepts Bishop Myers's view, treatment is obligatory unless it involves a significant burden, and so the presumption in favor of treatment stands until one determines the burdens of the treatment and evaluates its relative significance.

In the literature of which I am aware, the considerations necessary for settling this basic disagreement have not been brought forward. Some initial philosophical and theological arguments for and against each side have been published ([7], pp. 180-183; [8], pp. 16-17; [9], pp. 33-35; [47]; [62]), but these are neither sufficiently well developed nor sufficiently comprehensive theologically to settle the issue. In short, further investigation of the nature and scope of the duty to preserve life is essential for a resolution of this fundamental disagreement among the bishops ([12], p. 554) and within the broader Catholic community.

B. *The Burdens of Nutrition and Hydration*

The Bishops of Pennsylvania, in a statement that specifically addresses the issue of withholding nutrition and hydration from patients in PVS, indicate clearly the kind of thinking required if one begins with assumptions like those of Bishop Myers ([6], pp. 542-553). After a thorough discussion of the medical facts and the moral arguments, the Bishops conclude that, except when patients in PVS are unable to assimilate nourishment or are otherwise imminently dying even if nutrition and hydration are provided, withholding artificially provided nutrition and hydration from them is morally impermissible killing by omission, that is, prohibited passive euthanasia. Given this reasoning, a patient cannot direct beforehand that he or she be denied such measures; in effect, such a decision would be suicide, and those who cooperate by acting on such directions would be complicit in that sin ([6], p. 550).

The reasoning for this strongly restrictive conclusion is not compelling. However, a number of elements within it are worth noting. First, the Bishops make clear that providing nutrition and hydration is not required for all patients, nor for all patients in PVS, in all circumstances; there are cases in which such efforts involve a disproportionate burden or are strictly futile ([6], pp. 547-548, 550). This appears to mark one point of agreement among all the bishops who have addressed the issue ([12], p. 555; [36], p. 519). Its importance is that it undercuts restrictive arguments that rely on the premise that withholding food and water are inherently acts of killing ([8], p. 16) or that withholding them is always an unjustifiable failure to care for the patient.

Second, the Bishops comment helpfully on several distinctions prominent in the debate. They consider the moral significance of the artificial character of the provision of the nutrition and hydration. They note that virtually all feeding includes artificial elements and conclude that the artificial/natural distinction does not of itself carry moral weight. What is morally relevant, they say, is whether the effort to feed and provide water has any benefit and whether that effort involves undue burdens ([6], p. 547).

They also criticize the excessive reliance in the discussion on the distinction between treatment and care. They conclude that this distinction is not of fundamental moral significance, and that moral questions about treatment or care must be evaluated in terms of what is beneficial to the patient and what is excessively burdensome ([6], p. 548). Having posed the question in these traditional terms, the Bishops of Pennsylvania find it easy to answer. They do not see any burden in artificially providing nutrition and hydration to those in PVS, and they see a benefit: it prolongs life.

But the Bishops fail to consider the possibility of other burdens of the treatment besides the patient-centered burdens that, because of the patient's unconscious condition, they quite sensibly think do not obtain ([6], p. 549). In particular, they overlook the costs of the treatment, which are surely a central element in the wider public debate ([9], pp. 40-41; [36], p. 519). This oversight allows the Bishops to argue as follows:

> But if the pain of the inability to breathe or the pain of starvation and dehydration cannot be felt, then there is no reason at all to support the contention that the removal of nutrition and hydration is being done out of concern for the sufferings of the patient. It must, therefore, be based on something else; and what is that something else if not the decision that the life of this particular patient is not worth living? Sad to say, the intent is not to relieve suffering but to cause the patient to die ([6], p. 550).

This surely expresses one of the intentions that might motivate a decision to withhold nutrition and hydration from a patient in PVS. But one cannot soundly argue from the absence of one intention to the necessary presence of another. And it is the presence of the intent to end life that leads the Bishops to think that prior patient refusal of such treatment must be suicidal.

This deficiency of the Pennsylvania Bishops' argument is remedied in the statement of the United States Bishops' Pro-Life Committee. The Committee recognizes that some decisions to withhold nutrition and hydration are motivated by an intention to end life, but also notes that the relevant burdens of treatment include not only the possible physical and psychological burdens on the patient, but also economic and other burdens on caregivers. The Committee notes that tube feeding is not ordinarily expensive, and that what is expensive is the overall long-term care of severely debilitated patients. The Committee does not underestimate these costs, including the non-financial strains a family may face.

But the Committee worries that a decision based upon the intent to avoid the overall burdens of caring for a debilitated person may be morally suspect. They say:

In the context of official Church teaching, it is not yet clear to what extent we may assess the burden of a patient's total care rather than the burden of a particular treatment when we seek to refuse "burdensome" life support. On a practical level, those seeking to make good decisions might assure themselves of their own intentions by asking: Does my decision aim at relieving the patient of a particularly grave burden imposed by medically assisted nutrition and hydration? Or does it aim to avoid the total burden of caring for the patient? If so, does it achieve this aim by deliberately bringing about the death of the patient? (59], p. 708).

It is plausible to think that if the burden of artificially providing nutrition and hydration to patients is the cost, then the answer to the Committee's first question must be negative, at least in most situations in which the moral issue would arise. Hence, the answer to the second must be affirmative. As the Committee notes, received teaching does not have an explicit answer. Still, one can easily imagine situations in which deciding to avoid the costs of someone's overall care could be reasonable, and surely not homicidal. This situation might arise for an impoverished family living in a society that could not provide the needed social assistance. Thus, the affirmative answer to the second of the Committee's questions is not necessarily morally questionable and does not require an affirmative answer to the third.

At the same time, even when death is not intended, it seems difficult to justify withholding the total care of a debilitated and dependent person except under conditions of genuine hardship ([8], pp. 17-18; [9], pp. 40-42; cf. [7], pp. 177-180). Once again, therefore, there is a ground for a presumption in favor of providing nutrition and hydration for people in PVS. The Committee endorses such a presumption (59], p. 710).

In short, if one begins with the assumption that there is a presumption in favor of providing nutrition and hydration to patients in PVS because of the duty to preserve life, then one must seek to determine the burdens of the treatment and their significance. This investigation terminates too quickly if only patient-centered burdens are considered, thus raising the prospect that the decision to withhold nutrition and hydration in these cases is intentional killing. Further thought leads to a consideration of the costs of providing nutrition and hydration. But the burden here is not the specific costs of nutrition and hydration but of overall care. Thus, the U.S. Bishops Pro-Life Committee focuses the issue very helpfully: Is it permissible to stop all care for a person? On the assumptions shared by Bishop Myers, the Bishops of Pennsylvania, and the U. S. Bishops Pro-Life Committee, it is hard to see how an affirmative answer to this question is possible.

C. Advance Directives

The statements by the bishops surveyed in the preceding section also address the question of the legitimacy and advisability of advance directives. Although the discussion of advance directives by Catholic theologians and bishops is not nearly as developed and nuanced as that of the substantive moral questions raised by withholding life-extending treatments, several aspects are worth noting.

First, there is no objection to advance directives as such. While, with few exceptions ([15], pp. 188-189), there appears to be little enthusiasm for advance directives and little argument in favor of establishing them, there is no general opposition to them either. Rather, there appears to be a recognition that they have become part of the social and legal world within which medical decisions are made. Thus, the effort is to shape attitudes, legislation, and its implementation so that advance directives will be consistent with Catholic teaching on euthanasia and withholding treatment ([5], pp. 350).

Second, recent Catholic statements on this subject recognize explicitly that, within the limits set by Catholic moral teaching, competent patients are generally the final authorities in decisions about their health care, including those dealing with the termination of treatment. When patients are not competent to make such decisions, family members or other authorized proxies, not judges or health care personnel, should ordinarily make them. Although the authority of patients and their proxies in health care decisions is well established within Catholic teaching ([37], p. 277), the explicit recognition of this teaching in the context of the discussion of advance directives is a welcome addition.

However, the emphasis in the bishops' statements is much more on the moral limits of the right to refuse treatment than on its extent and implications. The basic limitation on the right to refuse treatment is that its exercise is governed by the prohibition against suicide and by the requirement that decisions to terminate treatment must be governed by teaching about proportionate and disproportionate treatments ([6], p. 550; [37], p. 277; [59], p. 710). Thus, the mere fact that a person does not want a given treatment is not a moral justification for him or her to refuse it or for others to accept that refusal.

It is hard to question this view of the moral responsibilities of competent patients or their proxies within the framework of Catholic teaching. However, the bishops' statements proceed very quickly beyond these responsibilities to those of physicians and health care facilities and to the content of relevant legislation. Physicians and health care facilities are not to cooperate in decisions that are not in accord with Catholic teaching; they should persuade the patient to act uprightly; and they should resign from the case rather than be guilty of complicity in suicide ([6], p. 550; [37], p. 277; [59], p. 710). The law should restrict advance directives so that people cannot wrongfully refuse treatments in advance ([6], p. 550; [55], p. 110).

This move from the responsibilities of patients or their proxies to those of physicians, health care facilitators, and the officers of political society surely requires nuancing. It is true that physicians and health care facilities are not simply the agents of patient desires; they must make their own moral assessments of the situation. It is also true that they should seek to persuade people not to perform seriously immoral acts. But accepting a patient's refusal of treatment, even when one thinks it ill considered or immoral, is not necessarily doing anything more than respecting the patient's authority in the matter. It is not choosing or intending that the patient's immoral decision be carried out, but recognizing the limits of one's right to interfere in someone's life. In other words, it does not necessarily involve the kind of complicity in evil that is absolutely excluded, what the Catholic tradition calls "formal cooperation."

Accepting a person's immoral refusal of treatment can be justified under some circumstances, for example, if the law requires it, or if a general respect for patient autonomy makes it prudent, or if one is not in a position to be certain that, for a particular patient, refusal of treatment is not in fact morally justified. One or more of these circumstances seems likely to obtain in virtually all decisions to terminate treatment in which a patient's wishes, whether stated at the time or in advance directives, are relevant to the decision. Thus, the bishops' worry that physicians and health care facilities will be wrongly complicit in immoral decisions is probably not justified.

Third, several of these statements suggest that advance directives that reject nutrition and hydration should the patient become permanently unconscious are morally unacceptable ([5], p. 350; [55], p. 110). As already noted, the Bishops of Pennsylvania hold that withholding nutrition and hydration from patients in PVS is in most cases killing. If so, any advance directive mandating that withholding would be conditional suicide, and acting on it would be prohibited euthanasia. But this view of the Bishops of Pennsylvania is mistaken. For there are burdens involved in providing nutrition and hydration to these patients, namely, the costs. As already noted, it is hard to justify a decision to forgo the costs of caring for a debilitated person, that is, a decision by others to refuse such care. But, as the U. S. Bishops Pro-Life Committee suggests ([59], p. 708), it is not clear that the decision by a patient to spare others the burdens of caring for him or her has the same moral implications. For a person's decision not to impose financial burdens on others is not as such suicidal, and so respecting that decision is not killing. Nor need it be breaking solidarity with that person, or abandoning that person, as one would be if one were refusing care on one's own initiative ([9], pp. 41-43).

This possibility has surely not been shown to be inconsistent with Catholic principles. Consequently, the bishops' exclusion of advance directives that mandate refusal of nutrition and hydration should the patient become permanently unconscious appears to overstate the implications of the received teaching.

V. ACTIVE EUTHANASIA

As the preceding sections make clear, the traditional Catholic opposition to suicide and euthanasia, that is, to intentional self killing or to the intentional killing of others, even at their request and for beneficent purposes, is assumed as the normative framework for dealing with decisions about the end of life. The challenge presented by highly publicized cases of physician-assisted suicide and by the movement to legalize this practice has led to several modest efforts by bishops and theologians to articulate the reasons behind the Catholic moral opposition to suicide and euthanasia, and to develop an appropriate public policy position to implement this opposition ([43]).

Two complementary reasons are most frequently proposed as the grounds for Catholic opposition to suicide and euthanasia. The first is that these acts are contrary to the sanctity or sacredness of human life ([30], pp. 25, 28). The second is that human beings do not have dominion over human life but only a limited stewardship ([5], pp. 347-348; [39], p. 258; [48], p. 361).

For many it may seem unclear why these considerations ground absolute prohibitions of suicide and euthanasia ([13], pp. 121-124; [45], p. 18). But as the notions of the sanctity of human life and the limited human dominion over life have developed within the Catholic tradition, the inference from these reasons to prohibitions against suicide and euthanasia are well-founded and anything but arbitrary ([1]; [41]; pp. 41-45; [47]). Sanctity of life does not simply mean that innocent humans should not be intentionally killed. For this notion primarily indicates something about the character of human beings and their relationship to God; it implies that they are not to be dealt with according to utilitarian calculation or the requirements of technology ([30], p. 28). Nor is affirming limited human stewardship over human life simply a more abstract way of saying that suicide and other intentional killing is wrong. For this affirmation indicates the limited role within God's providence of human discretion, a role whose details need not be supposed to flow from either divine fiat or the simple notion of stewardship ([1], pp. 95-96).

Therefore, the bishops who emphasize the sanctity of human life and the limited stewardship of human beings over human life are not simply reiterating "Thou shalt not kill," an effort that is hardly likely to persuade anyone not already convinced ([34], p. 199). And, while appealing to these reasons will not settle the question of whether or not Catholic prohibitions of suicide and euthanasia are absolute, sanctity of life and limited stewardship do present grounds, deeply entrenched in the Catholic conception of moral life, for thinking suicide and euthanasia morally bad. The further question of whether or not these prohibitions are absolute cannot be settled by narrowly bioethical considerations, but require resolution of the deep ethical disputes among Catholics about such matters as the nature of moral reasoning and moral principles.

When one turns from these fundamental moral considerations to questions of public policy, things grow more complicated and difficult. Recent Catholic writing by bishops and theologians recognizes this. The following factors are explicitly noted: the concern of people about how they will be cared for as they die, the power of the modern fascination with control and autonomy, contemporary individualism, the pragmatism of modern life, the secularization of the medical profession, and the sheer difficulty of making persuasive arguments ([34], p. 199; [38], pp. 300-301).

Despite the recognized difficulties and some disagreement about the absoluteness of the prohibitions against suicide and euthanasia, there appears to be a rare level of agreement among Catholic bishops and theologians in opposing granting legal status to physician-assisted suicide. The public policy arguments that reflect this consensus take some notice of the complicating factors listed above, particularly the first two. They seek not only to situate within a religious context the significance of a person's suffering and of the desire to exercise control over the end of one's life, but also emphasize that pain and suffering can be controlled, and that the most obnoxious prospects of a painful and undignified death can be rejected without choosing suicide or euthanasia ([5], p. 348; [13], p. 125; [34], p. 199; [41], pp. 45-46).

The substantive public policy arguments proposed by Catholics are neither directly theological nor paternalistic. They are based on the impact of physician-assisted suicide on others besides the person asking for help in ending his or her life and are referred to as "common good" arguments ([13], pp. 121-123; [30], p. 27). These arguments have no specific connection with the Catholic tradition, but are based on secular considerations that have shared force within various normative outlooks. Many of these arguments seem to be variations on Yale Kamisar's classical critique of legalized euthanasia, published over thirty years ago ([43], pp. 118-120). The common thread in these arguments against physician-assisted suicide is that the precedent set by allowing private killing unfairly puts others at grave risk ([14], pp. 476-480; [39], p. 258; [48], p. 360). A structurally similar argument is used to show that physician-assisted suicide is destructive of the role of the physician ([29], pp. 472-476; [41], p. 46).

The details of these arguments are complex, interesting and controversial. They will surely need development if they are to have impact on public policy as the debate over physician-assisted suicide develops. I will note simply one of the difficulties this material raises. The general concern about the negative impact of legalized assisted suicide on others contains many elements of what is called a "slippery slope argument." Such arguments are themselves notoriously slippery, and usually unpersuasive. Is there an argument here which is stronger than a prediction, based on guesses and historical analogies, about what the social impact of legalized assisted suicide will be?

Kamisar's original argument was not of the dubious slippery slope variety. He proposed as horns of a dilemma an unregulated system of voluntary euthanasia that would be unfairly dangerous and a strictly regulated system that would be too cumbersome even for those who wanted help in ending their lives ([43], pp. 118-119). The current Catholic arguments are not this well formulated, and they do not begin to consider the issues raised should proposed legislation move towards embracing the second horn of Kamisar's dilemma: what is a reasonable public policy response to proposals for a strictly regulated system that avoids unreasonable risks to the non-competent or the unwilling?

VI. BRAIN DEATH

There appears to be wide agreement among Catholic bishops, physicians, and theologians that total brain death, that is, the cessation of all brain function including brain stem function, is sufficient to constitute death, and that there are available clinical tests that, when properly used, show when this state of affairs obtains ([19]). Many Catholics have come to accept the idea that death occurs when the human body is no longer able to function as an integrated organism, and that the functioning of the brain stem is necessary for integrated organic functioning ([19], pp. 53-55; [27]; [53], pp. 24-31; [57], pp. 32-38).

This developing consensus reflects two interconnected concerns: (1) the distinction between brain death and persistent vegetative state, and more generally a rejection of redefinitions of death that allow a criterion of injury to the brain short of that which renders the entire brain incapable of function; (2) the need to guarantee that vital organs not be removed until a patient is surely dead, and in a manner that shows proper respect for the newly dead human being. I will consider these concerns briefly in turn.

Alan Shewmon's effort to defend, within the traditional categories of scholastic philosophy, a conception of death in terms of the destruction of neocortical function remains central to the Catholic philosophical debate about the difference between total brain death and conditions like persistent vegetative state. The most recent round of criticisms of Shewmon's position are no more philosophically conclusive than Shewmon's original argument ([53], pp. 16-23; [54], p. 59); [56]). But they point to the grounds within the Catholic conception of human beings which underlie the presumption that people who are permanently unconscious, but not totally brain dead, are living human persons ([6], pp. 544-545; [9], pp. 32-33). In particular, they point to the traditional Catholic conviction that a human being is a special kind of animal, namely, one with distinctive spiritual capabilities, and not a spirit housed for a time in a human body ([57], pp. 30-34).

The need to guard against the danger that vital organs will be removed before a person is really dead is starkly stated by Pope John Paul II. He details what he calls a "tragic dilemma": "[I]t is conceivable that in order to escape certain and imminent death a person may need to receive an organ which another patient who may be lying next to him in the hospital could provide, but about whose death there still remains some doubt" ([28], p. 210).

John Paul goes on to reject removal of vital organs from living persons, but adds that the conflict of values that define the dilemma may cause our moral vision to become clouded. Scientific research undertaken "in order to determine as precisely as possible the exact moment and the indisputable sign of death," can solve the conflict between the duty to respect life and the duty to save another's life.

Several aspects of this papal statement are noteworthy. First, the Pope does not so much as hint that the connection between the use of brain death criteria and the transplantation of vital organs should make us either reject brain death criteria altogether or embrace so stringent a definition of death that transplantation would be impossible ([19], pp. 49-50, 52). He plainly follows the judgment of Pius XII that the determination of the moment of death is a scientific and medical matter ([19], p. 53; [57], p. 34), and his dilemma would not arise if the most stringent definitions of death were assumed to be correct. Second, the Pope does not reject transplantation immediately upon the certain determination of death. Quite the contrary, he thinks that the latter possibility will make the dilemma disappear. Thus, Catholic concerns about the proper treatment of the newly dead and about the sufferings of relatives ([57], pp. 42-46) do not imply a rejection of transplantation immediately after death has been determined.

VII. TISSUE TRANSPLANTS

In recent years, Catholic discussions of organ transplants have been focused on the issue just noted, the certain determination of death before vital organs are transplanted, and on the use of tissue from aborted fetuses. Catholic teaching has set stringent conditions for the use of the remains of fetuses ([8], p. 11), including the certain determination of death. These conditions do not explicitly prohibit the use of tissue from electively aborted fetuses, and neither the Vatican nor bishops have taught specifically that they do. But, as a practical matter, several of the conditions appear difficult, if not impossible, to satisfy, and one, the requirement that complicity in deliberate abortion be avoided, appears in principle impossible to satisfy ([8], pp. 11-14).

Several recent articles underline these difficulties and develop the argument that complicity in deliberate abortion is impossible to avoid. The most important of the difficulties addressed concerns the requirement of informed consent. The central problem here is that the significance of consent by those who have decided to abort is questionable ([51], pp. 87-88). This is complicated by several possibilities that cannot be excluded if tissue transplantation from electively aborted fetuses becomes a standard part of medical practice. First, it seems impossible to prevent a woman's conceiving with the intent to abort for the sake of harvesting fetal tissue. Second, efforts to prohibit a woman's designating the specific recipient for the tissue from her aborted fetus may be difficult to enforce, and efforts to separate the decision to abort and the decision to donate the tissue are at best unpromising. Third, the prospects for decisively preventing the commercialization of tissue donations from deliberately aborted fetuses are bleak ([49], pp. 18, 27-29). To the extent that one or more of these possibilities is actualized to a significant degree, the possibility of undue coercion arises, and the contribution of this practice to the inducement of abortion becomes greater ([46], p. 15).

These articles also restate the standard concerns about complicity in abortion and answer several objections raised by secular moralists ([8], pp. 12-13). In particular, the articles argue that using tissue from fetuses deliberately aborted will legitimize abortion and provide an inducement to abortion by the promise of a benefit that will help redeem an otherwise bad situation ([46], pp. 15-16; [49], pp. 25-26; [51], pp. 85-86).

The new development in these articles is a detailing of the ways in which the enterprise of tissue transplantation must become involved in the carrying out of abortions. There are two aspects to this involvement. First, the financial incentives, the dynamism of the research, and the growing demand for tissue from deliberately aborted fetuses will likely lead to a close, symbiotic relationship between the abortion industry and the therapeutic enterprise ([46], p. 16; [49], pp. 25-26; [51], p. 86). Second, it will be impossible for the transplant effort to avoid intimate involvement in carrying out abortions because not all methods of abortion provide usable tissue, and abortions from which tissue is expected must be timed so that the tissue will be most useful ([3], p. 597; [49], p. 28).

In both these respects, there is a degree of complicity in abortion that transplant surgeons do not have in the deaths of those whose organs they harvest. Transplant surgeons make use of the results of tragic and sometimes wrongful deaths, but have nothing to do with the timing or manner of the deaths and are in no way suspected of wanting them to occur. However, when the deaths needed to provide a supply of materials for transplant are not accidental but deliberately caused, and when the transplant team helps arrange certain aspects of the death, then there is complicity of a kind that most would regard as wrongful if the death were a that of a child or adult and not of a fetus. In short, the Catholic prohibition of complicity in abortion seems to exclude the use of the tissue of aborted fetuses for transplantation. The complicity that will exist if the tissue transplantation enterprise comes to depend in a significant, institutional way on elective abortions may not be the most direct or most obviously wrongful form of involvement in others' wrongdoing. But it is surely sufficient for anyone who accepts the Catholic view of the moral standing of the fetus to reject it as simply wrong.[1]

St. Michael's College
Centre for Bioethics
University of Toronto
Toronto, Canada

NOTES

1. I am indebted to Richard Mansfield, J.D. for substantial research assistance in the preparation of this survey.

BIBLIOGRAPHY

1. Ashley, B.: 1992, "Dominion or Stewardship?: Theological Reflections," in K. Wildes *et al.* (eds.), *Birth, Suffering and Death: Catholic Perspectives at the Edges of Life*, Kluwer Academic Publishers, Dordrecht, pp. 85-106.
2. Barnet, R.: 1991, "Catholic Social Teachings and American Health Care", *Linacre Quarterly*, 58.2, 70-78.
3. Barry, R, and D. Kesler: 1990, "Pharaoh's Magicians: The Ethics and Efficacy of Fetal Tissue Transplants", *The Thomist*, 54, 575-607.
4. Bishops of Missouri: 1991, "On Ending Nancy Cruzan's Nutrition and Hydration", *Origins*, 21, 493-495.
5. Bishops of Oregon and Washington: 1991, "Living and Dying Well", *Origins*, 21, 345-352.
6. Bishops of Pennsylvania: 1992, "Nutrition and Hydration: Moral Considerations", *Origins*, 21, 541-553.
7. Bole, T.: 1992, "Why Almost Any Cost to Others to Preserve the Life of the Irreversibly Comatose Constitutes an Extraordinary Burden", in K. Wildes *et al.* (eds.), *Birth, Suffering and Death: Catholic Perspectives at the Edges of Life*, Kluwer Academic Publishers, Dordrecht, pp. 171-187.
8. Boyle, J.: 1991, "The Roman Catholic Tradition and Bioethics", in B. Andrew Lustig, *et al.* (eds.), *Bioethics Yearbook: Volume I: Theological Developments in Bioethics: 1988-1990*, Kluwer Academic Publishers, Dordrecht), pp. 5-21.
9. Boyle, J.: 1992, "The American Debate about Artificial Nutrition and Hydration", in L. Gormally (ed.), *The Dependent Elderly: Autonomy, Justice and Quality of Care*, Cambridge University Press, Cambridge, pp. 28-46.
10. Brandt, L.: 1990, "The Future of Health Care in the United States", *America*, 163, 272-274, 284-286.
11. Bueche, W.: 1991, "Destroying Human Embryos - Destroying Human Lives: A Moral Issue", *Studia Moralia*, 29, 85-115.
12. Bullock, W.: 1992, "Assessing Burdens and Benefits of Medical Care", *Origins*, 21, 553-555.
13. Cahill, L..: 1991, "Notes on Moral Theology: Bioethical Decisions to End Life", *Theological Studies*, 52, 107-17.
14. Callahan, D.: 1991, "'Aid-in-Dying': The Social Dimension", *Commonweal*, 118, 476-480.
15. Catholic Health Association: 1990, "A Patient's Right to Self-Determination", *Origins*, 20, 188-189.

16. Catholic Health Association: 1992, "Health Care Reform Proposal", *Origins*, 22, 60-63.
17. Christiansen, D.: 1991, "The Great Divide: Catholic Social Teaching and American Health Care", *Linacre Quarterly*, 58.2, 40-50.
18. Coughlan, M.: 1990, *The Vatican, the Law and the Human Embryo*, University of Iowa Press, Iowa City.
19. Diamond, E.: 1990, "Linacre Institute Position Paper: Determination of Death", *Linacre Quarterly*, 57.4, 46-58.
20. Diamond, E.: 1992, "Management of a Pregnancy With an Anencephalic Baby", *Linacre Quarterly*, 59.3, 19-23.
21. Fisher, A.: 1991, "'When Did I Begin?' Revisited", *Linacre Quarterly*, 58.3, 59-63.
22. Flaman, P.: 1991, "*When Did I Begin?* Another Critical Response to Norman Ford", *Linacre Quarterly*, 58.4, 39-55.
23. Ford, N.: 1990, "*When Did I Begin?* - A Reply to Nicholas Tonti-Filippini", *Linacre Quarterly*, 57.4, 59-66.
24. Heaney, S.: 1992, "Aquinas and the Presence of the Human Rational Soul in the Early Embryo", *The Thomist*, 56, 19-48.
25. Herranz, G.: "Vatican Report: RU-486: The Abortion Pill", *Origins*, 21, 28-33.
26. Hill, P.: 1991, "Changing Roman Catholic Attitudes Toward Termination of Life-Sustaining Treatments", *Linacre Quarterly*, 58.2, 51-59.
27. Jeffery, P.: 1992, "Brain Death: A Survey of the Debate and the Position in 1991", *Heythrop Journal*, 33, 307-323.
28. John Paul II: 1990, "Determining the Moment of Death", *The Pope Speaks*, 35, 207-211.
29. Kass, L.: 1991, "Why Doctors Must Not Kill", *Commonweal*, 118, 472-476.
30. Levada, W.: 1991, "Oregon 'Aid-in Dying' Proposal Opposed", *Origins*, 21, 25-28.
31. Malone, J.: 1991, "Oregon's Health Plan: Step Toward Medical Neglect"? *Origins*, 21, 270-272.
32. May, W.: 1992, "The Moral Status of the Embryo", *Linacre Quarterly*, 59.4, 76-83.
33. McCormick, R.: 1990, "The Embryo Debate: 3: The First 14 Days", *The Tablet*, 244, 301-304.
34. McCormick, R.: 1991: "Bioethical Problems in the Nineties", *The Catholic World*, 234, 197-204.
35. McCormick, R.: 1992, "'Moral Considerations' Ill Considered", *America*, 166, 210-214.
36. McHugh, J.: 1991, "Comments after Nancy Cruzan's Death", *Origins*, 20, 518-519.
37. Myers, J.: 1991, "Advance Directives and the Catholic Health Facility", *Origins*, 21, 276-280.

38. Murphy, T.: 1991: "Washington State's November Ballot: Euthanasia and Abortion", *Origins*, 21, 297-302.
39. National Conference of Catholic Bishops, Administrative Committee: 1991, "Statement on Euthanasia", *Origins*, 21, 257-258.
40. Oregon Catholic Conference: 1991, "State Health Care Rationing Plan Opposed", *Origins*, 21, 265, 267-268.
41. O'Rourke, K.: 1990, "Value Conflicts Raised by Physician-Assisted Suicide", *Linacre Quarterly*, 57.3, 38-49.
42. O'Rourke, K.: 1991, "Prolonging Life: A Traditional Interpretation", *Linacre Quarterly*, 58.2, 12-26.
43. Paris, J.: 1992, "Notes on Moral Theology: Active Euthanasia", *Theological Studies*, 53, 113-126.
44. Paris, J.: 1992, " The Catholic Tradition on the Use of Nutrition and Hydration", in K. Wildes *et al.* (eds.), *Birth, Suffering and Death: Catholic Perspectives at the Edges of Life*, Kluwer Academic Publishers, Dordrecht, pp. 189-208.
45. Peschke, K.: 1992, "The Pros and Cons of Euthanasia Reconsidered", *Irish Theological Quarterly*, 58, 14-24.
46. Post, S.: 1991, "Fetal Tissue Transplant: The Right to Question Progress", *America*, 164, 14-16.
47. Quay, P.: 1992, "The Sacredness of the Human Person: Cessation of Treatment", *Linacre Quarterly*, 59.1, 76-91.
48. Quinn, J.: 1992, "Defeat of 'Physician-Assisted Death Initiative' Urged", *Origins*, 22, 360-361.
49. Rae, S., and C. DeGiorgio: 1991, "Ethical Issues in Fetal Tissue Transplants", *Linacre Quarterly*, 58.3, 12-32.
50. Regan, A.: 1992, "The Human Conceptus and Personhood", *Studia Moralia*, 30, 97-127.
51. Ressler, M.: 1991, "Fetal Tissue Transplantation: An Ethical Analysis", *Linacre Quarterly*, 58.3, 79-94.
52. Shannon, T. and A. Walter, 1990, "Reflections on the Moral Status of the Pre-Embryo", *Theological Studies*, 51, 603-626.
53. Smith, P.: 1990, "Brain Death: A Thomistic Appraisal", *Angelicum*, 37, 3-35.
54. Smith, P.: 1990, "Personhood and the Persistent Vegetative State", *Linacre Quarterly*, 57.2, 49-58.
55. Stafford, J.: 1991, "Growing Euthanasia Mentality Seen", *Origins*, 21, 108-111.
56. Tardiff, A.: 1992, "The Thought Experiment: Shewmon on Brain Death", *The Thomist*, 56, 435-450.
57. Tonti-Filippini, N.: 1991, "Determining When Death Has Occurred", *Linacre Quarterly*, 58.1, 25-49.
58. Tonti-Filippini, N.: 1992, "Further Comments on the Beginning of Life", *Linacre Quarterly*, 59.3, 76-81.

59. U.S. Bishops' Pro-Life Committee, 1992, "Nutrition and Hydration: Moral and Pastoral Reflections", *Origins*, 21, 705-712.
60. United States Catholic Conference: 1992, "Criteria for Evaluating Health-Care Reform", *Origins*, 22, 23-24.
61. Wildes, K.: 1991, "Health Care Rationing and Insured Access: Does the Catholic Tradition Have Anything to Say"? *Linacre Quarterly*, 58.3, 50-58.
62. Wildes, K.: 1992, "Life as a Good and our Obligation to Persistently Vegetative Patients", in K. Wildes, *et al.* (eds.), *Birth, Suffering and Death: Catholic Perspectives at the Edges of Life*, Kluwer Academic Publishers, Dordrecht, pp. 145-153.

COURTNEY S. CAMPBELL

EMBODIMENT AND ETHICS:
A LATTER-DAY SAINT PERSPECTIVE

This essay will examine the perspectives of the Latter-day Saint (LDS) tradition on issues in biomedical ethics through the organizing theme of embodiment. This is a necessary feature for understanding the relationship of religious convictions and ethical values in this faith community because the tradition offers a distinctive interpretation of the existential and ethical significance of the human body. The tradition has rejected the philosophical and religious gnosticism of the body as a prison or tomb of the soul, the Cartesian dualism of mind and body, and the organic reductionism of modern science. The LDS theology of the body instead invokes themes of the body as temple or tabernacle, as teacher, and as gift. These theological perspectives are expressed in various ethical positions and moral practices relevant to health and medicine.

This connection between embodiment and ethics will be explored in a three-fold structure. First, the theology of embodiment requires attention to certain core convictions in LDS teaching about the nature of the cosmos, God, and the self. These convictions provide the basis for an understanding of the body that informs LDS practical teaching on issues such as preventive health, AIDS, abortion, genetic screening, care of impaired newborns, reproductive technology, end-of-life decisions about treatment termination and euthanasia, and organ transplantation. Such issues can become dilemmas within the tradition when the theology of the body conflicts with other central principles of family, relationality, and personal moral agency. Yet, ethics is itself a "dilemma" for the LDS tradition, an issue that will be examined in the concluding section of the essay.

I. A THEOLOGY OF EMBODIMENT

The Latter-day Saint tradition has historically affirmed a thoroughly materialistic and expanding cosmos. According to the canonical[1] writings of its founder, Joseph Smith: "There is no such thing as immaterial matter. All spirit is matter, but it is more fine or pure, and can only be discerned by purer eyes; We cannot see it, but when our bodies are purified we shall see that it is all matter" ([7], p. 266). This materialistic metaphysics, it should already be clear, has substantial implications for the theological significance of the body. The theological dualism of spirit-matter, or soul-body, which traditionally relegated the body to second-class status in the self, is simply collapsed on the LDS

B. Andrew Lustig (Sr. Ed.), Bioethics Yearbook: Volume 3, 43-67.
©1993 Kluwer Academic Publishers.

account. It is no longer possible to sustain a radical discontinuity between self (whether as soul, spirit, or mind) and body. Indeed, the body is essential to understanding of and knowledge about the nature of reality.

This account also provides the basis for two other very significant departures from central tenets in the biblical traditions. The first is an affirmation of a process cosmogony over against the conventional understanding of creation *ex nihilo*. LDS theologians have continually asserted that the creative activity of God is ongoing and should be understood as a process of "organizing" already existing material ("elements") rather than an act of creation out of nothing. The cosmic stuff or elements out of which comes the universe, the world, nature, and human beings are themselves "eternal" ([7], p. 182) and have existed, in certain respects, even prior to God. God fashions these eternal elements into a cosmos and world somewhat similar to the image of divine artisan or craftsman present in Platonic cosmology.

A second interpretative shift required by this materialistic metaphysics concerns the nature of God. While Christianity has at times discerned the significance of the body through the doctrine of the Incarnation, the LDS tradition has affirmed that embodiment is central to the identity and character of God. The canonical claim is: "The Father [God] has a body of flesh and bones as tangible as man's; the Son [Jesus Christ] also;. . ." ([7], p. 265). The tradition has therefore tended to interpret the biblical narrative of human beings as created in "the image of God" literally and physically. The *imago Dei* is not limited to the traditional Christian themes of reason or self-transcendence, but involves the fullness of a person, including his or her body. The radical discontinuity of God and persons due to the physical dimensions of the human self is therefore rejected in favor of an essential identity that includes both spiritual (e.g., love) and corporeal features. Indeed, this sense of relational identification is so deeply embedded in the tradition that it is fair to say that the LDS tradition views theology as an inquiry about what a person can become.

This implies, of course, that embodiment is integral to self-identity and self-understanding. LDS soteriology has articulated a four-fold process of "eternal progression" as part of the divine creative intention for human nature and destiny. This process can be seen as a grand "rite of passage", with various phases corresponding to what anthropologies of religion in general have termed a structure of separation-transition-liminality-reincorporation ([16]). Significantly, the existential significance of the body is presupposed at each step in this process.

The tradition refers to the first stage of individuated human life following the divine work of organization as an "ante-mortal" or "pre-mortal" existence. All persons who have lived, live now, or (importantly for the purposes of biomedical ethics) future generations who have yet to live, are held to have resided in a heavenly home or "first estate" with God. Human selves were distinctly individuated in this existence and entered into relationships and education about eternal truth and wisdom through a "spirit body", which as implied above, consists of a purer, refined matter, rather than an ethereal presence. Theological discussions have invoked passages in the LDS scriptures to indicate that this spirit body is identical in form, shape, and feature to the embodied self one is during mortal life ([3], p. 493).[2]

The human selves created in the image of God were created for the purpose of imitation of God (*imitatio Dei*). However, their capacities for progress in knowledge of truth, wisdom, creativity, and relationships were all limited by their lack of full bodily experience and expression. The "second estate" of human beings is therefore to assume a mortal body or body of flesh, which is accomplished through human procreation. Birth is a rite of passage that signifies the phase of "separation" from God and initiates the "transition" process. The human body as we know and experience it in mortality is thus viewed as both an essential symbol of this passage and a school for learning. All persons that lived with God in the pre-mortal life must pass through mortality and receive a mortal body to participate in the process of eternal progression. The body, then, is absolutely fundamental to a person's identity and salvation, and this view has significant implications for LDS practical ethics on procreation, contraception, abortion, care of impaired newborns, etc. Moreover, the body is a teacher of life experience and thus the tradition would invest great meaning in the common saying in medical discourse regarding the "wisdom of the body".

There is a very strong sense in which the fullness of the person is realized only in and through bodily experience. Indeed, the LDS canonical definition of "soul" refers not to a genuine or essential self or mind divorced from the body but to an embodied person: "The spirit and the body are the soul of man" ([7], p. 166). This gives the body the status of sanctity and holiness that is expressed in LDS discourse through metaphors of "temple", "tabernacle", or "sanctuary". Each of these, which invoke biblical images of venues for the dwelling place of God, convey attitudes of reverence and awe toward the body and require practices of purity and cleanliness. These are best displayed in attitudes and conduct regarding preventive health practices and sexual morality.

Death, which is understood as a temporary separation of spirit and body in LDS teaching, initiates the third phase of eternal progress. It is both a "transition" and a symbol of a rite of passage to the stage of "liminality", which in LDS discourse is referred to as the spirit world. A person enters this spirit world as a disembodied spirit and, depending on the nature of the deeds performed in moral life, may be given passage into a "paradise" to continue learning, service to others, and teaching, or assigned to a "prison", a state of affairs akin to traditional images of purgatory, in which education about truth and ultimate salvation is presented, but repentance (penance) is necessarily required.

There are some striking similarities between LDS images of this spirit world and the idea of Hades in classical Greek or Roman literature, such as

The Odyssey or *The Aeneid*. Just as the classical heroic figure, Odysseus or
Aeneas, journeys to Hades and there encounters and communicates with the
shadows of persons who have died previously, so, according to fundamental
LDS conviction, Jesus Christ, following his crucifixion and prior to his
resurrection, entered the spirit world and taught his message of salvation to the
gathered disembodied persons. The classical and LDS accounts of the heroic
journey to the underworld reflect, to be sure, substantial dissimilarities. The
first is that in the classical accounts, the virtuous and the vicious are largely an
undifferentiated group: death has leveled the moral differences of life. In the
LDS understanding, by contrast, the moral differentiation is retained so that
"paradise" and "prison" are distinctive in character and Jesus is portrayed
as teaching only among just persons. Secondly, Odysseus and Aeneas are
greeted with lamentations and mourning by the shadows of the dead who have
no hope of deliverance from their demise, while the message of Jesus offers
liberation and eternal life, which the just subsequently convey to the unjust. It
is this conviction that gives rise to the well-known LDS interest in genealogical
research and the significance of family relationships, which as I will discuss, has
substantial implications for reproductive ethics in the tradition.

The crucial point here is the canonical claim about why the message of
Jesus was so anticipated and received with joy: "For the dead had looked
upon the long absence of their spirits from their bodies as a bondage" ([6], p.
290). The experience of disembodiment is a deprived state of affairs; it is to
be incapable of fully expressing one's personhood That the absence of the body
is a form of bondage is a claim that runs directly contrary to philosophic and
theological views that hold the human problem attributable to the presence of
the body. The LDS account affirms instead that the body is a source of
freedom and that embodiment is empowering and enabling rather than limiting
and disabling.

This perspective is underscored by a prominent claim that the transition
stage of mortality, rather than the liminal stage of the spirit world, is the time
to prepare to "meet one's Maker," precisely because the body is necessary for
a person to engage in repentance for wrongdoing and sin. It is possible, the
tradition affirms, to engage in repentance and spiritual preparation in the spirit
world, but significantly more difficult because of one's disembodied state:
"When we go out of this life, leave this body, we will desire to do many things
that we cannot do at all without the body. We will be seriously handicapped,
and we will long for the body;. . . We will know then what an advantage it is
to have a body . . . We will find when we are dead every desire, every feeling
will be intensified. When clay is pliable it is much easier to change than when
it gets hard and sets" ([1], pp. 10-11).

The fulfillment of human progression involves entrance into the presence
of God (the phase of "re-incorporation" in rites of passage) in the form of a
resurrected person. Given the stress on the body in previous transitions, it is
no surprise that the LDS tradition conceives of the resurrection (which is

universal in scope) not as a symbolic spiritual presence, but rather as a literal reunion of body and spirit, both of which are required to realize a "fullness of joy". The bodily limitations persons do experience in mortal life, from severe abnormalities to impairments such as poor eyesight or even baldness are all to be alleviated in the resurrected body. We nonetheless retain our general bodily identity and characteristics: "The spirit and the body shall be reunited again in its perfect form; both limb and joint shall be restored to its proper frame, even as we are now at this time; . . . There shall not so much as a hair of their heads be lost; but every thing shall be restored to its perfect frame, as it is now, or in the body . . ." ([3], p. 236). This canonical claim has proved very influential in shaping the LDS approach to questions of organ transplantation.

The LDS theology of the body, then, views embodiment as essential to self-identity and integrity, rather than as incidental. We are our bodies in the most meaningful theological sense and this implies that a moral principle of respect for persons must be broadened to encompass respect and reverence for the body. The body is a source of personal empowerment; it is not the body but the absence of the body that is a form of bondage and limitation. I now wish to turn to some of the ethical implications of this theology of the body in the context of medicine by exploring the themes of body as temple or tabernacle, as teacher, and as gift.

II. THE BODY AS TEMPLE

A. *A Word of Wisdom*

The image of body as temple reflects what Mircea Eliade has referred to as a hierophany, a sacred space for dwelling place of the divine ([8], pp. 11-13). This basic image imposes on Latter-day Saints obligations of purity and purification and the avoidance of practices that are deemed unclean and polluting. The most prominent of these obligations is expressed in what is known as the "Word of Wisdom", a commandment regarding health practices ([7], pp. 175-76). The negative injunctions of this commandment, including proscriptions against wine, tobacco, coffee, tea, and addictive drugs, are held to be binding upon every member of the faith community. Additional positive stipulations concerning the consumption of appropriate foods, such as herbs, fruits, vegetables, and grains, as well as limitations on the consumption of meat, function more as counsels that allow agent discretion rather than as binding obligations.

Several lines of reasoning have been developed in the tradition to justify these requirements. A consequentialist approach has considered the substantial medical and social ills that afflict the United States due to alcoholism, drunk driving, workplace absenteeism, cancers, drug abuse and violent crime, and extensive patterns of meat consumption. By contrast, it has been noted by numerous commentators that Latter-day Saints characteristically rank among the healthiest of the nation's sub-communities.

Yet, one can reasonably argue that these negative consequences are the result of abuse rather than appropriate use of such substances and eating patterns. A moderate use of wine or coffee, for example, might not only have no substantial detrimental effects, but can, some studies suggest, even have practical, healthful benefits. From this perspective, the LDS insistence on prohibition rather than a rule of moderation seems excessively puritanical and an occasion of social embarrassment.

The reason for the prohibition must lie elsewhere than in personal or social consequences, and the more deontological line of reasoning in the tradition has invoked the theme of the integrity of the body as a temple. The use of such substances violates the sacrality of the body; the unclean intrudes upon the clean, and transforms a vessel of purity into that which is profane and polluted. Moreover, the intrinsic connection of self and body means that use of forbidden substances assaults and violates the person and not merely his or her physiological functioning.

A second response to the moderate usage argument reflects not only a temple image but also a teaching image. The experience of embodiment is an occasion for learning about and realizing discipline and mastery of self. That mastery is expressed not only in the capacity to make *right* choices but also in the ongoing opportunity to make *free* choices about right and wrong. The loss of free choice, as distinguished from making a wrong choice, implies that the agency of the person is incomplete. The concern, then, with even moderate use of certain substances is that their habit-forming addictive properties may over time produce involuntary actions and behaviors. The wisdom of the body consists partly in how we are educated to use and preserve our freedom to choose.

These required practices and this reasoning clearly have implications for issues in health care priorities, though with a very distinctive twist in the argument. Clearly, the general policy orientation of this approach would be towards preventive medicine and the promotion of healthy behaviors and lifestyles. One traditional criticism of a preventive orientation in health policy is that it involves, to greater or lesser degree, intrusions on personal liberties. It should be evident that this criticism would not be compelling in the LDS tradition, because personal freedom can be compromised or lost by an initial choice of riskier behavior. The question would be whether we should view freedom in terms of its durability as an aspect of character or as a feature of discrete choices. The moral burden of the LDS tradition would suggest the compatibility of freedom and preventive priorities rather than their conflict, in that right choices are necessarily intertwined with free choices.

B. *AIDS*

A second context of LDS discourse in which the theme of body as temple figures prominently is that of sexual morality. The normative requirement is expressed in the "law of chastity", which limits sexual relations to marriage and rejects other forms of sexual expression as "unholy and impure", language that is already embedded in the sacrality and purity of the body as temple. This has provided the framework, moreover, with which LDS ecclesiastical policy towards the issues of AIDS has been enunciated. For example, the "clear guidance" offered in two major policy statements about how AIDS may be avoided consists in principles of chastity, marital fidelity, and "reverence and care for the body, which is the 'temple of God' (1 Corinthians 3:16)" ([2]; [9], p. 11-5]).

The first public pronouncement on AIDS by an LDS leader occurred in April 1987 at the annual conference of church membership. That statement did not directly invoke of theodicy of AIDS as divine punishment for homosexuality, along the lines of some conservative denominations and approximately 43% of the American populace, according to surveys taken in late 1987. However, the frequent use of the language of "plague" to describe AIDS rather than the medicalized "epidemic" draws on a historical pattern of religious interpretation of widespread disease as a sign and symbol of divine judgment. Moreover, the pastoral emphasis in the statement on compassionate care for persons with AIDS cannot be easily disentangled from the tradition's negative moral attitude towards homosexuality. Thus, the statement advocated "Christlike sympathy for victims [of AIDS], innocent or culpable", and drew on the moral example of Jesus "who condemned the sin, yet loved the sinner" ([10]). Although not inconsistent with the principal epidemiological patterns of AIDS in the mid-1980s, the dominant sin of culpability presupposed in the discussion is that of homosexuality.

Subsequent formal policy statements reflect a broader horizon of medical concern, identifying illegal intravenous drug use and sexual intimacy with infected persons (without distinguishing heterosexual or homosexual relations) as modes of transmission, along with perinatal transmission and exposure to infected blood. Nonetheless, the moral language of "innocent" victims of AIDS continues to be retained in official discourse, and indeed a form of preferentialism in attitude and disposition, if not in practice, emerges: "We express great love and sympathy for all victims, but particularly those who have received the virus through blood transfusions, babies afflicted from infected mothers, and innocent marriage partners who have been infected by a spouse". The statement also invokes a theodicy of compensation in the afterlife for those persons who experience present suffering, pain, and injustice "not of their own doing" [2].

These distinctions between innocence and culpability, between those who will receive eternal compensation for injustice and those who, implicitly, are responsible for their own suffering have not gone unchallenged by lay scholars in the tradition. Writing in the magazine *Sunstone*, Stephen C. Clark criticizes the judgment-laden language of ecclesiastical statements and contends their moralizing tone makes the advocacy of compassionate care muted and condescending. Indeed, the distinctions may have precisely the opposite effect of the intended practices of care, instead engendering "intolerance and bigotry". Clark therefore commends to his LDS audience the approaches of other Christian denominations that have acknowledged institutional complicity for the epidemic (because of teachings on sexuality) and have made institutional commitments to use financial, educational, and caregiving resources to prevent the spread of AIDS and provide effective support to persons with AIDS [6].

It is clear that AIDS has occasioned a reconsideration of traditional LDS attitudes towards homosexual orientation and behavior in some circles. However, the general stance of the ecclesiastical leadership is that the movement for gay and lesbian rights reflects a "campaign to make spiritually dangerous life-styles legal and socially acceptable" [13]. However, Clark's concern that LDS teachings on the connection between AIDS and homosexuality would produce a climate of intolerance and bigotry does not seem to have been borne out. The official ecclesiastical policy that persons who have AIDS are to be treated with "dignity and compassion" ([9], p. 11-5) seems instead to have been the guiding rule embedded in practice. Some wards (the LDS equivalent of parishes) have developed "AIDS Projects" to provide emotional, social, and spiritual support for persons with AIDS, and these projects have been described by one ecclesiastical leader as displaying the essence of "the gospel of Jesus Christ-caring for people who are really in need" ([15]).

AIDS confronts the LDS tradition, no less than other denominations, with a series of vexing theological and pastoral issues. It is fair to suggest that the direct experience of church members with AIDS-infected persons has thus far been so limited that the theological and practical questions are not prominent in the religious consciousness of the tradition. The ongoing response of the tradition will nonetheless continue to be informed by principles of purity, reverence for the body, and compassion.

III. THE BODY AS TEACHER

We have already seen that the LDS theology of the body makes birth an absolutely essential soteriological rite of passage. I now want to explore the moral meaning of this rite of passage for LDS teaching on the issues of abortion, genetic screening, care of impaired newborns, and reproductive technology.

A. *Abortion*

LDS teaching on abortion presents what appears as a very deep paradox. The tradition has, on the one hand, consistently affirmed a very conservative position on abortion; even if abortion is permitted in certain exceptional circumstances, it is not ever to be solely the private choice of the pregnant woman. This opposition is commonly rooted in an affirmation of the sanctity of life and its correlative obligation that prohibits acts of killing. Yet, the tradition has also never adopted any official stance on a threshold criterion – e.g., conception, quickening, viability, birth, etc. – for the presence of the human person. In addition, LDS ritual practices have always differentiated between miscarriages or stillborn births and neonatal deaths. The moral position can thus seem inconsistent with both LDS ritual and metaphysics.

The theology of embodiment provides insight into this paradox. The imperative that follows from this theology is that procreation is a moral necessity so that *earthly tabernacles* (in the parlance of the tradition) may be provided for those spirit beings that currently reside in the pre-mortal existence. There then emerges a pro-*birth* bias in the tradition, quite irrespective of when it is that spirit and body unite to form a *soul* or person. Birth is a necessary means of access to experience and knowledge that cannot be obtained in an unembodied or disembodied condition. This provides a basis for a theology of the body as teacher. We learn experience not only through the body but simply by virtue of having a body.

In an important sense, this account avoids the controversial question of when human life begins that the moral discussion of abortion typically founders on. Yet, the parameters of the debate then shift to other questions that are no less difficult to resolve. Given the strong pro-birth orientation of the tradition, it is reasonable to ask how any abortion could be valid. A more conservative, absolutist rationale for the immorality of all abortions would be difficult to construct. It is in fact possible to claim that the current ecclesiastical teaching on abortion constitutes an absolute prohibition with an allowance for some *exceptions* (noted below) based on compassion and sympathy.

However, it is conceivable that the theology of embodiment could generate the almost diametrically opposite conclusion. That is, since the tradition has not claimed that unembodied spirits who are deprived of a bodily tabernacle by abortion are thereby deprived for all eternity of ever experiencing bodily life, but has rather tended to suggest that such spirits will receive another *chance* at mortal life, then it seems reasonable to ask why any abortion would be deemed a morally grave decision. This conclusion would simply require an assumption that unembodied persons remain in the heavenly queue for future earthly vessels, rather than being consigned to some prison for the unembodied, and that their bodily life and experience is deferred but not lost. This position is readily coherent with a view that birth is the decisive threshold of humanity and avoids the knotty problem of explaining what happens to the spirit of the unborn upon abortion.

Moreover, on this view, abortion might be seen as a humanitarian effort to ensure a safe passage from unembodied to mortal life and to enhance the quality of one's mortal experiences, which themselves are a transitional step to eternal life. In the context of LDS soteriology, abortion might seem reasonable to ensure that a person is not disadvantaged by the circumstances of his or her birth.

This perspective would also have some significant implications for questions of wrongful birth or wrongful life, and even of social eugenics. The LDS tradition would not agree with the philosophical claim that abortion of a possible or potential person is not a form of harm because possible persons do not exist, except in the imagination. The person does exist as a real presence in the pre-mortal world, and abortion does constitute a form of harm or injury because it prevents the person from obtaining a body necessary to experience mortal learning and wisdom. Yet, it could be plausibly argued that it is better for the person to be born into one set of (familial, economical, educational, etc.) circumstances that would enhance the quality of mortal life than into another set of circumstances that would be relatively deprived by comparison. The tradition has already clearly validated this kind of reasoning in asserting that it is preferable for spirit persons to be born into the context of an LDS home life, a theological rationale that has encouraged the large families one characteristically finds in LDS congregations.[3] Thus, while the tradition could not adopt the precise reasoning of a wrongful life claim, that is, "It is better that I not have been born", it does seem committed to claiming something very close: "It would be better that I not be born *now*".

Notwithstanding the quite different directions the pro-birth position could go, the tradition has historically been consistent in ruling out abortion in all but exceptional cases, most commonly when continuing a pregnancy to term will jeopardize the life or health of the expectant mother. Recently, some modifications to this traditional allowance have occurred, influenced in part by sensitivity to situations of unconsented-to pregnancy as well as by new medical technology. Thus, the policy promulgated under a 1989 revision of ecclesiastical guidelines permits abortion in instances of pregnancy resulting from rape or incest or when "the fetus is known . . . to have severe defects that will not allow the baby to survive beyond birth" ([9], p. 114).

This policy was reaffirmed in January 1991 in the midst of heated controversy over a very restrictive abortion bill proposed in the wake of the Supreme Court's decision in *Webster*. The state of Utah is approximately 75% LDS in population, so it is no coincidence that the bill was a virtual mirror of ecclesiastical policy. The bill would have prohibited abortion unless the woman's life were threatened, the pregnancy resulted from rape or incest, or a physician determined that a child would be born with physical or mental defects deemed incompatible with sustained survival. (A modified version of the bill was approved but deemed unconstitutional upon judicial review.

To opponents, including women's rights groups and the American Civil Liberties Union, the noticeable similarities seemed to present a blatant violation of the establishment clause of the First Amendment. However, the public statement issued by ecclesiastical leaders disclaimed responsibility for the bill, affirming: "The Church of Jesus Christ of Latter-day Saints as an institution has not favored or opposed specific legislative proposals or public demonstrations concerning abortion". The statement also sought to rebut the alleged violation of church-state separation by distinguishing between institutional roles and the responsibilities of "citizens to let their voices be heard in appropriate and legal ways that will advance their belief in the sacredness of life" ([5]). What is also striking about this statement is that it represents the first public pronouncement in which abortion is said to be "justified" rather than permitted as an "exception", although the grounds for justification are left unspecified.

B. *Prenatal Screening*

The compassionate exception or justification based on severe fetal defect implicates indirectly the moral status of prenatal genetic screening. Since this issue is nowhere else directly addressed in ecclesiastical policy, a few comments are appropriate here. It is not entirely clear what the practical impact of this exception would be. A moral casuistry to identify those severe abnormalities that would fall under the permission has not been undertaken. Moreover, given the soteriological significance of birth, it would seem important that abortion not be performed if the baby is expected to "survive . . . birth", even if survival cannot be sustained beyond birth, as might be the case with instances of anencephaly that could be detected *in utero*. The exception seems to be so limited as to be almost vacuous.

The existence of the exception presupposes use of prenatal genetic screening methods of some form, such as chorionic villus sampling, amniocentesis, or ultrasonography, and the question arises as to how resort to genetic screening coincides with the tradition's pro-birth orientation. In short, what is the context presupposed by the exception? Prenatal screening is obviously used to detect many conditions, both for "severe defects" and for genetic diseases in which a child could live for several years beyond birth and even into adulthood, as well as for sex selection. One question is whether the genetic information disclosed by screening could be restricted to only the most severe abnormalities, or whether information about abnormalities that would clearly not be justified by the genetic exception would also be disclosed and thereby create a desire or need for abortion.

The exception may also reflect an example of a "trickle up" direction in the formation of ecclesiastical policy, in which embedded practices shape policy. The LDS tradition has never articulated a direct stand regarding amniocentesis. This ecclesiastical silence may appear surprising in light of the pro-birth orientation, which would seem to require moral disapproval of amniocentesis. Although this is not true in every case, ecclesiastical silence is frequently interpreted as a signal for persons to make their own decisions about moral questions in collaboration with relevant family members and informed medical professionals.

The process may have occurred in the LDS community following the widespread availability of genetic screening technologies in the mid-1970s. LDS physician and historian Lester E. Bush has compiled several accounts of LDS couples seeking out genetic counseling and screening, and in some instances relying on the information disclosed by amniocentesis to opt for selective abortion, as well as the use of amniocentesis by practicing LDS physicians. The rates of abortion for fetal indications in Utah are lower than the national average of 80%, but still fairly high at 65% ([Bush]). The genetic exception to the prohibition of abortion may then reflect a pastoral accommodation to a practice to which some couples and professionals already resorted in the absence of specific guidelines. It is, in any event, difficult to discern a consistent principled rationale for the exception, other than on grounds of compassion for the family.

C. *Care of Impaired Newborns*

I have claimed that LDS theological convictions about embodiment require a pro-birth orientation, which is to be distinguished from both a pro-vitalist and a pro-choice position in the context of abortion. This distinction is even more necessary when considering the question of selective non-treatment of impaired newborns. This issue has not been addressed directly in ecclesiastical policy and only rarely in scholarly articles, even though personal narratives frequently appear in popular LDS literature or in community discussion groups. A general guideline about termination of medical treatment may be applicable to the situation of seriously impaired newborns, though its stated context is terminal illness at the typical end of the life cycle: "When dying becomes inevitable, it should be looked upon as a blessing and a purposeful part of eternal existence. Members should not feel obligated to extend mortal life by means that are unreasonable" ([9], p. 11-6).

The reference to an eternal context for understanding the place of death and dying, coupled with a deeply-embedded theodicy of ultimate justice for the handicapped in the tradition, could in principle converge to support a presumption in favor of non-treatment of seriously ill or even moderately impaired newborns. This argument would rely on a set of distinctive LDS assumptions, which include a denial of some basic theological tenets in the Christian tradition, such as the doctrine of original sin and the practice of infant baptism.

Three points seem central to establishing this presumption. The first claim is that a central purpose of the life passage we call mortality is the obtaining of a physical body, the earthly tabernacle. This is achieved for any newborn, normal or impaired, through birth. A second claim is that accountability for actions and the capacity for sin presupposes a developed moral agency that is held to be present in children at around eight years of age rather than at birth.

LDS children are typically baptized and confirmed shortly after their eighth birthday. It follows from this that children who die from illness (or accident) before the age of moral accountability, or impaired or handicapped persons who may live beyond eight years of age but never achieve the mental and moral capacities of that threshold are not held responsible for their actions and in a theodicy of compensation are understood to be recipients of eternal salvation. The canonical claim is that "all children who die before they arrive at the years of accountability are saved in the celestial kingdom of heaven" ([7], p. 286).

It is not as though such children (biologically or morally) receive a free passage, however. A third claim is that the experiences and trials of mortality are unnecessary for such persons because they have already proved their fidelity to God and learned sufficient truth in their first estate or pre-mortal existence. Echoing a theme that occasionally surfaced in medieval Christian art and architecture, in which anencephalic children were portrayed as angels of God, the LDS tradition affirms that seriously impaired newborns and handicapped children are especially beloved of God, to the extent that the only required condition of salvation is that they obtain a mortal body. Thus, the tradition again comes down with a strong pro-birth, but not necessarily vitalistic, orientation and indeed the theological claims would tend to support a fairly liberal policy of non-treatment for impaired newborns whose dying is inevitable, even if it is not imminent.

Two LDS practitioners have developed a version of this theology of non-treatment through consideration of a hypothetical case of a comatose 4-year-old boy (Sam) who had sustained significant and apparently permanent brain damage secondary to respiratory failure. The boy was capable of unassisted breathing but unable voluntarily to take nourishment. Val D. MacMurray and Kim Ventura argue that a decision about continuing or discontinuing treatment first requires a determination of options and consequences and a process of clarifying basic values; a consideration of relevant canonical passages or authoritative statements by ecclesiastical leaders; and an assessment of both the needs of the family and those of the child. The evaluation of the child's best interests turns precisely on the theology of embodiment: "What are Sam's needs? Sam has acquired a mortal body and firm place in a family with the potential of being together forever . . . Barring a [divine] manifestation to the contrary, we would [decide] to release Sam's spirit, since his condition simultaneously denies him both any conscious experience of mortality and the progression available to disembodied spirits" ([12], p. 282).

Several large leaps of faith are required for this theodicy of compensation to be intellectually compelling and pastorally consoling. However, for those who do make the leaps, it does hold a powerful pastoral impact. It is not at all the case that a child born with impairments or the premature death of a healthy child is an occasion of joy for a family. The emotional trauma and the sense of loss are experienced deeply and profoundly. Still, the language of "tragedy" does not quite seem to fit the theological reality of such situations. Instead, families often invoke the language of "blessing" or "gift" to refer to their impaired child, and the compassionate care they offer to such children is a moving witness to the immense depth and capacity for love of the human spirit.

There are nonetheless some serious questions to be asked of this perspective. One concerns how the cumulative effect of the theology of embodiment and the theodicy of compensation is not one of abandonment and medical neglect that could be construed as a form of child abuse. It is important to distinguish the LDS tradition from other views that would refuse medical assistance entirely and rely on expectations of divine or spiritual healing. The tradition does affirm healing as a spiritual gift, and commonly a person who is ill will request the ritual of "administration to the sick". At the same time, it has embraced rather than declined medical interventions, drawing on two basic assumptions about the nature of medicine in relation to religion.

The first assumption is that the capacities of modern medicine and the powers of medical technology are themselves gifts of healing that derive ultimately from the same divine source as spiritual healing methods. More fundamentally, there is a basic conviction in the tradition that medicine, and the science upon which it is based, are a complement rather than an antagonist of the religious community. The tradition discerns an ultimate harmony and convergence between science and religion that plays itself out in a trusting attitude towards medicine and the moral integrity of medical professionals.

The second assumption derives from the faith *and* works soteriology of the tradition. The faith expressed in healing rituals of administration to the sick and in prayer should be accompanied by and may be effectuated through the works of medicine. Thus, an impaired newborn should receive sufficient medical attention to alleviate pain and discomfort, and procedures to remedy the impairment should be contemplated. However, though death should not be hastened, life should not be prolonged merely for its own sake.

As a second challenge to the pro-birth orientation, it may also be susceptible to the critique of standard pro-life positions, namely, that it offers more support and protection to prenatal than to neonatal life. The validity of the critique depends on the cogency of its underlying assumptions. The LDS tradition would not accept the closed historical paradigm presupposed in the criticism and would instead claim that decisions about treatment or non-treatment must be contextualized in an eternal perspective. In that context, it may well be morally preferable (though not obligatory) to allow a seriously impaired child to be allowed to die, not because non-treatment would terminate a burdensome life, but rather to liberate the child to new occasions for knowledge and progress in the world of disembodied spirits.

Moreover, the tradition would not affirm, contrary to the presuppositions of the critique, that the moral character of a society is best gauged by the extent of state protection and support for neonatal life. That itself reflects an abdication of moral responsibility by persons, families, and communities. Families, both immediate and extended, as well as compassionate and nurturing communities, have the primary responsibility of stewardship for children; in such contexts, the commitment of care for newborn life should be extensive. The LDS popular literature is in fact replete with narratives of adoption of children from unwanted pregnancies and of children with various handicaps. This form of community responsiveness and interdependence would be seen as morally preferable to state mandates and as expressive of the moral character of church as the *body of Christ*.

This leaves the question of the ethics of selective non-treatment of impaired newborns somewhat unresolved in the tradition. The underlying theological convictions about the body and salvation could clearly support a presumption in favor of non-treatment, at least for seriously impaired newborns, but the practice of the tradition is by and large to err on the side of prolongation of life. A necessary task facing the tradition is to develop a moral casuistry to determine under what circumstances it would be permissible to withdraw or withhold life-sustaining treatment from impaired newborns.

D. *Reproductive Technology*

We have already portrayed how the theology of embodiment entails a pronounced procreative imperative. This in turn has significant ramifications for questions of reproductive technology. Although there is no adequate empirical data, anecdotal evidence suggests that infertility is a feature of married life for an increasing number of LDS couples. It can be an especially wrenching experience for such persons because of the various ways in which the tradition emphasizes that personal identity and welfare in both mortal existence and eternity are bound up with parenting. The tradition is so family-conscious that it sometimes has been accused even by its adherents of "familiolatry" (family idolatry), and persons who are single or married but childless report perceptions of isolation and unintended stigmatization. Thus, the force of the procreative imperative is experienced just as acutely among those persons unable to procreate as among those capable of complying.

In this context, reproductive technologies of artificial insemination, in vitro fertilization, or surrogacy might well be seen quite literally as a godsend. The procreative imperative coupled with the necessity of providing earthly tabernacles to the innumerable unembodied spirit persons would appear to provide a very strong positive rationale for the widespread availability of reproductive technology. Yet, the tradition has at best given lukewarm approval to reproductive technologies, and then only within certain limits, and these have the effect of imposing significant restrictions on access. These limits draw primarily on fundamental commitments about the nature of family and of relationships.

We have previously seen how the tradition's teaching on reproductive "choice" allows for a possible distinction between the necessity of birth and the timing and circumstances of birth. While this distinction seems to have minimal significance in the context of abortion, it appears to be overriding relative to the moral assessment of reproductive technology. There is in current ecclesiastical policy no positive recommendation of any reproductive technology; deference to the decisions of married couples about AIH or IVF using the married couples' gametes can be inferred by ecclesiastical silence. Meanwhile, use of third party gametes for AID is "discouraged" and in the case of IVF, "strongly discouraged". The condemnation becomes even stronger in the situation of attempts by single women to conceive a child through AID, which are "not approved" and may bring upon the woman forms of ecclesiastical discipline ([9], p. 114).

What is clear is that the circumstances of a family with clearly delineated relational lines is deemed the preferable context for use of reproductive technology if that course becomes medically necessary. That approach is not inconsistent with the screening criteria of many infertility clinics, although certainly not as pervasive as during the late 1970s and early 1980s. Nonetheless, the stated rationale for drawing the line of ecclesiastical silence at married couples may invite challenges of arbitrariness. The concern about use of third party gametes in the case of AID, IVF, and surrogacy is that this practice "may seriously disrupt family harmony". Of course, it also may not; the family seems a very adaptable and resilient social relationship, as illustrated by the capacity of many families to welcome nonrelated persons into their homes through adoption. Moreover, given the powerful connection between personal identity and parenting in the tradition, it can also be argued that the inability to conceive either naturally or through technological means itself creates significant strains in family life. The concerns for family stability and cohesiveness are at least relevant to a decision about reproductive technology, but insofar as the mutual relationship of the couple does not lead to recriminations or jealousies about the child, there would seem to be no principled reason for an absolute prohibition on AID, third-party IVF, or even surrogacy. The language of "discourage" rather than (as with single women) "not approved" suggests acknowledgement of familial flexibility and adaptability, and this is explicitly reinforced in the cases of AID and IVF by recent policy statements that "this [i.e., use of third party gametes] is a personal matter that ultimately must be left to the husband and wife, with the responsibility for the decision resting solely upon them" ([9], p. 11-4).

This line of reasoning, of course, could well lead to the same conclusion about the access of single women to reproductive technologies. If not offering the ideal context for raising children, single women have certainly demonstrated the capability to provide a nurturing, stable home life. In short, the ecclesiastical prohibition in this area looks not unlike a "family values" criticism of a Murphy Brown scenario.

The ecclesiastical rationale for this prohibition draws, however, as much on a theology of relationships as it does on an idealized understanding of family. In the tradition, special relationships are understood to have eternal duration; that is, death does not sever the relationships of family, friendships, and community. The canonical claim is "that same sociality which exists among us here will exist among us there [heaven]; only it will be coupled with eternal glory, which glory we do not now enjoy" ([7], p. 264).

The eternal nature of family relationships is realized in the LDS tradition's most sacred ritual of "sealing", one that is performed in specially-constructed temples rather than in congregational churches. In the sealing ritual, spouses enter into a covenant of fidelity to each other, of obedience to God, and of care and nurturance to present or future children. These mutual promises are verified by an appointed leader who is authorized to "seal" the covenant for "time and all eternity".

Yet, as this covenant presupposes a mutual relationship of husband and wife, the ritual is denied to single persons. The assertion of ecclesiastical leaders that artificial insemination of single women would "frustrate the eternal family plan", Lester Bush has observed, presupposes this ritual context. "The church will not allow a child to be sealed eternally to only one parent", regardless of whether the context is reproductive technology, adoption, or divorce. Thus, the prohibition is not premised so much on family values for mortal life as it is a soteriological understanding of the eternal breadth of family.

Reproductive technology, it is clear, holds substantial implications for core convictions of the LDS tradition. It is in fact one area of contemporary biomedical technology in which ecclesiastical policies have tended to express reservations or prohibitions rather than implicit approval or support. Yet, these policies, especially on AID and IVF, have actually evolved in a more approving direction as questions of safety and efficacy have been resolved, as infertility has been medicalized, and as reproductive technology has been integrated into the mainstream of medical practice. There are limits to this moral evolution imposed by a context of ritual practice and a theology of relationships, and it can be expected that a more restrictive attitude on surrogacy would be forthcoming should this become an issue for the LDS community rather than a social policy question. However, in the context of AI and IVF, ecclesiastical reservations ultimately give way to the decisions of conscientious couples about the shape they wish to give to their families and their eternal relations.

IV. DEATH: THE BODY AS GIFT AND BURDEN

Mortality in the LDS perspective is that transitional passage in a person's existence in which knowledge is learned and relationships are created and sustained through the experience of embodiment. The body is a gift of God and of parents through which all the events of mortality, whether for joy or sorrow, pleasure or pain, happiness or suffering, are mediated "for your experience, and for your good" ([7], pp. 243-44). The faith community is not promised immunity from life reversals, misfortune, injustice, pains of the body, or sufferings of the spirit, nor the ultimate leveller of death, but rather that the "trials" of mortality are to be an occasion for learning the lessons of life about self and others. It is this context that frames the tradition's response to the burden of the body experienced in dying and death.

If birth is the passage of the self from unembodied to embodied life, death is but a similar passage to disembodied life. Theologically, death means the separation of body and the spirit that had been united as soul at birth and that will be re-united for eternity in the passage of resurrection. The effort to identify some bodily organ as the seat of the soul along the model of Descartes's pineal gland, would not be followed by the tradition, since soul is the embodied person. At death, a person's spirit, this consists of the same form and characteristics as the physical body, is separated from the body in its entirety.

A. *Persistent Vegetative State (PVS)*

This account leads to some puzzles when confronting the possibilities of life-prolonging medical technology. Although certainly not unique to the LDS tradition, the condition of persistent vegetative state (PVS) presents significant perplexities. One possible argument would be that the condition of PVS signifies that the separation of body and spirit has already occurred. The person is already dead theologically, even if not legally or philosophically. There would then be no hesitation about discontinuing life-prolonging treatment.

Another possibility would be that the presence of irreversible coma inhibits any learning prospects. The person may not be dead, but since the possibilities of progression are so substantially limited, it would be permissible to forgo further medical treatment.

Yet, while ecclesiastical policy allows treatment to be withdrawn or withheld when the means are "unreasonable," this policy also presumes that dying is "inevitable", which is precisely the medical dilemma encountered in PVS. Death is inevitable only when a decision to forgo treatment has been made, but can be forestalled for many years with continuation of treatment. Thus, for some in the tradition, the presence of unassisted bodily functions, such as circulation and respiration, would be a sufficient reason to continue life supports.

This diversity exists in the tradition in part because ecclesiastical policy has not undertaken a moral casuistry to elucidate the meaning of "unreasonable means". Rather than identifying any criteria or designating particular life-sustaining means as unreasonable under certain conditions, the tradition has deferred responsibility to patients and families in collaboration with competent medical advice. Nor has any policy guidance been forthcoming about the propriety of advance directives. The general pattern again seems to be that in matters of termination of treatment, ecclesiastical silence signifies that the decision is a matter for personal free agency within the parameters allowed by law.

B. *Euthanasia*

It is highly improbable, however, should physician-assisted suicide or active euthanasia become a legal option, as considered recently in California, Oregon and Washington, all of which have substantial LDS communities, that the tradition would be silent on such alternatives. It is instructive that, in the context of widespread national discussion about legalized euthanasia, the tradition seems to have at least begun the casuistical discussion necessary. In 1989, a policy on *euthanasia* was first articulated, as distinct from earlier policies on the prolongation of life. Euthanasia was defined as *deliberately putting to death a person suffering from incurable conditions or diseases* and declared to *violate the commandments of God* ([9], p. 11-5). It is likely that this statement is not intended to address directly the social policy debate but is meant to provide pastoral guidance to the faith community, whose members can be confronted with the torment and suffering of their terminally ill relatives.

It is important to identify what the wrong of euthanasia consists in, because it is not immediately evident just what divine commandments are violated. One prime candidate would be the rule prohibiting killing or respect for the sanctity of life. Yet, if euthanasia is the moral equivalent of homicide, it would seem that the condemnation would be accompanied by a statement that participants would be subject to ecclesiastical discipline, as is the case with abortion. Indeed, abortion is not even considered killing under current policy, but rather is analogous to or *like unto* killing. If the rule against killing is violated by euthanasia, it would seem, then, that euthanasia is a graver wrong than abortion.

However, following the pattern of the policy on abortion, it might be argued that euthanasia is also only *like unto killing*, because it is relevantly dissimilar to those acts thought to violate the rule against killing in the following manner. At least in the form of euthanasia most frequently defended by advocates, the person requests and consents to his or her own death. Moreover, the motive for euthanasia is characteristically portrayed as mercy killing rather than malevolence. If euthanasia is best seen as analogous to, but not identical with, killing, then it could be argued that, as with abortion, euthanasia could be permissible under certain exceptional cases. This is essentially the reasoning offered by supporters of legalized euthanasia within the tradition.

This approach suggests, however, some other possible reasons for the wrongfulness of euthanasia in the tradition. The appeal to a person's consent to death might be considered suspect for the same reason the tradition condemns an act of suicide (while not holding the person blameworthy). That is, suicide or euthanasia is not a choice to which a rational person can voluntarily consent. Euthanasia might be viewed as wrong because it violates or at least is inconsistent with a principle of personal free agency.

The difficulty with this rationale is that the LDS theology of death can certainly make death as a passage to new life preferable than mortal existence. Death can arguably be said to be a rational choice in the sense of coherence with a religious paradigm. However, the problem of euthanasia might not be so much with the choice of death as with its *timing*; the tradition has appealed to various canonical passages to affirm that each person has a "time appointed to death" in the plan of God. Euthanasia then might violate the sovereignty of God over life and death. The difficulty here is that the timing of death is very much conditioned by the use of medical technology. To make the principle of divine sovereignty the decisive consideration can push in the direction of technological fatalism, which the tradition has seemed to reject by allowing unreasonable means to be discontinued.

If the prohibition of euthanasia cannot be successfully grounded in the moral logic of personal freedom, an alternative approach could challenge the appeal to mercy by the proponent of euthanasia. The argument could claim that compassionate care requires family and professionals to be present to the terminally ill person in his or her suffering rather than eliminating suffering by eliminating the sufferer. Moreover, the appropriate response of the patient to suffering is to express the virtue of "endurance", in keeping with a central principle that fidelity to God requires a person to "endure to the end". The suffering borne by the body is not itself sanctified, but it can be a means to sanctifying the person. Suffering is understood in the tradition as an occasion for being tutored in obedience and fidelity and for the purification of the self In submitting to suffering and enduring it in fidelity a person engages in the imitation of Christ (*imitatio Christi*). Thus, while the tradition does not say so explicitly, its approach to suffering reflects themes embedded in the claim of Roman Catholicism that through suffering a terminally ill person may participate in the passion of Christ.

A related point may critique the labeling of a person with a terminal condition as "hopelessly" ill and therefore a candidate for assisted suicide or active euthanasia The context of "hopelessness" and "hope" requires specification for this claim to be compelling. Such language reduces the patient to a medical condition, and may neglect other sources of hope, including affirmation of one's life experience and expectations regarding death. The presence of the caregiver is itself a sign of hope to the patient.

The ecclesiastical ground for prohibiting euthanasia then may rest not only in the paradigm of unjustified killing but also in what it means to live out the religious life according to the virtues of faith (fidelity), hope, and love (compassion). Euthanasia may be a concern not only because of a principle regarding killing but also because of what it displays about a person's moral character. The prospects for continued policy discussion and possible legalization of euthanasia will likely inform both ecclesiastical perspectives and practices within the faith community.

C. *Organ Transplantation*

The discussion of determination of death and termination of treatment inevitably leads to questions of organ donation and transplantation. The history of LDS discussion on this issue reveals a gradual liberalization in favor of respecting the decision of the individual and family that both presupposes and is limited by the organic integrity of the body. During the period when organ transplantation was largely experimental research rather than validated therapy, an informal prohibition was instituted, attributable in part to unresolved medical questions about safety for donors and efficacy for recipients, and in part to unresolved theological questions about the implications of a transplant for a resurrected body. The development of immunosuppressive therapies in the late 1970s helped resolve many of the medical issues and clearly established transplant as therapy. Not coincidentally, the ecclesiastical and theological perspectives shifted significantly. The informal prohibition gave way to a formal policy that held that "willing" one's organs for purposes of transplantation was a matter of personal choice. Meanwhile, articles and narratives about successful transplants appeared in LDS popular literature that cited canonical claims about the perfectly restored nature of all resurrected bodies as sufficient reason to think that organ donation would not jeopardize one's prospects for eternal progress. Such a question, of course, would not even arise, let alone make sense, in a context (non-religious or religious) where the body was not understood to be essential to self-identity and integrity. It is nonetheless striking that organ transplantation has not received a more positive endorsement at the level of ecclesiastical policy. The tradition places tremendous emphasis on altruistic ideals of sacrifice and service to others, and it might be thought that such ideals could find few better mediums of expression than the gift of one's body to others in a transplant of vital organs. Yet, the policy statement invokes the legalistic language of "willing" organs rather than the religious-moral language of "donation".

One possible reason for the reluctance to fully embrace organ donation is a concern to protect the free choice of the donor, whether of the person or of family members, so that they will not experience duress either from the dire need of the recipient or from religious motivations. It is instructive that many of the personal narratives in LDS popular literature relate instances of enhanced relationships through living related donors. Given the eternal nature of family relationships in the LDS perspective, a concern about duress can seem very compelling. The moral integrity of donation itself presupposes a voluntary decision.

At another level, such reluctance may reflect an ongoing concern about the integrity and reverence owed to the body. The issue here might best be expressed by recalling Paul Ramsey's critique of Protestant agapism as a rationale for organ donation. Ramsey argued that such a justification, "because of its freedom from the moorings of self-concern, is likely to fly too high above concern for the bodily integrity of the donor". Ramsey instead commended the approach of Jewish ethics in its "concern for man's embodied existence" and its "joyful affirmation of the integrity of the flesh" ([14]). That orientation to the body, I have argued, is central to the LDS theology of embodiment and therefore shapes the tradition's more conservative conclusion on organ transplants.

This concern for bodily integrity would in all probability override the concern for voluntary choice should a commercial organ market become an option in future social policy. Such a policy would transform understandings of the body and its transplantable organs and tissues into objects of "property", commodities that can be alienated. Because the body is essential rather than incidental to self-understanding and moral integrity, commercial alienation of the body through an organ market might well be ecclesiastically discouraged or disapproved. Such a market may be seen as lacking the requisite reverence for the body and expressing not only the alienability of the body but also alienation from the body and thus also from one's self

V. SOME CHALLENGES AND DIRECTIONS

As should be evident from this discussion, the LDS tradition has been somewhat sparing in developing ecclesiastical positions or recommendations on the array of questions that constitute contemporary biomedical ethics. While the most sustained attention has been given to core matters of life and death, such as abortion or the right to die, even these issues are treated rather cursorily, leaving many basic questions, such as the timing of embodiment (abortion) or disembodiment (death), unanswered. Nor have scholars in the tradition devoted much reflection to the ethical issues embedded in medicine. This is a significant oversight, since anecdotal evidence suggests such questions are encountered with increasing frequency in the lives of persons and their families. The tradition may have failed to provide the kind of pastoral direction many of its adherents need, and more importantly, want. Moreover, by and large, the tradition has not engaged in social policy debates on issues such as abortion, reproductive technology, or euthanasia, and has left other deep social questions, such as resource allocation and the setting of health priorities, to citizen activism within the political process.

Yet, this reticence is not accidental, but itself reflects central convictions about ecclesiological identity. First, with the exception of three general leadership bodies, the ecclesiastical affairs of the LDS Church are administered through a lay clergy. This represents the LDS commitment to a "priesthood of all believers" (though currently ordination is limited to males twelve years of age and older), but it also means the tradition has no body of professional theologians who specialize in ethical questions. It is instructive of the state of discussion that the recently-issued *Encyclopedia of Mormonism*, a four-volume work surveying LDS doctrine, history, scripture, and culture in over 1,200 articles contains virtually no entries on medical ethics [11]. Thus, resources for decision making and ethical discourse tends to default to the general ecclesiastical leadership or to individuals and their families in their own particular situations of moral perplexity.

Secondly, ecclesiastical policy tends to be limited to short position statements without either normative defense or casuistical explication. The broad patterns of the ecclesiastical approach have been to offer general guidance that allow for personal self-governance, to engage in reactive ethics by avoiding declarations until scientific and medical questions are resolved, and to place broader questions of social justice in the providential responsibility of God. These patterns are consistent with LDS values of respect for personal moral agency, trust in the generalized wisdom and expertise of the scientific and medical communities, (which ultimately reflects divine knowledge), and "strict neutrality" in political issues. This last value is also supported by a deep conviction of eschatological or millenarian compensation for injustice. The same patterns that support a generalized approach of ecclesiastical silence simultaneously reinforce the substantial authoritativeness attributed to any ecclesiastical pronouncement. In this respect, the tradition reflects a strong emphasis on hierarchical or trickle-down ethics.

Third, these patterns also allow for a trickle-up context for ethical decision-making, although this seldom issues in sustained ethical discourse. This occurs for at least four identifiable reasons: (1) When confronted with an apparent moral dilemma, the most common popular response is a resort to prayer. There is a profound confidence that the answers to life's riddles, as well as biomedical perplexities, can be realized through prayer, and Latter-day Saints who display fidelity to God are assured that they will receive "divine inspiration or revelation" to solve apparent dilemmas. (2) The situations of moral choices experienced by individuals are typically understood to be unique and particular to the involved persons. This restricts the possibility of a generalized ethical framework applicable across situations and culminates in a form of relativism at the level of situational decisions (though this may be corrected for by the absolutism assured through prayer). (3) As implicit in these first two reasons, the tradition manifests a pronounced suspicion of reaching moral closure through reason alone. This does not mean that rationality is completely excluded from moral choices, but it does assume a subordinate role. A commonly invoked pattern in pastoral sermons is that a person confronting a choice (moral or otherwise) should come to his or her

own conclusion through methods of study and dialogue, and then seek
confirmation of that decision through prayer and inspiration. (4) Latter-day
Saints are not encouraged to be politically quietistic. The canonical admonition
that all persons are to be "anxiously engaged in a good cause, and do many
things of their own free will, and bring to pass much righteousness . . ." ([7],
p. 105) is frequently invoked as support for civic involvement and activism.
However, coupled with the stance of strict institutional neutrality in the political
process, it becomes evident that persons who are so engaged in civic affairs and
social policy are (or should be) present in the debate as citizens rather than as
representatives of the LDS Church. In policy contexts, then, the relevance of
religious convictions on matters of social justice may be minimal or indirect.

There are some important lessons to be gained from this analysis. It is,
first of all, important to recognize that the position of religious traditions on
questions of medical ethics are deeply embedded in and interwoven with
fundamental metaphysical, theological, and ecclesiological convictions. It is
difficult to sever the metaphysical-moral relationship in discourse internal to a
tradition and unfair for critics external to a tradition to consider only a
normative conclusion on a given issue and neglect the metaphysical context out
of which the normative stance arises.

The LDS tradition does not, except indirectly, propose that its ecclesiastical
positions be adopted in social policy, so a critique of those traditions offered
from the standpoint of generally accessible reasons may not be compelling
(assuming the critic could construct a morality independent of assumptions of
time, community, and human nature). Nonetheless, it is not evident that the
tradition could meet criteria of internal coherence. There are thus two major
challenges presented for scholars and interpreters of the tradition that suggest
new directions for ethical discourse on medicine. The first is to identify the
norms and principles that underlie and substantiate the normative conclusions
presented in current ecclesiastical policies. The second is to establish a closer
connection between principles and practices by developing a moral casuistry.
This essay hopes to have offered an initial contribution to both these tasks. It
is to be hoped that continued discussion along these lines will help identify and
resolve some of the current tensions between ecclesiastical authoritarianism and
individualism, or between absolutism and relativism, and thereby enable
Latter-day Saint ethics to be embodied in a genuine and vital moral tradition
of ongoing argument.

Oregon State University
Corvallis, Oregon, U.S.A.

NOTES

1. The Latter-day Saint tradition has an "open canon", which currently consists of *The Holy Bible* (KJV), *The Book of Mormon*, *The Doctrine and Covenants*, and *The Pearl of Great Price*. The four books are referred to as "the standard works", that is, the "standard" by which religious and moral truth can be measured.
2. For ease of expression and clarity, in subsequent discussion of the pre-mortal existence I will use the language of "unembodied" experience, although this is not completely true on the LDS view for the reasons mentioned.
3. This was also one of the influential justifications given for the community's experience with plural marriage during the 19th century.

BIBLIOGRAPHY

1. Ballard, M.: 1969, in "Three Degrees of Glory", as cited in S.W. Kimball, *The Miracle of Forgiveness*, Bookcraft, Inc., Salt Lake City.
2. Benson, E.: 1988, "First Presidency Statement on AIDS", *Ensign* 18:7, 79.
3. *The Book of Mormon*: 1986, The Church of Jesus Christ of Latter-day Saints, Salt Lake City.
4. Bush, L., Jr.: *Health and Medicine Among the Latter-day Saints: Science, Sense and Scripture*, forthcoming.
5. "Church Issues Statement on Abortion": 1991, *Ensign* 21:3, 78.
6. Clark, S.: 1992, "And They All Prayed On", *Sunstone* 16:2, 62.
7. *The Doctrine and Covenants*: 1986, The Church of Jesus Christ of Latter-day Saints, Salt Lake City.
8. Eliade, M.: 1959, *The Sacred and the Profane*, Harcourt Brace & World, New York.
9. *General Handbook of Instructions*, 24th ed.: 1989, The Church of Jesus Christ of Latter-day Saints, Salt Lake City.
10. Hinckley, G.: 1987, "Reverence and Morality", Ensign 17:5, 46-47.
11. Ludlow, D. (ed.): 1992, *Encyclopedia of Mormonism*, Macmillan Publishing, New York.
12. MacMurray, V., Ventura, K: 1983, "Decision Models in Bioethics", in D. Hill, Jr. (ed.), *Perspectives in Mormon Ethics*, Publishers Press, Salt Lake City, 253284.
13. Packer, B.: 1990, "Covenants", *Ensign* 20:11, 84.
14. Ramsey, P.: 1970, *The Patient as Person*, Yale University Press, New Haven, 187.
15. Roberts, S.: 1990, "Pastoring the Farside", *Sunstone* 14:1, 17.
16. van Gennep, A.: 1960, *The Rites of Passage*, University of Chicago Press, Chicago.

PRAKASH N. DESAI* AND B. ANDREW LUSTIG

HINDU AND INDIAN DEVELOPMENTS

INTRODUCTION

It has been two years since the publication of Volume One of the *Bioethics Yearbook*, a short time in the life of an ancient civilization. Except for specific developments on several issues that will be reported in Section II of this essay, only a modest amount of reflection in bioethics has transpired since 1990 in Hindu thought or in Indian medical practice. Yet the same two years have been a long time in the life of a people in cultural transition. India has been torn by interreligious and communal strife which, although not new, has recently increased dramatically in ferocity and intensity. Strife between the Hindu and Muslim communities has engulfed most of India, and places that previously had been known for their inter-faith amity have been engulfed in flames.

In Section I, we will suggest that the failure to respect human dignity lies at the heart of such conflict. By implication, we will recommend that the concept of human dignity must be central to bioethical discussions as well. By human dignity we mean the conviction that human beings, *qua* human beings, are inherently worthy of respect. In Section II, we will briefly trace a number of recent developments on specific topics in bioethics.

I. VIOLENCE IN INDIA: A PROBLEM OF HUMAN DIGNITY

Sanctity of human life has been one of the highest values in contemporary religious and bioethical thought. Equality and justice, even as the Communist world has collapsed, have been reasserted as pivotal values in bioethics as well as in the delivery of health care services. Although bioethicists have been relatively silent about traditional values that conflict with or constrain human dignity and autonomy, cultural pluralism is not simply a matter of tolerance. While each faith tradition has historically espoused the well-being and dignity of its believers, each has often been inimical toward the sanctity of life of believers of another God. Our own times have not been any more tolerant.

The violation of human dignity is not a new problem in India. For example, the inferior status of women and untouchables in a hierarchical society have long been matters of explicit reflection by social reformers and progressive thinkers. But recent Hindu-Muslim conflicts (intensifying in part because traditional mechanisms for conflict resolution have broken down) heighten our awareness of the pervasive failure to respect human dignity. Moreover, the

B. Andrew Lustig (Sr. Ed.), Bioethics Yearbook: Volume 3, 69-82.
©1993 Kluwer Academic Publishers.

decade-old confrontation between the Sikhs and the Indian state, still unresolved, confounds the story, because secessionist fever adds a further ingredient to the social maelstrom.

Two years ago, the essay on Hindu developments, while acknowledging the reality of communal tension and reporting on the problems faced by women in India, tended to focus on narrower issues. The recent strife in India, however, requires us to look in greater detail at the larger social dimensions of communal and religious conflict. The remainder of our discussion in this section, therefore, will offer a brief account of the religious influences at work in India's history, especially in the ongoing violence since the time of India's independence, in the hope that increased understanding of the past will illuminate the present situation of conflict ([14];[15]).

A. *A Brief History*

1. *The Early Phase.* From antiquity, trade across the Arabian Sea between Arabia and the West Coast of India had flourished. Muslim traders followed similar routes, thus following an established tradition of rich exchange on the Malabar coast. The first military incursion occurred in 712 C.E., when Mohammed ibn-Kasim conquered Sind (the extreme Western part of what was then India and is now Pakistan) for the Caliphate and later overran other neighboring territories. The next major invasion was carried out by Mohammed of Ghazni, who sacked many Northern regions of India. After razing the temple in Mathura c. 1018, Mohammed's most severe blow to Hindu pride, etched in collective memory, was his destruction of the temple of Somnath in 1026. In 1191, Mohammed of Ghur marched beyond the Punjab into the land of the Rajputs and defeated them. That era was characterized by atrocities committed upon the populace, destruction of temples, desecration of Hindu idols, forcible conversions, and wholesale plunder. The Hindus, plagued by internal divisions, were rarely able to offer united opposition.

2. *The Middle Phase: The Moghul Period.* Babar, with his conquest of Delhi in 1526, established the Moghul Empire in India. The Moghul Empire was consolidated through conquests and alliances throughout India, especially by Emperor Akbar, who was known as a generous ruler. Akbar adopted an attitude of toleration toward Hindu rulers and the general populace and attempted a religious synthesis by founding a new religion, *Din-i-ilahi*. The greatest glories of the Moghul Empire were achieved under the benevolent rule of Akbar and his immediate descendants. For example, Shahjahan, a grandson of Akbar, commissioned the building of the Taj Mahal. Nonetheless, the Moghul dominance was short-lived. Less than a hundred years later, in 1738, Nadir Shah, invading from Iran, sacked Delhi and Agra, sparing neither women nor children and repeating earlier plunders. Nadir's invasion signalled the loss of power and prestige of the Moghuls and marked the beginning of the end of

their empire. The last Moghul emperor, Bahadur Shah, who participated in the revolt against the British in 1857, died in exile.

3. *Defiance of The Moghul Empire*. During this phase, the subcontinent spawned a new religion. A long history of invasions and hostile incursions into the Northwestern territories had martialized the people of that region. Contradictions within the Hindu faith and Islamic influences led to the foundation of Sikhism, which soon became a symbol of defiance of the Moghul empire. Sikhs wore their body-hair unshorn, thus obliterating caste distinctions, and carried a ritual knife, the Kirpan, to symbolize their willingness to defend their honor.

The Sikh shrines (*Gurudwaras*) were built to house religious texts containing the teachings of the founding gurus. Later gurus established an independent state and massed a formidable army, thus cementing the Sikhs' cultural and political identity.   Ironically, the people who chose to obliterate caste distinctions conspicuously distinguished themselves from other Indians.

A second major resistance to the spreading Moghul empire came from the South. A local Maratha Chieftan, Shivaji, challenged the Empire by carrying out several successful raids against neighboring Moghul occupations. Shivaji is celebrated today by the Hindu militants who call themselves the Shiv-sena (army of Shivaji). Shivaji's legendary exploits emboldened the Peshwas to found still another kingdom in the area immediately south of Bombay.

4. *Late Phase: Western Rule.* With the entry of European powers into India, for a time Hindu-Muslim problems receded from prominence. Vasco da Gama, who came in search of "Christians and spices", opened Indian markets to Portugal, Holland, France, and England [15]. During the next 250 years, the British triumphed and become the rulers of India. Although Christianity had been an established presence in India for many centuries, missionary activities dramatically increased. The patterns of Christian proselytizing were not unlike the earlier waves of Islamic conversion, and Hinduism found itself again on the defensive. The spread of Islam had provoked a variety of Hindu responses, including an intensifying of the devotional tradition of *Bhakti*. Likewise, Christian efforts at conversion prompted the formation of new social and religious movements in Hinduism. Some emphasized monotheism or rejected image worship; others called for social reform, rejected the caste system, or championed the cause of women [6].

The emergence of the Indian National Congress brought the Muslims and the Hindus together in the struggle for freedom. Nonetheless, a section of the Muslim leadership saw in the rise of the Congress a danger to their own prospects for dominance in Indian affairs. The Muslim League, founded in 1906, was a development that plagued India for decades by playing into the British strategy of "divide and rule". Mahatma Gandhi would struggle in vain for a way to end the animus between the two communities. Ultimately the partition of India caused an unparalleled migration of peoples and left a trail of rage, revenge and destruction, with at least a million persons dead.

5. After Independence. In fashioning a coalition in the struggle for freedom, Mahatma Gandhi had aroused the masses and inducted rural communities successfully into the independence movement. While Gandhi appealed to rural sensibilities through his simple and spartan life, he also challenged villagers to permit the untouchables to enter the mainstream of society. At his invitation, women had already joined the movement in great numbers, thus helping to lower the social barriers against their public participation. Gandhi also included Indian Muslims. In this respect, he offered a model of inter-faith dialogue, although his prestige subsequently suffered in the aftermath of partition with the forcible eviction of Hindus from Pakistan.

The spirit of dismissing ethnic and religious differences in public life was championed by Jawaharlal Nehru, Gandhi's political heir and the first prime minister of India. In founding the Indian nation-state, Nehru emphasized secularism, and the first Indian constitution enshrined the principle with special protection for the untouchables. The restoration of human dignity thus provided a cornerstone of the new constitution.

During the struggle for independence, political leadership under a Hindu banner had sought unsuccessfully to achieve dominance, although Hindu groups continued to exert influence on the periphery. The murder of Gandhi by a member of a Hindu nationalist group, the Rashtriya Svayumsevak Sangh (RSS), effectively ended its influence, but other political parties, holding obvious Hindu sympathies, have held sway in various parts of India since that time. During the last decade, the Bhartiya Janata Party (BJP) has assembled a coalition and advanced the claim that the state of India should renounce its secular character to extol and embrace the Hindu faith of the Indian majority [14]. Hindu advocates have argued that the ruling Congress party is pro-Muslim, that Muslims have too much say and sway in Indian politics, and that Muslim votes are won by pandering to narrow interests.

These perceptions have been strengthened by a peculiarly Indian definition of secularism. A "secular" spirit in India does not dictate that Hindus and Muslims are treated alike under the law, but rather that each religious community is governed by its own religious law in matters of personal codes. Hindu fundamentalists have seized upon this as evidence of India's pseudo-secularism, while others agree that such "toleration" functions regressively, especially on such issues as the status of women.

In the aftermath of the British decision to partition India, certain Hindu factions had insisted on complete transfer of population. The mayhem that occurred after the partition intensified that call. Persistent questions about the extra-territorial loyalties of Muslims have also been sounded whenever tensions have arisen between India and Pakistan. To a civilization already wounded, Pakistan has come to represent a loss of pride more than a loss of territory.

There is another way in which the Hindu civilization has been wounded, this time from within. Over fifteen percent of the Indian population belongs to the underclass of the so-called "untouchables", with another seven percent "tribals". Both groups are outside Hindu orthodoxy, as compared with a Muslim population of twelve to thirteen percent. Even among the remaining two-thirds of India's population, only a third are the so-called high castes – *Brahmins, kshatriyas* and *Vaishyas*. The rest form another layer of the underclass, largely poor, serving the upper castes. Over the centuries, both Christian and Muslim converts have tended to come from the underclass. However much the Hindus may rail against such conversions, those who have been kept on the margins of social, economic, and religious life have flocked to other faiths where they might recover their dignity and self-esteem.

Everyday endemic violence against untouchable men and women continues to bleed the Hindu spirit. Rape, blinding, flogging, and burning alive are not uncommon. Those who wave saffron flags of Hindu wisdom and sanctity have often failed to take cognizance of what Hindu tradition has wrought upon the untouchables. The promise held by a secular constitution of an independent India to alter the lives of the untouchables and the tribals has delivered them neither from social or economic tyranny nor from indignity.

Nonetheless, India has committed herself to change and to guaranteeing human dignity under a secular state. Since independence, the pace of social and economic change has been impressive. The country is now fully self-sufficient in meeting its own agricultural needs. In the area of health, India has reduced maternal and child mortality by nearly half. Mass movements to eradicate illiteracy and communicable diseases have been launched. Ambitious projects to stem the population explosion and supply drinking water within a reasonable distance to all have also been launched. Universal vaccination of infants and pregnant mothers have been implemented for more than half the population.

At the same time, a number of troubling aspects of Indian social and economic life persist. The rate of population growth, urban growth, and growth in the number of children continues at a staggering pace. The Hindu-Muslim problem, as well as the poor status of the untouchables, is confounded by the volatile combination of heightened economic expectations and competition for scarce resources. The secular constraints against violation of human dignity are as yet not well enough rooted in the culture to withstand such pressures.

The rightful demands of women, both individually and collectively, further erode confidence in the system. Traditional values regarding appropriate marital partnerships and family connections are increasingly challenged. Assigning women to a protected and subordinate role is ever less acceptable, especially in the urban middle class. Although male dominance continues, large numbers of women in the labor force, especially in mid-level and professional jobs in urban areas, bring increasing pressure for change. Dowry deaths tragically represent the reassertion of cultural cruelties, but the age of information does not permit easy cover-ups. Women in politics and leaders of the women's rights movement speak to the conscience of the nation as they expose sham amniocenteses for purposes of sex selection, female infanticide, child marriages, and bride burning (see *Yearbook*, Vol. 1, pp. 48-54).

To those issues may be added the problems engendered by the Sikh separatist movement. A secessionist campaign in Kashmir exemplifies anew the Hindu-Muslim divide; the majority Muslim community in Kashmir is asking for self-determination. Hindu militants, and even many moderates, express a sense of revulsion toward the further fragmentation of India and a recurrence of the same passions that followed partition in 1947. In the wake of the desecration of the Sikh Golden Temple and the assassination of Indira Gandhi, the body-politic of India has been severely weakened. Political assassinations on the subcontinent have become commonplace. Angry confrontations leave little room for reasonable negotiations. Indeed, violations of human dignity are too often protested through acts of violent retribution.

B. *Is There a Way Out?*

Is there a way beyond the Hindu-Muslim impasse? Can anyone succeed where the Mahatma had failed? All around the world, problems of ethnic cleansing, communal hatred, and disenfranchisement of minorities defy solutions. One may legitimately ask why expressly religious voices are not rising to stem the tides of violence and why the call to restore dignity and civil rights is not a part of every sermon.

A. Nandy has suggested that the erosion of Indian selfhood under foreign subjugation was facilitated by the wish to emulate and identify with the aggressor, since a master best accomplishes his dominance by stripping the slave of his dignity [7]. We may say that assumptions of a false self impoverish the true self. To hold on to the past or to be seized by a revivalist spirit does not restore dignity, but to wallow in self-contempt certainly erodes selfhood. And wounded pride, irrespective of the source of injury or the degree of self-deception, is ready to explode into narcissistic rage.

Of course answers for India will have to come from India, and there are no simple or easy solutions. But no dialogue can begin without acknowledgment of the past. Inhumanities and atrocities that occurred during the Islamic invasion and Muslim rule must be confronted and accepted. Retribution is no answer; it is "ethically grotesque" [14]. Shifting economic and social patterns have exacerbated the long-standing conflict between Hindus and Muslims. In addition, new realities of foreign rule, trade and industry, urbanization and the breakdown of village life have contributed to animosities between the two communities. The lingering effects of the partition of India and the creation of Pakistan as an avowedly religious state must also be acknowledged. Nevertheless, a solution must emerge from the religious leadership on both sides.

Systematic violations of human dignity have occurred for centuries in India, directly sanctioned by the hierarchical arrangement of the Hindu society. Those on the lower rungs of the social order have been denied the opportunity to participate in the religious life of the tradition by being denied education and maintained in illiteracy. For a variety of reasons, the lot of women has been only slightly better. In addition, Hindus historically have not permitted Muslims full participation in communal life.

Hindu leadership, therefore, must develop the full range of appropriate responses required to overcome the systematic violations of human dignity that remain. Hindu leadership must be ready to adapt to and implement fully the norms of a democratic society. Moreover, Hindus must atone for their treatment of Muslims as outcasts, and for the treatment of the outcasts themselves. They will be required to reinterpret their scriptures to accord new respect to the untouchables, to women, and to Muslims.

Hindus and Muslims in dialogue also must acknowledge their respective strengths and leave it to each community to examine its own weaknesses and deficiencies. At its best, Islam has stood for universal brotherhood, "a simple caste-less dignity . . ., strong preference for simple rituals, the distaste for priestly barriers between man and God, and [a] strong legal sense" [12]. Hindus, on the other hand, have enjoyed an unfettered spiritual inquiry and equally unfettered private quest for God. But Hindus must come to come to terms with their antiquated notions of purity and pollution, hierarchy and order, which often conflict with human dignity. Similarly, Muslims must learn to deal with people who worship a different God, a people not "of the Book". For if India becomes a nation-state of the Hindus, as Pakistan has become a Muslim state, India will be condemned to communal strife and constant erosion of human dignity. A recommitment to Gandhi's vision of tolerance and respect for democratic ideals offers the only way to peace.

II. OTHER ISSUES

In Section II, we report briefly about developments in India on a number of other bioethical topics during the past two years. These issues, while not discussed in expressly religious terms, pose challenging questions that call for response from the Hindu community. For this reason, they are included in this theological yearbook. To some extent, the discussion here amplifies I.C. Verma's essay on recent Indian developments in Volume Two of the *Yearbook, Regional Developments 1989-1991*.

A. *Issues of Public Health*

1. *Oral Polio Vaccine to Continue*

The World Health Organization has consistently advocated relying upon oral polio vaccine as the most efficient and cost-effective way to control polio in developing countries. Thus, recent discussions advocating the introduction of a high-cost injectable polio vaccine as part of India's universal immunization program provoked significant controversy. In 1992, the Health Ministry of India, heeding the WHO recommendations, decided not to introduce the injectable vaccine, ending the controversy over its use for the time being [8].

2. *Ban on Some Anti-Diarrheal Drugs*

In October 1992, the World Health Organization issued a report recommending a ban on certain anti-diarrheal drugs commonly prescribed for children. The report notes that certain binding agents (diphenoxylate, loperamide, streptomycin, neomycin, kaolin, and pectin) used in the drugs may actually aggravate diarrhea, interfere with the action of antibiotics, and, in high doses, even induce coma or death.

The report has provoked serious controversy in the Indian press. A number of pharmaceutical companies have labelled the proposed blanket ban "unfair" and insensitive to the particular difficulties of controlling children's diseases and conditions in developing countries.

In response to the WHO report, the Directorate General of Health Services has appointed an expert committee to study the findings on anti-diarrheal drugs [5].

3. *Blood Policy*

On October 15, 1992, India's Supreme Court called on the Union Government to respond officially to a proposal by a citizens' lobby meant to develop a national policy on transfusion. The citizen group, called Common Cause, recommends centralized oversight of blood banking and transfusion and a central authority to develop guidelines, grant licenses, and monitor transfusion technology. Specifically, the proposal urges an end to the sale of blood in six months, "to be replaced by voluntary donation" [4].

4. *The Use of the Norplant Contraceptive.*

Norplant, a contraceptive inserted into a woman's body that prevents conception for five years, is scheduled to be introduced into India's family planning programs in several centers, despite significant opposition from a number of women's groups. Three years ago, plans to introduce Net-en (an injectable contraceptive) into family planning programs were thwarted when a number of women's groups filed petition in the Supreme Court to prevent its dissemination.

In their petition, those groups made the following points: (1) the Government was conducting trails without informed consent. Women recruited for the trial were not informed about Net-en, its possible side effects, or the purposes of the trial; (2) trials of Net-en were to be conducted on women belonging to the lower strata of society who were totally unaware of the trial and its ramifications; and (3) women seeking abortion were also recruited for the Net-en trial, with their participation made a precondition for medical termination of pregnancy.

In response to arguments from those groups, the Court granted a stay against the introduction of Net-en which is still in effect. Nonetheless, the Government is "proceeding with trials for testing Norplant" [16]. 100 medical colleges and 20,000 women are presently enrolled. In light of the history of Net-en, and the dangers of abuse from undersupervised and poorly directed trials, a number of commentators argue that the same concerns posed by Net-en arise with Norplant, and that, at the present time, proceeding with trials is unreasonable and unfair [16].

5. Contraceptive Technologies and AIDS

Responding to a request by the Union Health Ministry for a "fool-proof condom to combat AIDS in India, the World Health Organization, in May 1992, recommended new standards for condoms suited to the particular climatic and demographic factors in India [19].

6. The Use of Synthetic Vaccines

An International Conference on Synthetic Vaccines, held in New Delhi in the first week of December 1992, concluded that genetically engineered vaccines and products developed abroad cannot be introduced into India without further safety trials conducted in India. Dr. S. Ramachandran, the Chairman of the Global Children's Vaccine Initiative, made the following recommendations:

If a vaccine has already been tested, approved, and is in use abroad, limited field trials would do. With a totally new recombinant vaccine, several other factors covering the local population and the environment will have to be taken into account [18].

Dr. Ramachandran observed that a number of vaccines likely to be introduced during the next ten years will be so-called "cocktail" vaccines, which protect recipients of several diseases at the same time. Despite the promise of such vaccines, Ramachandran noted that their use will require even more stringent and complex safety regulations [18].

7. *A Call for Increased Research on Health Systems*

In a five-day conference sponsored by the National Institute of Health and Family Welfare (NIHFW), held in New Delhi from December 14-19, 1992, a number of speakers urged that health systems research should set a few major research priorities, including research on national health programs, health services research, and a ranked assessment of the health care needs of most Indian citizens.

Two speakers offered important perspectives on the need to focus health systems research on aspects of Indian life and culture that are traditionally underemphasized by tertiary medical care in the private sector. Dr. Aloke Mukhopadhya, the Director of the Voluntary Health Association of India, called for health system research to "understand the ethos and the cultural milieu" of Indian health care delivery as central aspects of improving quality of care [13]. Professor P.L. Trakroo, head of NIHFW's Department of Communication, emphasized the need to "evolve strategies for ensuring public scrutiny of the health system" [13]. In addition, Professor Trakroo outlined the "great potential" in "traditional ways of healing and curing," a potential that has been poorly recognized or integrated into India's health care delivery. Trakroo and Doctor N.S. Deodahr, a health consultant from Pune, both pointed out that although the vast majority of Indian health services are "curative" in nature, the "preventive" aspects of health care continue to receive low priority in health system research and in medical practice [13].

B. *The Use of Amniocentesis for Sex Selection*

"The Prenatal Diagnostic Techniques (Regulation and Prevention of Misuse) Bill" was introduced in September 1991. I.C. Verma describes the purposes of the bill as follows:

> It proposes to prohibit prenatal diagnostic techniques for determining the sex of the fetus leading to female feticide ... The bill provides for: (i) prohibition of the misuse of prenatal diagnostic techniques for determination of [the] sex of [the] fetus, leading to female feticide; (ii) prohibition of advertising of prenatal diagnostic techniques to determine sex; (iii) permission and regulation of the use of prenatal diagnostic techniques to detect specific genetic abnormalities or disorders; (iv) permitting the use of such techniques only under certain conditions by registered institutions; and (v) punishment for violation of the provisions of the proposed regulation [17].

A 21-member Joint Parliamentary Committee was formed to gather evidence and pursue fact-finding from several voluntary organizations and a number of hospitals in Bombay during the spring of 1992. The voluntary organizations the Committee interviewed include the Forum Against Oppression of Women, the Family Planning Association of India, and the Forum Against Sex Determination and Preselection. The Joint Committee was scheduled to make its recommendations to make the legislation "more meaningful and effective" in late 1992 [19].

C. *Issues of Population Growth*

In several reports issued in 1992, population control was judged to be the most pressing challenge facing India in the next two decades ([1];[3];[10];[11]). A number of factors were stressed as central to a comprehensive effort: contraception and family planning information, increase in female literacy, growth in employment opportunities for women, and general "enhancement" of the social status of women.

Two elements from the reports are noteworthy. First, the Indian state of Kerala exemplifies the close relationship between positive changes in female literacy and social status and the increased acceptance of the small family as a norm. Kerala has a female literacy rate of nearly eighty-seven percent, double that of its nearest competitor, the state of Tamilnadu. By contrast, in the four northern Hindu states, less than thirty percent of the women can read. Kerala's infant mortality rate is less than 25 per 1000 live births, while in the four northern states, the mortality rate is four to five times greater [10].

In light of such statistics, the Indian government has suggested a number of changes in its family welfare program, with emphases on provision of information, increased efforts at literacy training, and more effective communication networks, especially for presently undeserved rural areas. The Government message would be to "associate family welfare with planned parenthood and not just with the adoption of contraception" [10]. Special emphasis would be placed on improving quality of life for families through effective family planning. In addition, the government study recommends special efforts to communicate with the forty percent of the population presently not reached by any form of mass media. In that outreach, particular emphasis would be placed on traditional forms of communication, including traditional art forms and folklore [10].

The Population Crisis Committee (PCC), a private non-profit public interest organization based in Washington, D.C., issued a 1992 report entitled "India's Family Planning Challenge: From Rhetoric to Action" [1]. According to the PCC, although the Indian family planning is "by no means a failure", the stabilization of population is "not yet on the horizon" [1]. The PCC report locates India's difficulties with overpopulation primarily in the northern states and identifies three primary obstacles to effective family planning: low female literacy, high infant mortality, and poor administration of planning efforts. Moreover, the report is critical of the "single-minded focus" on sterilization at the field level of family planning efforts [1].

In a related development, Dr. Nafis Sadik, the Executive Director of the United Nations Population Fund, addressed a United Nations expert group meeting of Family Planning, Health, and Family Well-Being hosted by the

Indian Government in Bangalore on October 26, 1992. Sadik noted that a number of significant practical improvements must be made to control population growth more effectively, especially emphasis on expanding educational opportunities, increasing literacy, and enhancing the status of women. Sadik also raised doubts about two tenets of the "conventional wisdom" on population control. First, Sadik observed that improvements in economic status are not necessary preconditions of successful family planning, because many poor communities in fact adopt family planning if they learn to "trust the system" [3]. Second, Sadik said that religion is not a hindrance to family planning; even the Vatican calls for "responsible parenthood", although the "natural" method it recommends is difficult for many to follow [3]. Among leading religions, Sadik noted that Hinduism and Buddhism both support planned parenthood [3].

D. *Organ Donation and Transplantation*

At the Fifth Asian Pacific Congress of Nephrology on December 13, 1992, R.L. Mishra, the Union Health Secretary, announced that the Government of India has decided to prohibit "gifts" of organs from unrelated donors, except in unusual circumstances where "special bonds of affection" can be established by independent review. Mishra restated the Government's opposition to commercial trading of organs as unacceptable in civilized society. In order to increase the supply of solid organs for transplant, while decreasing the temptation to traffic in organs, Mishra noted that the Government would seek to coordinate national efforts for voluntary donation [2].

E. *Health Care Economics*

A symposium on "Health Care Economics", held on September 4, 1992, focused on the epidemiological and demographic problems that thwart the provision of health care in India. S.L. Rao, the Director-General of the National Council of Applied Research, commented on several aspects of India's "poor record" in health care. He noted that the northern states "lag significantly behind other states" according to most indices of development. Rao also profiled the gender-based inequality of women in India. Among children, the survival rate for girls was significantly lower than that for boys. Not surprisingly, female mortality was significantly higher in the 15-34 age group among women of child-bearing years. Finally, Rao offered several observations about Indian health expenditures. According to 1991 statistics, India spent 5.5 percent of GDP on health programs, a figure higher than a number of other developing countries, including Pakistan, Sri Lanka, and Indonesia. Nonetheless, Rao observed that the results of such spending remain uneven. He recommended that the Government should re-order its priorities toward prevention and public health and fund ongoing studies of the efficacy of public health delivery systems [9].

III. CONCLUSION

In this essay, we have addressed a number of concerns that are central to understanding bioethics developments in India during the last two years. Section I, while not focused on specific issues of bioethics, emphasized human dignity as a value central to the resolution of recent religiously inspired violence in India. Section II chronicled a number of recent developments on a range of topics that, although not the focus of expressly religious discussion, nonetheless invite increased reflection and study by Hindu and other religious leaders in India.

University of Illinois Medical Center
Chicago, Illinois, U.S.A.

Center for Ethics, Medicine, and Public Issues
Baylor College of Medicine
Houston, Texas, U.S.A.

*Dr. Desai wishes to thank Ivan Pavkovic, M.D. and Bhawani Prasad, M.D., for their many useful suggestions.

BIBLIOGRAPHY

1. Bose, A., 1992: "Population Crisis Committee's Report", *Financial Express*, October 6.
2. "Gifting of Human Organs to Be Banned", 1992: *The Times of India*, December 14.
3. "Global Summit on Population in 1994", 1992: *The Times of India*, October 24.
4. "Government Given More Time on Blood Policy", 1992: *The Times of India*, August 16.
5. Irani, M., 1992: "The Drug-Ban Debate", *The Sunday Times*, October 25.
6. Kothari, R., 1970: *Politics in India*. New Delhi: Orient Longman, pp. 21-97.
7. Nandy, A., 1983: *The Intimate Enemy: Loss and Recovery of Self Under Colonialism*. Delhi: Oxford University Press.
8. "Oral Polio Vaccine to Continue", 1992: *The Times of India*, October 28.
9. "Poor Record in Health Care", 1992: *The Statesman*, September 5.
10. "Population: Challenge for the 90s", 1992: *The Independent*, July 11.
11. "Population Growth Rate Falls", 1992: *The Hindustan Times*, October 24.
12. Prasad, Bhawani "Roots of the Communal Divide". *The Business and Political Observer*, New Delhi Edition, April 26, 1991.
13. "Research in Health System Stressed", 1992: *The Times of India*, December 16.
14. Sen, A., 1993: "Threats to Secular India", *New York Review of Books* April 8, pp. 26-32.
15. Spear, P., 1961: *India: A Modern History*. Ann Arbor: The University of Michigan Press, pp. 94-181, pp. 310-446.
16. Srinivas, K., and Kanakamala, K., 1992: "Introducing Norplant: Politics of Coercion", *Economic and Political Weekly*, pp. 1531-1533.
17. Verma, I., 1992: "Bioethical Developments in India: 1989-1991", in B.A. Lustig (sr. ed.), *Bioethics Yearbook*, Volume 2, Kluwer, Dordrecht, pp. 309-341.
18. "Warning Against Blind Use", 1992: *The Statesman*, December 12, p. 5.
19. "WHO Submits Standards for 'Fool-Proof Condoms", 1992: *The Independent*, May 19.

JUDITH A. GRANBOIS AND DAVID H. SMITH

THE ANGLICAN COMMUNION AND BIOETHICS

In this report, we survey policy statements, monographs, commission reports, periodicals and other materials that, in some sense, represent the views of the member churches of the Anglican Communion on questions of biomedical ethics. In the interval since publication of the first volume in this series, we have gained improved access to church offices around the world. We have identified helpful respondents in the Anglican churches of Australia, New Zealand, Canada and England. (We reported on developments in the churches in Scotland and Wales in the last volume, and we have no additional information for this writing.) We have no knowledge of statements that may have been published in India, Africa or Asia, however.

Consistent with the editorial policy of the Yearbook, we have allowed ourselves more freedom for editorial comment than in our first report of 1991. A fuller sense of our perspective may be found in two other works ([37] and [38]).

I. UNDERSTANDINGS OF HEALTH AND HEALING

Several themes recur in recent Anglican statements about health and healing: an expanded understanding of health, a renewed interest in mental health, and a new emphasis on "holistic" health.

First, some national churches have stressed an understanding of health that is not limited to merely physical aspects, but includes social and psychological components as well. For example, *Faith in the City*, a 1985 report by the Archbishop of Canterbury's Commission on Urban Priority Areas, states:

Health care is much more than the treatment of ill-health. Underlying the problem of <u>disease</u> is the more fundamental problem of <u>unease</u> which has its roots in factors such as anxiety, low personal esteem, broken relationships, and the stress of poverty, deprivation, unemployment and bad housing ([3], p. 270).

Second, a renewed interest in issues of mental health is apparent. For example, Resolution D-088a, adopted by the Episcopal Church of the United States of America (ECUSA) in 1991, encourages Episcopalians to become knowledgeable about mental illness to reduce stigma and stereotypes; encourages support for persons with mental illness, recognizing their abilities and gifts; encourages development of programs to equip clergy and laity for ministry to those who have mental illnesses and their families; and calls for

B. Andrew Lustig (Sr. Ed.), Bioethics Yearbook: Volume 3, 83-115.
©1993 Kluwer Academic Publishers.

advocacy for public policy into causes and treatment of mental illness ([24], pp. 822-3).

The Church of England's interest in mental health is reflected in an article entitled "Mental Health in Society" in *Crucible*, the quarterly journal of the Board for Social Responsibility. In the article, Arthur Hawes provided a historical summary of treatment for mental illness and identified gaps in services. He outlined the church's appropriate responses as advocacy for the vulnerable and powerless, education to develop pastoral care and change public attitudes, and support and care for the mentally ill [19]. In 1992, the Board for Social Responsibility published *Community Care and Mental Health*. The report summarizes relevant British legislation and raises concerns about funding for services to mentally ill persons, lack of facilities, homelessness and the impact of mental illness on families and friends of affected persons [11].

The General Synod of the Anglican Church of Canada endorsed an official statement on the church's ministry to the mentally retarded in 1980 (Act 41). The statement called for the church to "be involved" in efforts to provide financial assistance and support for racial minorities, handicapped persons and the economically deprived "to maintain for itself and its members a stated position as messengers of the Gospel of God's love for all human beings" ([1], p. 1).

Third, some attention has been paid to the notion of a "holistic" approach to health. The Church of England sounds that note in *Faith in the City*:

The Church needs to promote a broader understanding of the meaning of health. This must be concerned with more than the absence of disease. It must concern the significance of the Biblical concept of "Shalom" and wholeness: for the care we take for the quality as well as the length of people's lives ([3], p. 271).

In its report to the 1991 General Convention (ECUSA), the Standing Commission on Health describes the model of modern biomedicine as "based on the idea that the body is a machine and that disease can be understood by analyzing the functioning of the different body parts down to the molecular level" ([40], p. 183). Acknowledging the remarkable medical progress that has resulted from reliance on this model, the Commission argues that "overall health has not improved significantly," citing the problems of chronic diseases, escalating costs, static life expectancies, and new problems such as AIDS, substance abuse and suicide.

The Commission supports two strategies to correct this oversimple stress on scientific medicine. One is personal responsibility. Resolution A-098 stresses preventive medical care, healthy diet, regular exercise and avoidance of substance abuse. Resolution A-094a recommends establishment of guidelines for healthy Christian living and support for those in the field of health care. The other response, described in the Commission's report, is religious: pastoral counseling, prayer, meditation and laying on of hands. The Commission commends a new, holistic approach to health:

The goal is spiritual attunement, our ability to be in touch with the meaning and purpose of our lives, a deep understanding of our relationship to ourselves, to nature and to God, which will make us more loving and caring persons dedicated to the art of living ([40], p. 184; see also [15]).

In keeping with that emphasis, Resolution A-062 affirms Christian healing as a ministry to the whole person and an essential expression of the gospel and urges each diocese to find ways to promote knowledge of Christian healing and assist those involved in ministries of healing.

In opting for a broader definition of health, these documents note the many social determinants of ill health and stress the overlap between health care and the concerns of the church. They do not stress the importance of biomedical research or the distinction between health and well being.

II. NEW REPRODUCTIVE TECHNIQUES

Several branches of the Anglican Communion have addressed the moral issues raised by techniques of assisted reproduction. In general, the various bodies have endorsed artificial insemination and in vitro fertilization within marriage but have expressed reservations about techniques that employ gametes from a third party (i.e., artificial insemination by donor and surrogate motherhood).

In 1982, the Board for Social Responsibility of the General Synod of the Church of England named a five-member working party to submit evidence to the government's Committee of Inquiry into Human Fertilisation and Embryology (the Warnock Committee). In his foreword to the working party's report, the Rt. Rev. Hugh Montefiore, Bishop of Birmingham, remarked: "The advent of new medical techniques in the field of human fertilisation and embryology had produced new problems which not merely raised ethical issues but which required theological elucidation" ([8], p. iii).

The working party summarized the "major areas of debate" as:

(a) The status of the fertilised human egg or early embryo, and the protection it should be given . . .

(b) The nature of the marriage bond, and the effect of it on the introduction of a third (or even fourth) party . . .

(c) The nature and extent of divine providence and human responsibility ([8], p. 2).

Anglican discussions of the problems raised by technological reproduction tend to cluster in these three areas.

A. *Status of the Embryo*

Surveying debates about embryonic/fetal status in the early Christian literature, the authors of *Personal Origins* note,

The Christian tradition sought to answer moral questions in the light of what was then known about early embryonic life. It is because that tradition was formed before contemporary advances in knowledge . . . that we are required to examine again what we believe about the nature and status of the early human embryo ([18], p. 23).

Today, conflicting viewpoints on the status of the embryo emphasize either the continuity of the human subject or the possession of certain attributes, primarily the phenomenon of consciousness, that determine personhood. Tracing the disagreements between the two camps, the document points to one important point of agreement and finally reveals the authors' failure to agree.

[T]he two schools of thought . . . both acknowledge that the human status of the unborn child is something which must be discerned, quite apart from our wishes or our decisions, as a reality which simply commands our recognition as of right . . . Some of our contemporaries have hoped to avoid the question of the embryo's status altogether . . . The implication of this manoeuvre would seem to be that human status is not so much discerned as conferred; that social practice is sufficient of itself to validate or invalidate the claims of any pretender to humanity. The authors of this report, though by no means of a common mind as between the two Christian approaches which we have tried to describe, are agreed in finding this solution unsatisfactory ([8], pp. 33-34).

The authors can agree that the status of the embryo is not a question of human definition, but something to be discovered and that the process of discovery or "discernment" is difficult. They fail to agree, however, about what that status is.

The Episcopal Church of the United States of America (ECUSA) has contributed little to the discussion of this specific issue in recent years. In preparation for the 1991 General Convention, the Standing Commission on Health pondered a variety of techniques of assisted reproduction, including induction of ovulation, in vitro fertilization, embryo transfer, gamete intrafallopian transfer, use of donor gametes, and surrogacy [33]. The Commission's report to the General Convention briefly discussed infertility and reproductive technology.

In its report, the Commission pointed to a number of practical issues associated with assisted reproduction, including high cost and low success rates. The report also discussed embryo freezing and "the fate of surplus embryos," which "constitute potential human life and thus should be treated with respect." The Commission concludes that freezing embryos "would seem to be permissible" if they are used for attempts at conception and "may be permissible" if they are used for "research to improve fertilization technology." The Commission cautioned against donation or sale of frozen embryos to infertile couples, however ([40], p. 189).

In its study of IVF, the Canadian church conducted a more thorough examination of the ethical issues raised by the disposition of frozen embryos. At the 1989 General Synod, the Doctrine and Worship Committee was asked to prepare a position paper on the subject for approval by the National

Executive Council. In an interim report, Phyllis Creighton, convener of the task force that explored these questions, directed the church's attention to the forthcoming recommendations of the Royal Commission on New Reproductive Technologies, which were due to be released in October 1992. She recommended that the National Executive Council name a working group to develop a response to the Royal Commission's recommendations and suggested that ecumenical collaboration might be helpful.

Tracing the ethical debate that surrounds the practice, Creighton observed, "The moral status – that is, the value and rights – of human life at its beginnings cannot be read off the biological data" ([18], p. 5). Her review of Roman Catholic and Anglican teaching led her to reject "the deliberate creation of embryos for research" as demeaning to embryonic life. She concluded,

Anglican recognition that unborn human life has a high but not absolute value, and the need for beneficence towards humanity in response to God's providential love might ground morally the use of embryonic life for important research on the mechanisms of fertilization and embryonic development or transfer, if it could be accomplished in no other way and might yield knowledge of wide benefit, providing the basis for treatment or prevention of embryonic loss or grave abnormality. The goal would be enhancement of embryonic life ([8], p. 8).

Citing feminist critics, Creighton issued a series of caveats about IVF, citing the low success rates experienced by couples undergoing the procedure, the pain and emotional cost to women, possible adverse effects of drugs on women and fetuses, and the significant financial expense, which raises questions of distributive justice in medical care. Her prescription for Christians confronting these issues is as follows:

Our faith must inform our reasoned judgements: from theology can come moral insights of relevance. We need moral imagination, and soberness that begins in awe. We know that our procreative powers are a gift from God and that every human life is of inestimable value, so we must strive for the fullest respect for the embryo as the earliest life form of humanity, reject reductionist notions of it as mere tissue, oppose its consumption by adults or children for prolonging their own lives, protect it in its frozen state of suspended animation. We must steady our gaze on the fundamental human values and press moral questions ([18], p. 22).

According to unofficial reports (official documents are not yet available), the 1992 General Synod referred the "Interim Report on the Disposition of Frozen Human Embryos" to the National Executive Council for dissemination and directed the NEC to appoint the working group recommended by Creighton (Resolution C-28, [44]).

In 1984, The Most Reverend Dr. P. F. Carnley, Archbishop of Perth, discussed the beginning of human life in his column, "From the Archbishop" in the *Anglican Messenger*, a provincial newspaper for Anglicans in western Australia. The column grew out of the Archbishop's remarks on "Miracles, Morals and Medicine," presented to the national conference of the Royal

Australian College of General Practitioners. The address apparently caused a stir.

In his column, Archbishop Carnley stressed the distinction between conception and fertilization; conception should be understood "less as a *moment* and more in gradual and continuous terms as a *process*." [emphasis added] Fertilization progresses to conception only when the embryo is successfully implanted in the lining of the uterus.

Discussing "soul-talk," the question of when the embryo is endowed by God with a soul, Archbishop Carnley observed that a claim that the soul is given at the moment of fertilization raises the "embarrassing" question of what happens to the soul in an embryo that divides to produce twins. The fourteenth day after conception, when implantation occurs, is a dividing line. Prior to that point, the embryo should be treated with the respect due human genetic material. However, the "condemnation of all IVF procedures as involving the inevitable killing of "conceived human individuals' is . . . unhelpful and, indeed, reprehensible." On the basis of this argument, Archbishop Carnley concluded that both the freezing of fertilized ova and experimentation upon embryos under the 14-day limit are both permissible if carefully controlled ([12], p. 4).

Archbishop Carnley revisited the subject in the February 1991 edition of the *Anglican Messenger*, addressing "the sinister side of the Human Reproductive Technology Bill," which was about to be debated in the Western Australia Parliament. Acknowledging the good intentions behind the bill, he expressed grave concern over a provision that would ban research on human reproduction "based on the belief that it is 'generally unacceptable in our community.'" The Archbishop forcefully opposed "the prospect of unwittingly hampering advances that may be of ultimate value to human life by anti-deluvian [sic] legislation." He encouraged all Anglicans to enter the discussion as possible "agents of enlightenment in the community."

The Archbishop agreed that embryos should not be permitted to grow in vitro for longer than 14 days. However, he argued, by banning diagnostic testing on genetic material in the 14 days before individuation may be said to have occurred, the proposed legislation would create the anomaly of prohibiting diagnostic procedures that medical practitioners are legally able to perform on the fetus after conception when it is to be accorded the status of a human individual ([13], n.p.).

In the May 1991 *Anglican Messenger*, Archbishop Carnley again addressed the issue of the moral status of the embryo, reaching back to the arguments presented in his 1984 column.

Insofar as the proposed Human Reproductive Technology Bill is based on the contention that the developing embryo is to be accorded the status of a conceived human individual from the moment of fertilisation onwards, it is based on a piece of medieval mythology ([14], n.p.).

Citing Roman Catholic theologians Karl Rahner and Bernard Haring in support of his view, he concluded that abortion cannot justifiably be described as termination of a human life until after conception is complete ([14], n.p.).

These materials reveal important differences of emphasis on the status of embryos within recent Anglican statements. The tone of Archbishop Carnley's remarks in Australia differs from that in the recommendations of Phyllis Creighton in Canada. She is more cautious, he, more eager to challenge conservative views. It is noteworthy that none of the statements adopts the view that the embryo falls completely outside the zone of respect owed to human beings – a view vigorously defended by the then Anglican Joseph Fletcher thirty years ago. None of the recent statements absolutely precludes use of embryos of up to 14 days gestation for research purposes. We do not mean to suggest that a consensus exists, merely to observe that on this issue the ongoing argument may be focused within certain broad parameters. Differences in tone may reflect differing political and rhetorical contexts.

B. *The Nature of Marriage*

Considering techniques of assisted reproduction inevitably raises questions about religious understandings of marriage. *The Book of Common Prayer* places primary emphasis on the relational aspects of marriage, the "mutual joy" of husband and wife and "the help and comfort given one another"; the procreation of children is in a sense a separate – but no less desirable – benefit of marriage, "when it is God's will." On those terms, interventions to bring about procreation are to be regarded as an attempt to pursue a proper end, but only within marriage, where "relational" and "procreational" goods should be and remain linked.

1. *Third-Party Techniques of Conception*

Thus, several branches of the Anglican Communion have recorded their concerns about the use of third-party techniques of conception. *Personal Origins* clearly expresses uneasiness in the Church of England. Referring to long-standing Christian traditions that take the view that marriage should lead to parenthood, the document sanctions "attempts to relieve childlessness" as a means of "assist[ing] marriage to fulfill one of its natural ends" ([8], p. 35). Motivated by "a fundamental concern" for "the preservation of the good of Christian marriage, as instituted by God himself, and for the welfare of children, who are to be brought up in the fear and love of the Lord" ([8], p. 41), it asserts the desirability of holding together the "procreational and relational 'goods' of marriage." ([8], p. 36).

The document reports a divided mind on the use of AID, however.

For here there is a question of introducing genetic material from outside the union altogether. What, then, is left of the procreative end of the marriage? . . . [H]ere procreation is separated from relationship completely, at the genetic level, even though the connection between the two is preserved at the social level ([8], p. 39).

In contrast to its ambivalence on AID, *Personal Origins* clearly rejects surrogate motherhood, in which "the Christian institution of the family is fundamentally endangered," and concludes "that it cannot be morally acceptable as a practice for Christians" ([8], p. 41).

Similarly, in its report to the American church's General Convention in 1991, the Standing Commission on Health pointed to a number of issues that are related to the nature of marriage. Like the Church of England's working group, the Commission affirmed the use of techniques of assisted reproduction that help husband and wife to conceive, noting that Protestant communities, in general, have raised no objections in the context of marriage. The 1991 statement is consistent with previous ECUSA pronouncements on this subject. However, in an action that may reflect some lingering unease about high technology interventions in the process of conception, the 1991 General Convention passed a resolution (A-101a) recommending that married couples who are considering external fertilization and embryo transfer seek professional and pastoral counsel and consider adoption as an option ([24], p. 773).

Considering reproductive techniques that rely on a third party outside the marital dyad, the Commission's 1991 report echoed concerns explored in its previous statements. Again, the Commission stated that these practices raise "issues of lineage, legitimacy, parenthood, family and identity. . . [and] could damage the child and/or the parents [through] custody battles, marital stress, incest, identity problems and psychological trauma" ([40], p. 189).

These issues were discussed in reports of the Commission and its forebears in 1982, 1985 and 1988. The 1991 General Convention, like past General Conventions, declined either to approve or to condemn reproductive techniques that involve third-party gametes.

The Episcopal Church of the United States of America has wrestled with the issue of surrogacy at least since 1973. In that year, the Joint Commission on the Church in Human Affairs issued a warning about the practice, based on concern about exploitation of the surrogate mother:

[T]he use of a host uterus to obtain the gestation of a child outside the family almost necessarily involves the treatment of the second woman as a mere object. ([22], p. 595)

The Standing Commission on Human Affairs and Health compared AID and surrogate motherhood in its 1982 report, again finding the latter more troubling. The Commission cautioned against the possibility of exploitation in even stronger language:

Certainly, the natural mother must experience all the emotional, psychological, and physical changes associated with child-bearing that will force strong ties to the newborn, while, at the same time, she is being treated as a mindless child-bearing animal by the prospective recipient parents ([41], p. 133).

In its 1988 report, the Commission stated, "At the present time, we cannot affirm surrogate motherhood as a moral option for members of this church" ([42], p. 159). In 1991, however, the Commission articulated a neutral position:

The Standing Commissions on Human Affairs and Health of the Episcopal Church have expressed grave doubts about these methods of having children, but the General Convention has neither approved nor condemned these practices that have potential both for good and evil. Being wary of absolutes and open to change has been an unstated policy of this Church. We value this openness. If we attempt to overcontrol – to prohibit the unfamiliar – we stifle creativity and make it impossible for anyone to give us anything new. It seems inappropriate at this time either to affirm or denounce surrogacy or use of donated sperm, ova or embryos ([40], p. 188).

Reservations about AID are also apparent in the official statements of the Anglican Church of New Zealand. The Public Affairs Unit of the church's Social Responsibility Commission and its predecessor body, the Provincial Public and Social Affairs Committee, have articulated their positions on several occasions. A 1984 church statement on "In Vitro Fertilisation" asserted that "there is nothing inherently wrong with the process of IVF. . . [which] (like other advances in medical science) can quite properly be seen as part of God's ongoing creative and redemptive purpose" ([2], n.p.). The statement, however, expressed concern about several issues raised by the use of donors in the process. It urged the development of legislation that would clarify the legal rights of children conceived by IVF, but concluded that, given "proper guidelines" and the preservation of the integrity of the marriage relationship, government should not raise obstacles to the use of donors. The statement continued:

We have doubts about the wisdom of unmarried persons using IVF and are opposed to its availability for unmarried single women because the model of parenthood to be encouraged involves both a mother and a father. We are also concerned about possible excesses in experimentation. In all cases, the ethical guidelines for IVF should be clearly laid down and be available for public scrutiny. These guidelines should cover such matters as the storage and disposal of gametes, consent and counselling of the parties, and the use of donors. We find the guidelines of the British Medical Association highly satisfactory, ([2], n.p.).

The statement also addressed pastoral issues, encouraging couples to consult with their clergy on issues of motive, strength of character needed to face the procedures and their possible failure, and the implications inherent in the use of donors. Although it strongly encouraged any couple to seek such counsel, it firmly concluded: "The couple and their medical advisors must make the final choice" ([2], n.p.).

In its "Submissions to the Justice and Law Reform Committee On the Status of Children Amendment Bill 1986," the Provincial Public and Social Affairs Committee of the Anglican Church in New Zealand clearly reiterated its preference that all children have two legal parents and endorsed legislative attempts to clarify the legal status of children conceived by AID [29]. Although the Committee expressed disquiet about the availability of the technology to persons in de facto relationships, it concluded that "the marital status of the parents should not be a barrier to the application of the new rules about a child's status" ([29], n.p.).

The committee issued an additional statement entitled "Surrogate Motherhood: A Christian Perspective," which declared: "Because birth technologies are so new, the Church is not yet in the position to make a definite statement on whether to fully support or discourage surrogate motherhood. Christians will have widely different viewpoints" ([30], paragraph 7). In a section on pastoral care, the report acknowledged the strains on a marriage that can be caused by infertility and encouraged open discussion of all relevant issues to enable the parties to make informed and responsible decisions. It strongly opposed businesses that might seek to take advantage in this emotionally sensitive arena:

profit-making, blatant commercialism and marketing of children by agencies and large corporations are quite a different proposition. Christians would ethically oppose such practices as not in keeping with the dignity of the creation of human life and the unique value of each individual. It may follow from this that the Church should support moves to make the commercial arranging of surrogacy illegal ([30], paragraph 8).

The report continued:

Surrogacy does meet a deep human need. Private arrangements are going to occur in spite of legal controls. On one hand legal prohibitions may drive it underground, yet on the other hand laws offer protection for all parties involved. If strict laws are made, it is important for the child's sake that the parents are not classified as criminal and that the consequences do not interfere with parenting and child care ([30], paragraph 17).

The committee also expressed concern about the possibility that financial need could force women into entering surrogacy arrangements, about the dangers of childbirth for the biological mother, and about the consequences of the "commissioning" parents' rejection of the child.

The Anglican Church of Canada also has studied the impact of assisted reproduction on traditional understandings of marriage. At its June 1975 meeting, the General Synod requested that the Primate reappoint the Task Force on Human Life to conduct an official study and report on the issues raised by AID. Under the leadership of Phyllis Creighton, the task force produced a report entitled *Artificial Insemination By Donor: A Study of Ethics, Medicine, and Law in Our Technological Society.*

The task force's statements reflect ambivalence of thought and feeling. In a discussion of ethical issues, the report stated that a majority of task force members believe AID

may be a fully acceptable medical treatment [and] a humane response to legitimate human need which in the absence of readily adoptable children cannot at present be met in any other way. We accept it largely because we see children as a precious and real fulfillment of a couple's love, and in faithfulness to the belief which Christians share with many others that children are a blessing enriching marriage and society ([17], 61).

However, the report also described the task force's divided views on the moral acceptability and social desirability of AID. Although no members considered AID "clearly morally wrong" or believed that it should "be made illegal or unavailable," the report continued,

Some of us have serious personal reservations about A.I.D., based on our understanding of Christian teachings about marriage and about human nature. Holding that for Christians marriage is a joining, before God, of two persons in a mutual life, we believe that a married couple denied the blessing of children may yet live creatively in true self-giving, and together find fulfillment as they serve God by reflecting his love within the family of man ([17], pp. 61-62).

The report recorded the doubts of some members about the morality of semen donation, based on the belief that a man should accept "full responsibility for the life which his sperm creates"; others believe that "donation of sperm is humane and responsible." Some members believe that "neither the church nor society ought to stress that woman's fulfilment lies only or chiefly in maternity" ([17], pp. 61-62).

The task force encouraged counselling for those seeking AID in order to select "only mature couples who have fully come to terms with their feelings and whose marriage shows the strengths needed to cope with the extra psychological burden which A.I.D. imposes." The report called for teams conducting the procedure to include various experts of both genders and endorsed extended follow-up of families. Donors should "be carefully selected, with a view to eliminating those with serious medical or genetic risk, or undesirable motivation." The task force reached no consensus on the issue of secrecy – whether children or other family members should be told about the procedure ([17], pp. 63-64). Seconding the concerns of the church in New Zealand, the report called for legislation to remove all "legal doubts about the effect of A.I.D. on the status of both the marriage and the child" ([17], pp. 64-65). The report was received and commended for study in the church and the Community at the 1977 meeting of the General Synod.

In May 1987, the National Executive Council of the Canadian church passed a resolution asking the Doctrine and Worship Committee to examine the practice of surrogate motherhood. A task force convened in response to that charge produced a book, *Whose Child is This? Ethical, Legal, Social, and Theological Dangers of Surrogate Motherhood* [4]. The 1989 General Synod passed resolutions accepting the report and commending it to the church and community for study and action (Act 70) and urging that surrogate motherhood be discouraged, that surrogating contracts be unenforceable and that commercial surrogacy be banned (Act 112). In a third resolution, the General Synod affirmed the institution of marriage, asserted that "the absence of children in itself does not compromise the integrity and value of a marriage," and asked "all couples . . . to consider the reality of various limitations for example, fertility, personality, or genetic impairment which may make children for them either impossible, hurtful or simply unwise" (Act 71; [4], p. 101). The task force's statements are unequivocal in their opposition to surrogate motherhood.

Human beings must be treated as ends, not means. The humanity of women must not be subordinated to their reproductive capacities. Nor may children be deliberately created for sale. These two grave ethical flaws are inherent in surrogate motherhood. The buying and selling of human beings, for whatever purpose, incorporates the evil present in slavery and is just as offensive. The acquisition of children through payment reduces them to a market commodity. The worth of a human being is not defined by exchange value. We reject a value system that promotes the commodification of persons and their relationships ([4], p. 93).

The moral issues arising from IVF, AID, and surrogate motherhood were extensively discussed in Australia in the 1980s. In 1984 the Social Responsibilities Commission of the Anglican Church of Australia published an anthology of essays entitled *Making Babies: The Test Tube and Christian Ethics* [27]. Introducing the issues raised by "reproductive technology," the Rt. Rev. Oliver Heyward, Bishop of Bendigo and chair of the commission, defined the primary question: "At what stage does human life begin?" He reported the commission's deliberations on that issue, dating from 1981. In 1982, the commission approved IVF and embryo transfer (ET) only for married couples using only their own gametes, called for limiting the number of embryos fertilized to "such number of ova as are necessary to accomplish a successful pregnancy," rejected compulsory amniocentesis as part of IVF and ET, stipulated professional counseling, and rejected experimentation beyond IVF and ET with human embryos ([27], pp. 2-3). In a 1983 statement, the Commission declared its reservations about AID, but, noting that the practice was likely to continue, it recommended guidelines that restricted AID to married couples, called for professional counseling and informing "AID children of their true origins," and supported legislation that would regulate "all aspects of AID" ([27], p. 4). Bishop Heyward quoted a position paper issued by the government of Victoria in 1983, citing its emphasis on the interests of children who are born through reproductive technology.

In another essay, William A. W. Walters, an associate professor of obstetrics and gynecology at Monash University, explored the ethical issues associated with IVF technology, including the status of the embryo, consent for the embryo, the impact on marriage, the status of children conceived by IVF and cost implications [45].

Among other topics, individual authors explored questions related to social policy formulation, the biblical perspective, moral status of the embryo, family issues, pastoral care and legal implications of the new technology.

As in the case of the status of embryos, we can see some convergence on these issues: Despite the more accepting tone of the most recent American statement, surrogate motherhood is consistently condemned throughout the

Anglican Communion. AID, however – the most common and technologically easiest form of gamete donation – usually divides the collegial bodies asked to comment on it. The reason for this division may lie in the fact that surrogacy obviously involves a thinking, talking and feeling third party – the surrogate mother – whereas the sperm donor seems to be, and in many ways is, impersonal. Moreover, surrogacy raises issues of personal and political immediacy, in contrast to AID, where the issues are more speculative, the benefits clearer and the possible problems, especially in the short run, harder to verify or quantify. To what extent should Anglicans agree that infertility creates a need that must be met? That question naturally leads to the next topic.

C. *Humanity and Nature*

Clearly, moral issues associated with reproduction raise larger questions about human nature and destiny and about the appropriate constraints, if any, on interventions in the reproductive process. Confronting the profound challenges to traditional understandings of nature and God's purposes posed by developments in reproductive technology, a working group of the Church of England outlined two responses, which need not be mutually exclusive. The first is "to welcome the changes in thought and experience" in a spirit of

readiness to accept new knowledge and more accurate ways of understanding the natural order . . . We are in the midst of a journey whose beginnings lay in creation and whose end is to be realized in the hope given to us in Jesus Christ. The Christian task. . . is a constant search to turn both knowledge and practice to good ends. In terms of the Divine purpose, we must seek it through a developing process which is shaped towards some ultimate good, but not yet achieved goal ([8], p. 17).

The second response is to reflect on what may have been lost, including

any serious sense of the boundaries of natural law and of the purposes for which things are created by God. We run the risk of over-estimating human abilities and our place in relation to nature. We fail to consider that God may have set limits in the natural order which we, if we are to remain faithful in our stewardship of the world, should respect and not seek to breach ([8], p. 17).

The text of the working group's report sets human reproduction in the context of an Anglican understanding of the natural world. The statement is based on a number of fundamental principles, including the belief that the universe was created by a sovereign God for a purpose, which implies the existence of a natural law. Human beings do not have absolute dominion but are obligated to respect the integrity or order that exists in nature; they are constrained by their obligations as "stewards and trustees of what God has made and maintains" ([8], p. 18). Christians are not to fear the new, including scientific discovery, but are to seek in all things God's providential care, trusting in the promise of redemption.

The writers reported no consensus on whether specific new techniques of reproduction are licit, given this understanding, or whether they represent human overreaching. They note the profound significance of human beings' physical embodiment: Because we are spirits *in* the body, called to fellowship with the Holy Spirit, our bodies are intrinsically valuable and may not be treated as mere instruments. Some of these theological claims would seem to point to restrictive policies, but the authors of *Personal Origins* do not draw the inferences. We note some of their relevant observations elsewhere in this report.

III. ABORTION

Constitutional protection of a right to early abortion in the United States, established by *Roe v. Wade* [34], has been the center of controversy since 1973. Qualifying or compromising policies have been established by executive actions of the Reagan and Bush administrations (e.g., U. S. Department of Health and Human Services 1988 regulations of the family planning program funded under Title X of the Public Health Service Act, upheld by the U. S. Supreme Court in *Rust v. Sullivan* [35]); U. S. Supreme Court decisions (*Webster v. Reproductive Services* [46], *Planned Parenthood of Southeastern Pennsylvania v. Casey* [28]); and a variety of initiatives in state legislatures.

Against that background, the 70th General Convention of ECUSA, meeting in 1991, considered two resolutions on abortion. The original text of Resolution C021 (Woman's Right to Choice), proposed by the Committee on Social and Urban Affairs, called on the 70th General Convention to "express its unequivocal opposition to any legislative, executive or judicial action . . . that abridge [*sic*] the right of a woman to reach the informed decision about the termination of pregnancy and that would limit the access of a woman to safe means of acting on her decision" ([24], p. 160). Resolution C037 contained similar language but added a clause opposing abridgement of abortion rights for minors. In the event, General Convention did not adopt Resolution C021, but simply reaffirmed the 1988 resolution on abortion.

The 70th General Convention did, however, adopt an amended resolution opposing legislation that requires parental notification or consent for minors who seek abortions unless the law includes a nonjudicial bypass (C037s). The nonjudicial bypass is necessary in situations when parents cannot be notified or when "family dysfunction" places minors at "serious physical, psychological or emotional risk." In such situations, the resolution continued, minors should have the power to make informed decisions with the "notification of some other responsible adult with experience and/or professional expertise, such as a clergy person, teacher, guidance counsellor, mental health professional or other family member" ([24], p. 839).

These resolutions are the latest in a series that dates at least to 1967, which are summarized in Volume 1 of this yearbook and by David A. Scott [36]. Scott criticizes General Convention resolutions on abortion as

confused in their goals, their intended audience, and their language. Marred by tensions in logic, the resolutions avoid fundamental issues related to abortion and fail to identify standards which should guide moral conscience . . . The limitations connected with resolutions raise the question of whether this form of communication should be the means by which the church seeks to educate the conscience of its members ([36], p. 56).

In place of General Convention resolutions, which, he says, are "not the best medium for the church to form Christian conscience" ([36], p. 57), Scott urges more serious attention to moral teaching on abortion that can be found in articles and books by Episcopal theologians or ethicists, seminary courses and resources produced by diocesan study committees. He advocates teaching through pastoral letters by bishops, which would allow more thorough exploration of the issues and would take seriously the bishops' roles as moral teachers and "administrators of the discipline of the church" ([36], p. 67).

The Public Affairs Unit of the Social Responsibility Commission of the Anglican Church of New Zealand addressed the issue of abortion in both its "Submissions to the Justice and Law Reform Committee on the Crimes Bill 1989" [32] and its "Submissions to the Social Services Committee on the Contraception, Sterilisation and Abortion Amendment Bill 1989" [39]. The former document concluded that "the question of abortion is regarded as a matter for the conscience of each person, informed by the law and the teachings of the Church and where appropriate, worked out in conjunction with the person's spiritual advisors" ([32], paragraph 5.1). In the latter submission, the committee declared its opposition to both abortion on demand and a virtual ban on abortion, urging "equitable provision of services and counselling" throughout the country and expressing its support for "a simplified and more accessible system, as the existing one can be discriminatory and demeaning" ([39], n.p). Because the most frequently cited legal ground for abortion is the health of the mother, the committee proposed that doctors be carefully scrutinized and held accountable for their recommendations and actions. The report went on to recommend high-quality counselling, "free from persuasion, available early in the process and with good follow-up to minimize long-term effects" ([39], section 3, paragraph 4).

The Anglican Church of Canada also has reflected on abortion. In General Synod resolutions of 1973 and 1980, the church strongly rejected "abortion on demand" while recognizing that abortion may be necessary in some circumstances ("risk to a pregnant woman's life or serious impairment of her health").

In 1988, the Canadian Supreme Court struck down section 251 of the Criminal Code, which had established a legal right to abortion in Canada. The court's action opened a public debate on the issue. In response, Archbishop Michael Peers, Primate of the Anglican Church in Canada, convened a three-member task force, which he asked "to study what actions need to be taken to uphold our Church's stand on abortion in relation to changes in the abortion law, and to report its recommendations" ([43], p. 5).

The task force's report, *Abortion in a New Perspective*, was endorsed by the National Executive Council and the House of Bishops in 1988 and remains the official position of the Anglican Church in Canada.

The document offered far-reaching recommendations, beginning with the following prologue:

As Anglicans, we insist that abortion be seen for what it really is – the taking of a life that otherwise, in the normal course of events, would come to be – and that to resort to it lightly or casually is to degrade our humanity, to deny the responsibility and responsiveness of human nature. Accepting that abortion is sometimes a tragic and needed choice for a woman, and recognizing that it always demands a serious response from the community, we make the following recommendations, to address the legal vacuum we have identified, as well as the moral task and the social agenda ([43], p. 17).

The task force recommended that the church

i)   urge that . . . legislation establish procedures to make abortion available equitably across the country as a therapeutic measure for women whose pregnancies endanger their life or their physical or mental health.

ii)   propose that administrative procedures put in place should
a) promote responsible decision-making on the part of all those involved – the woman, her partner, where possible, and the medical personnel, and
b) provide assistance to the woman in examining alternatives, including securing social or financial supports to meet her needs in housing accommodation, child care, employment or retraining, welfare benefits or income support, as well as consideration of adoption of the baby expected.

iii)   request that the procedures require
a) a one-week delay between the woman's initial consultation on the possibility of an abortion being advisable, and the agreement that it will be done
b) counselling by a social worker or other recognized, trained counsellor be available for her
c) consultation with and approval of a second physician
d) the two signed medical opinions, with reasons, to be submitted in writing with notification of the abortion to appropriate provincial authorities, without identifying directly or indirectly the woman for whom the abortion has been procured
e) a record of both the number of abortions and the factors conducing to them to be compiled across the country and published at regular intervals, as information needed for the community to identify and resolve the difficulties that lead women to seek termination of their pregnancies.

iv)   request that the conscientious right of health care personnel to refrain from participating in abortion procedures be guaranteed, including protection from demotion, suspension, or discharge from employment ([43], pp. 17-18).

The report resisted any attempt to make even first trimester abortions "available on demand"; acknowledged that late abortions may sometimes be necessary for the sake of the mother's life but stated that abortions should not be allowed if the fetus is viable; and opposed abortion because of genetic defect in the fetus or in cases of incest or rape ([43], pp. 18-19).

The task force further recommended that the church "tackle with renewed commitment its own task of helping people to develop awareness of personal and social conscience"; encourage the use of available educational resources on abortion and sexuality; use family education programs to "encourage both men and women to take responsibility for their own sexuality and their God-given gift of the power to procreate"; and "foster responsible attitudes towards contraception and abortion" ([43], pp. 19-20).

In the third section of the report, "Social Action," the task force proposed a series of recommendations on many topics that, they believed, have an impact on abortion issues, including adequate, affordable housing; fair wages and pay equity; maternity and family benefits; a guaranteed annual income; adequate child care; emotional support for single parent families; "educational and retraining programs to keep pregnant women and new mothers in the mainstream of society; intensified efforts to collect child support; protection of "children and women from sexual abuse, domestic violence, sexual harassment, pornography, rape, and other forms of violence used against them"; training in nonviolent conflict resolution; improved sex education programs, including coverage of contraception; development of family planning services; comprehensive women's health centers; and expanded government funding for contraceptive research.

Lastly, we commend to the church and community, as a matter of spiritual necessity, first, a renewed discussion of the meaning of sexuality. . . and secondly, a renewed reflection on the wonder and awe of being alive, on the goodness and preciousness of life, on children as a blessing entrusted to our care ([43], pp. 20-23).

Addressing the church's response, the report concluded,

While addressing urgent needs for social and economic reforms, the church must not forget her primary calling to be a reconciled people, ministering the love and grace of Jesus Christ to those caught in the pain and brokenness of abortion. From one perspective, poverty and sexism are vying for the death of an unborn generation – abortion is a tragic arena in which the war between classes and sexes is being waged. In this war, how do we turn our weapons of destruction into instruments for peace? Through a genuine commitment to partnership and mutuality modelled in communities transformed by hope. Let us not lose heart as we seek together to respond with the love of Christ to the challenge of "restructuring our society" through justice, so that no woman feels she has to "restructure her womb" through emptying it ([43], p. 23).

Of the Anglican statements on abortion we have seen, *Abortion in a New Perspective* strikes us as the most thorough exploration since the Church of England's *Abortion: An Ethical Discussion* [16]. Its recommendations at the level of public policy will be controversial, but they are reasonably related to the vision of abortion developed by the task force.

In contrast, ECUSA's 1988 resolution on abortion, reaffirmed in 1991, specifically *rejects* legislative "solutions."

We believe that legislation concerning abortions will not address the root of the problem. We therefore express our deep conviction that any proposed legislation on the part of national or state governments regarding abortions must take special care to see that individual conscience is respected, and that the responsibility of individuals to reach informed decisions in this matter is acknowledged and honored ([23], pp. 683-684).

While we discern no consensus in the Anglican Communion at the public policy level, it is clear that many member churches agree in treating abortion as an action with a "tragic dimension, calling for the concern and compassion of all the Christian community" ([23], p. 684), an action that has moral gravity. At the same time, the denomination declines to issue a blanket prohibition, reserving the decision – and assigning responsibility – to those most intimately involved.

IV. EQUITABLE ACCESS TO HEALTH CARE

Issues of equity and social justice arouse the concern of Anglicans in a number of contexts, including health care. The Social Policy Committee of the Board for Social Responsibility (Church of England), charged with an examination of the modern welfare state in Britain and an evaluation of proposed models for reform, articulated the theological basis of this concern.

Christian scripture and tradition assert that we humans share a common life and nature. This means not only that we have the same physical nature as a member of a species, but also that we have a common human nature with its glories and its weaknesses, sin and death. In theological terms all human beings are in solidarity with the first human beings and with each other.

This means two things in particular. First, it is the basis for the Christian stress on the unique worth of each individual person. We may not treat some as of more value than others . . . Second, it is the basis for our sharing together in community, in a life of mutual service and obligation ([9], p. 17).

It is probably not coincidental that this report was commissioned during an extended Conservative government, which stressed privatization and clearly intended major reforms in the National Health Service. In this context, the Committee completed a comprehensive review of the welfare state, which included an assessment of the National Health Service. Noting real achievements in health as in other areas, the Committee nonetheless documented class-related disparities in health status, access to hospitals and use of the health service. It called for political and social priorities that recognize the interdependence in human life, again citing a theological basis for its conclusions.

The Committee sounded three primary themes in its report. The first was human interdependence and fulfillment through community. Unacceptable approaches may favor the independence of some members of the Community at the expense of others, or create problems of overdependence; the ideal society is one in which persons both give and accept help. The second theme is a reminder of God's concern for justice and protection of the poor or disadvantaged. Third, the Committee contends that all forms of social organization are imperfect. Thus,

Christians live between the ages, impelled to look at their own lives, to be concerned with those who are the losers and to challenge the present order. In this sense the kingdom of God is still to come. The call of God's kingdom is not just addressed to individuals but to nations ([9], p. 126).

Finally, the report set out for consideration a series of five models or approaches to providing welfare services, assessing the strengths and weaknesses of each alternative: private enterprise and charity; the state as "safety net"; the state as primary funder; the state as primary provider; and the state as exclusive provider.

In 1989 the government published a white paper, *Working for Patients*. The Board for Social Responsibility responded with a report, which, confusingly, has the same title as the white paper. Stressing the central importance of health and healing in the Christian tradition, the response raised questions about the increased size, cost and complexity of the National Health Service (NHS) and "whether the needs of the person who is ill have become secondary to the effective functioning of the organisation, and the interests of the people who work within it" ([10], p. 2). The response does not dispute the need for reforms in the NHS, but it raises several questions about some of the specific proposals for reform advanced by the white paper: 1) issues of timing, consultation and lack of clarity; 2) concerns about the effect of the proposals on patient care and physician-patient relationships; 3) areas outside the scope of the white paper's recommendations, including preventive medicine and community care; and 4) the balance between high technology medicine and routine care. The report affirms needed reforms, but does not endorse changes instituted merely to save money or to pander to inadequate models of health and health care.

Issues of social justice in health care have not escaped the attention of the church in the United States, but here the political context is very different. In its report to the 1991 General Convention (ECUSA), the Standing Commission on Health drew attention to critical problems in access to health care in America. Pointing to the U.S. failure – unique among industrial democracies – to provide universal health care, the Commission asserted,

We believe in a Gospel that demands our concern for those in need including the sick, a Gospel that reminds us that it is a problem of faith if we allow millions of our neighbors to be excluded from even the most basic health care ([40], p. 185).

Noting pending proposals to address these issues, the Commission described the task of the church:

Our Lord's call to feed the hungry and give drink to the thirsty implies that we have a duty to help provide adequate health care to all in our nation. At the same time we should expound the Christian vision that physical health is not an end in itself, and that our primary goal in this life is not to postpone death but to prepare for the life to come. In this spirit the church should support all those who are trying to devise a system of equitable health care delivery for all citizens, with emphasis on preventive care and if necessary a certain form of rationing of health care ([40], p. 186).

The 1991 General Convention adopted a number of resolutions related to access to health care. Resolution A-099 "decries the inequitable health care delivery system of the United States of America and calls upon the President, the Congress, Governors and other leaders to devise a system of universal access for the people of our country" ([24], p. 610). Resolution A-010 asserts "the right of all individuals to medically necessary health care, including long-term services"; encourages the Church at all levels to "advocate for legislation for comprehensive medical benefits" ([24], p. 764).

Resolution C027 supports increased funding for the Women's, Infants', and Children's program to include all pregnant women, pregnant teenagers and children under five years of age, and Resolution D059 urges that Norplant implants be funded through Medicaid.

Universal access to health care does not seem to be a controversial goal for Episcopalians, or for Americans in general, for that matter. Divisions will become apparent as the debate opens over rationing resources, designing mechanisms for health care finance and organizing delivery structures. The differences in emphasis between Anglicans in England and Episcopalians in the United States concerning access to health care are entirely predictable, given their national settings and cultural differences. Watching their engagement with ongoing discussions in their home countries will be of considerable interest.

V. ORGAN DONATION AND TRANSPLANTATION

Anglicans generally affirm organ donation. In that spirit, Resolution A-097, adopted by ECUSA at its 1991 General Convention, "recommend[s] and urge[s]" Episcopalians to consider the opportunity to donate organs after death so that others might live, and to communicate their decisions to their families, friends, churches and attorneys. In past statements, church bodies have cautioned potential recipients of organ transplants against overzealous attempts to avoid death, which may contradict the tradition's teachings [42].

The use of fetal tissue for research and transplantation constitutes something of a special case. The topic has been contested territory in recent years in the United States. In 1988, the U. S. Department of Health and Human Services imposed a moratorium on federal funding for research using fetal tissue from elective abortions. In May 1992, the Bush administration announced plans to establish a fetal tissue bank, collecting tissue from miscarriages and ectopic pregnancies but excluding tissue from induced abortions. Critics have questioned the feasibility of the proposal, and President-elect Bill Clinton has announced that he will rescind the moratorium, which remains in force at this writing.

Resolution A-096a, adopted by General Convention in 1991, addresses some of the issues surrounding the use of fetal tissue. The resolution rejects conception for the purpose of providing fetal tissue for therapeutic or research uses and rejects the use of fetal tissue aborted for profit. It calls for continued discussion during the next triennium on "the use for therapeutic or research purposes of tissues from healthy fetuses, aborted to save the life of the mother" ([24], p. 384).

A task force of the Anglican Church of Canada briefly addressed this issue in its recommendations on legislation governing abortion:

Because of current scientific developments in the use of fetal cells and tissue, for example for the treatment of Parkinson's disease, severe anemia, or diabetes, and the possibility of deliberate abortion for such purposes – fetal farming – we believe that legislation is needed to ban commercial transactions in human genetic material, and to identify protections for the right of the unborn ([43], p. 19).

VI. WITHDRAWING OR WITHHOLDING TREATMENT

On Dying Well, a seminal Anglican document on euthanasia, was the report of a working party established in 1970 by the Board for Social Responsibility and published by the Church of England in 1975. The report's discussion of theological considerations begins by observing,

Moral debate is carried on in the language of rights, principles and interests. When Christians join in the discussion they will often use the same language. . . Nevertheless, differences exist . . . For the Christian . . . moral reflection and decision are embedded in his total relationship to God, and moral language is delicately interwoven with religious language. Freedom is set within a context of obedience, responsibility within a context of divine invitation and grace ([6], p. 15).

On this understanding, it cannot be asserted that human beings' lives are entirely their own, to dispose of as they will. They have "a divinely offered future and destiny," and they "belong to God, 'in whose service is perfect freedom'" ([6], p. 16). However, human beings have free will, and they are obligated to exercise their freedom responsibly. Thus, the church recognizes and approves human agency in decisions to begin a new life or to refuse to prolong a life that is ending.

Based on the concept that all life is a gift from the God who created all things, we owe respect to life and must not destroy it unnecessarily. Death is more than an obviously natural event; it must be illuminated not only by the doctrine of Creation but by the doctrine of Redemption as well.

> Because death is the destruction of man himself and of all his powers, the faith which conquers death must be a faith which throws itself entirely on the being and love of God, a faith which finds a meaning in death, not in anything which man himself can achieve, nor indeed in the nothingness of final extinction, but only in what God can and will achieve . . .

> For the Christian, then, death signifies the ultimate helplessness of man before God and his ultimate dependence on God . . . It is this insight, it seems, which prompts the almost universal Christian feeling that suicide is wrong ([6], pp. 19-20).

On these terms, suicide – and perhaps voluntary euthanasia – might be interpreted as "the expression of a refusal to trust in God, an embracing of death for its own sake, a form of self-justification, a desertion to the enemy" ([6], p. 20).

On the other hand, however, "If my disintegration as a human being occurs before death, is there still any sense in speaking of my dying as either action or passion, self-determination or waiting on God?" ([6], p. 21). The working party's answer is to point to the value of human life, in which suffering and pleasure are inextricably mixed. Suffering is "part of the pattern of becoming human," and the hope of the resurrection demands faithfulness to God ([6], pp. 21-22). Further, a single human life can never be understood or evaluated in isolation. We live our lives in a web of relationships with others, who must also be valued. *Agape* may be "better expressed and more deeply nourished by the careful accompanying of a person in his dying than by any established practice of voluntary euthanasia" ([6], p. 22).

The working group analyzed a number of case studies in an effort to explore the contributions to terminal care that can be provided by adequate medical support and loving family members. Its conclusions approved withholding treatment in order to allow terminally ill patients to die; providing drugs to relieve pain and suffering, even if they shorten the patient's life; and deliberate killing only in extreme and extraordinary cases where adequate care is not available. It did not find justification for a change in British law to permit euthanasia.

In 1982, the Board for Social Responsibility released a statement that asserted:

> The Church of England upholds the Christian moral tradition that all human life is sacred. There are however two positions which should be distinguished. It can be morally legitimate not to seek to preserve life at all costs, as if existence were the main or only end to be achieved. On the other hand, a deliberate intention to kill must be condemned. There is an overriding moral responsibility to relieve pain and distress, even though this may shorten life, as well as to provide nursing and other care ([7], n.p.).

Debate on the issue is continuing in the Church of England. For example, *Crucible*, the quarterly journal of the Board for Social Responsibility, recently published a two-part article by Russell Blacker, Consultant Psychiatrist in Liaison Psychiatry at Royal Cornwall Hospital, Truro [5].

Blacker argues that contemplating circumstances in which we ourselves would not wish to live requires a degree of projection, in which we imagine ourselves in the situation of another and respond either with compassion or disgust. Projection, however, requires a certain distancing or dehumanizing, which may affect our sense of responsibility to others.

Pointing out that the debate about euthanasia often revolves around handicapped persons, he notes that our conceptualizations emphasize their disabilities and impairments, assigning a value that is not "based on any innate quality they may possess themselves, but according to someone else's assessment of their apparent worth" ([5], p. 19). From assigning value to measuring cost is a dangerously short step, according to Blacker, and the next step may be endorsing *involuntary* euthanasia.

In the second installment of his two-part article, Blacker provides an historical perspective on suicide and euthanasia. He draws a distinction between a patient's licit action in "shaping" his or her own death and the giving of treatment that "creates" a death, which is homicide. He raises the question of whether euthanasia might be justified by exceptional circumstances, such as situations in which the intellect is affected (e.g., anencephaly, "persistent organic stupors" and dementia).

Judaism, Islam and Christianity teach that men and women are given the special dignity of being created in the "image of God". . . This raises an important question. . . [C]an the divine image be so debased by brain damage that we can say that the creation identity has either not been met, will never be met or has been irretrievably lost? ([5], p. 79).

He concludes by describing the possible content of legislation that might legalize euthanasia in the United Kingdom, sounding a cautionary note by citing the experience of Holland and expressing concern about the possibility of prompting "altruistic suicide."

The Board for Social Responsibility is currently deliberating issues of euthanasia, the prolongation of life, living wills (which are not binding under current British law) and the church's ministry to the dying. In addition, the House of Bishops has considered a study of assisted suicide. Further publications may issue from these efforts.

In the American Episcopal Church, questions of euthanasia and related issues were most recently discussed at the 1991 General Convention, which adopted a number of germane resolutions. Resolution A-093a sets forth principles and guidelines related to forgoing life-sustaining treatment. The resolution affirms the "sacredness of all human life" but acknowledges death as "part of the earthly cycle of life," transformed by the resurrection of Jesus Christ "into a transition to eternal life." It rejects euthanasia as "morally wrong and unacceptable," but concludes that the process of dying need not be prolonged by "extraordinary means." In cases of persons who are comatose and without "reasonable expectation of recovery," Episcopalians are urged to seek the assistance of the church community's advice and counsel and its sacramental life. The resolution stipulates respect for individuals' rights to make informed decisions about their care and express provision for "withholding or withdrawing life-sustaining systems" with appropriate safeguards against abuse. The resolution encourages church members to execute advance directives "during good health and competence" as a "loving and moral act." Acknowledging the right of medical professionals to refuse to honor requests for termination of treatment on moral or religious grounds, the resolution calls on medical care givers promptly to disclose their policy on withholding or withdrawing treatment to patients and surrogates ([24], pp. 383-384).

Resolution C008, reaffirming a resolution adopted in 1982 (C-2a) and the position taken by the Standing Commission on Human Affairs and Health in its 1988 report to General Convention, endorses living wills and encourages physicians and patients to discuss and execute this "beneficial document." The resolution urges patients, families, medical care givers and legislative bodies "to show aggressive commitment" to allowing peaceful death in a setting that enables the patient to maintain control and dignity, free from the intrusion of unwanted and inappropriate technology, and also from intolerable suffering because of under/use of available pain medication, including narcotic drugs. The resolution concludes by calling for further study of issues posed by quality of life concerns and care for the dying, particularly the "rightness of refusing life-saving therapy" and the questions of inappropriate prolonging of life and sustaining persons in a "permanent vegetative state" ([24], p. 387).

These resolutions are consistent with official statements of other church bodies in the Anglican Communion. The Public Affairs Unit of the Church of New Zealand's Social Responsibility Commission made submissions to the government's Justice and Law Reform Committee on the Crimes Bill 1989. In the document, the Commission recommends no liberalization of the laws governing euthanasia; liberalization, the report states, would raise many more questions than it would resolve.

When will euthanasia be permitted? Only when a person is in pain? Only when dying? Must there be consent? Or does the logic of euthanasia not also justify paternalistic euthanasia of those who are incapable of consenting or are not prepared to consent on reasonable grounds? How can we be sure that consent is genuine? Who should perform the act? Doctors, police, family. . . We also point out the difficulty inherent in the common phrase "right to die" – if there is such a right, then upon whom rests the correlative duty to fulfil that right? To impose a duty to kill is a horrific prospect [32].

The issue of euthanasia also has attracted the attention of Australian Anglicans. The Reverend Dr. John Morgan published an article entitled

"Euthanasia and Death in Contemporary Debate" in *Church Scene*, the national Anglican weekly newspaper. Morgan refers to the American and Dutch experience with this issue, specifically the Washington state initiative, the work of The Hemlock Society in the United States, the actions of Dr. Jack Kevorkian, the debate engendered by the article "It's Over, Debbie" in the *Journal of the American Medical Association*, and Holland's experience following a decision that physicians would not be prosecuted in assisted suicide cases provided that specific procedures are followed. A Voluntary Euthanasia Society exists in Australia, but the idea has not yet gained a firm foothold, according to Morgan. In two Australian states, "right to die" legislation provides a legal right to decline medical treatment.

Morgan calls for a middle ground between euthanasia and all-out technological intervention.

We need to avoid the tyranny of either a "life at all costs" view, or one that is based on quality of life considerations alone . . . A too easy rejection of life – an opting out – even when physical existence is burdensome – flies in the face of the gift of creation and the love spent by God in Christ. We are certainly not required [sic] – and indeed should not – deploy all our medical technology and know how in trying to save physical life as an end in itself when the battle for life submerges the possibility of our fellowship with God and each other. But neither should we opt for a quick fix via euthanasia ([25], pp. 5-6).

Morgan points out the ethical dangers of making "blanket decisions for classes of person in the way in which a so-called 'regulated euthanasia policy' seeks to do."

At its June 1975 meeting, the General Synod of the Anglican Church of Canada asked the Primate to reappoint The Task Force on Human Life to study and report on "the issues related to death and dying including the extension of life by mechanical and other means." Study groups established throughout Canada reported their discussions, and the task force submitted an interim report to the General Synod at its 1977 meeting. The report was revised and published in 1980 under the title *Dying: Considerations Concerning the Passage from Life to Death*.

In this book, the task forces makes several specific recommendations. It urges that the Church

take every possible opportunity to influence those involved in care of the dying by providing active and continuing moral and spiritual guidance . . .

recognize its responsibility to provide educational programmes to foster a better understanding of the needs of the dying patient, of those responsible for the patient's welfare, and of the next of kin [which] should focus on . . . [t]he elaboration, in the continuing education of clergy, of their special role with the dying patient and with their immediate families . . . [e]quipping the laity for effective ministry to the terminally ill in conjunction with the medical team and for service in volunteer home-care programs of hospitals . . . development in the Church and in society at large of a more realistic and wholesome attitude to and acceptance of the dying process and of death itself ([47], pp. 70-71).

The report calls for public policy initiatives, including support and encouragement of persons and institutions that provide care for the dying, advocacy for the development of small units for the care of terminally ill patients, and the expansion of home care programs. The report sparked debate in both the 1977 and the 1979 General Synods, which reached no conclusions; hence, the book stands as a study document and not as a policy statement. Now out of print, it is the most recent statement on issues of death and dying from the Anglican Church of Canada.

More recently, the church in Canada has begun to explore the issues of living wills, euthanasia, and protection of physicians from criminal liability for carrying out the terms of living wills. These issues are currently under discussion.

Thus, on the record, the Anglican churches favor withholding or withdrawing treatment for terminally ill persons and support hospice care. They have not endorsed positive or voluntary euthanasia or a right to suicide, although we can anticipate increased Anglican interest in these matters as the debate intensifies, at least in the United States. Anglican bodies have given relatively little attention in recent years to the issues surrounding honest communication with terminal persons or to the definition of death.

VII. HIV/AIDS

ECUSA's Joint Commission on AIDS was established by the 69th General Convention in 1988 "to focus the Church's attention on the theological, ethical, and pastoral issues of AIDS, and to develop recommendations and strategies to increase AIDS awareness throughout the Church" ([21], p. 2). In its report to the most recent General Convention, the Commission asserted, "The Episcopal Church is an acknowledged leader in the response of the international faith community to the HIV/AIDS pandemic." The Commission attributed the church's leadership role to "the traditional liberality of the Episcopal Church in taking seriously the Gospel call to honor the integrity of all people by seeking to minister to those most marginalized in the world," to the leadership of Presiding Bishop Edmund Browning and to the efforts of church organizations ([21], p. 4).

As a reflection of the church's pastoral concern for persons affected by HIV/AIDS, the 70th General Convention adopted no fewer than ten separate resolutions related to HIV/AIDS. Four resolutions attacked discrimination against persons with AIDS or HIV.

Resolution A-003 endorses the Executive Council resolution that prohibits discrimination on the basis of HIV infection or AIDS. It recognizes church entities that have adopted similar policies and calls on remaining church-related organizations to do so no later than December 15, 1992. Finally, it calls on every diocese to establish an HIV/AIDS task force to advocate for "all affected by HIV/AIDS" ([24], p. 775).

Resolution A007a adopts "Ten Principles for the Workplace" as the standard for Episcopalians and asks church-related entities and organizations to "review, discuss and decide" whether to adopt the principles. The resolution also asks Episcopalians to share the principles with management in their workplaces and urge their adoption. The "Ten Principles" begin by asserting that persons with HIV/AIDS are "entitled to the same rights and opportunities as people with other serious or life-threatening illnesses." The principles also call for employment policies that recognize scientific findings about transmission of the virus, that comply with relevant laws and regulations against discrimination, that protect confidentiality of medical information, and that provide appropriate education and training of employees ([24], p. 774).

Resolution A008a urge baptized members of the church to speak publicly against legislation at all levels that discriminates against persons with AIDS or HIV, encourages improved access to services for marginalized communities and calls on the HIV/AIDS Ministry Office to prepare and disseminate anti-discrimination information.

Resolution B025 calls for an end to HIV/AIDS-based restrictions on foreigners' travel to and within the United States.

A second group of resolutions relates to testing, medical care and research. Resolution A009 affirms and encourages early intervention and anonymous testing, counseling and medical treatment for HIV. Resolution D-096a calls on the U. S. Congress to include issues affecting women and children in the design and funding of research, treatment and experimental protocols and asks Congress to require health agencies to define HIV/AIDS-related conditions in women and children that will allow them access to treatment and assistance. Resolution A-006a encourages the National Council of Churches, Anglican Consultative Council and World Council of Churches to address the global epidemic and the church's response.

Finally, a pair of resolutions urges educational efforts focused on adults (A-004a) and youth (A-005a). Both stress the need for sensitivity to "cultural and sexual diversity and [the incorporation of] current events" ([24], p. 386). A third resolution (A002) encourages identification, affirmation, encouragement and publication of HIV/AIDS ministries, "particularly those initiated and sustained by gay and lesbian people and people of color, as a significant segment of the total ministry and evangelism of this church" ([24], p. 762).

In March 1987, the Anglican Church of New Zealand published a brief statement on AIDS prepared by the Provincial Public and Social Affairs Committee. In language both passionate and pastoral, the statement encourages loving ministry toward all who are in need. It repudiates the tendency among "some Christians" to

adopt the Old Testament view that there is no neutral zone; only life or death, good or evil, sin or punishment, blessing or curse . . . The Christian accepts the reality of both the dark and light side of the human condition and seeks to move forward to bring hope in all circumstances ([31], p. 1).

According to the statement, "True compassion is not limited by circumstance. It is of the greatest importance to recognise that caring response is given out of love and is not restricted by one's lik[e] or even one's dislike for the other" ([31], p. 2). The report also quotes *AIDS -Some Guidelines for Pastoral Care*, a booklet published in 1986 by the Board for Social Responsibility of the Church of England:

[T]he bedside of a gay AIDS patient is not the place for [the care giver] to work out his or her anxiety about sexuality; this needs to be done elsewhere. The prime responsibility of caregivers is not to obtain agreement on the boundaries of what is acceptable behaviour, but to reveal God's love for . . . each individual (quoted in [31], p. 2).

The report concludes with questions:

Is it not the job of the Church to take a stand against superstition, misconceptions, denigration of the individual? An important factor in our individual response is to decide what kind of God we worship: the God spoken of in the Old Testament or the God who revealed Himself to us through Christ's ministry? ([31], p 2).

In 1989, the Church of England National Council for Social Aid published *Responding to AIDS*, described as a "consultative document." The Council was organized in 1969 to assume the work of the Church of England Temperance Society and the National Police Court Mission. Its mission was to promote improved community services for "offenders and persons addicted to drink, drugs or gambling" ([26], frontispiece).

In his Foreword, The Rt. Rev. Colin Docker, Chairman of the Council, asserts:

As members of Christ's Church, we have a responsibility to address the vital social issues of today and, with due regard to basic Christian teachings and values, to construct appropriate responses. The compassion with which all Christians should respond to social needs must not be restricted or withheld because these needs are seen by some to be an occasion for proclaiming moral truths ([26], no page number).

The Council begins by providing factual information on the etiology, transmission, impact and prevention of AIDS, emphasizing the practical needs of persons with AIDS and assessing society's response. Observing that discussion within the church has tended to focus on issues relating to sexual preference rather than on practical responses to those with HIV or AIDS, the council asserts, "We believe that people with AIDS should be welcomed, helped and cared for with love and understanding whether or not they believe or act according to traditional Christian teaching and values" ([26], p. 1).

In its discussion of "The Implications of AIDS for the Church," the booklet enumerates a variety of contributions that the church could make, including counsel for the dying and bereaved, volunteer assistance, and initiatives in housing and hospice care. The Council cautions about the need for the Church to exhibit "great sensitivity" in public debate.

[T]he impression is often given that deeply held religious convictions opposed to homosexuality must be abandoned before a caring response is possible . . . there is a genuine danger that the fundamental issue of how the Church should care for people with AIDS could be confused by debates on AIDS which focus on theological arguments about homosexuality. We believe that it is important to separate concern for people with HIV infection from the debate about homosexuality ([26], p. 16).

The Council offers proposals for a Church of England Workplace Policy on AIDS, which emphasize responsibility on the part of HIV employees, support for initiatives to raise awareness and educate about HIV, nondiscrimination in employment and recruitment, and confidentiality. The document concludes with "examples of good practice," citing a hospice, an education and training program, and a residential program, among others.

These documents could usefully be complemented by statements from other branches of the Anglican Communion, especially the churches in Africa, but relevant materials, if any, are not available to us. Church bodies in the United States, New Zealand and England have supported acceptance, care and compassion for persons with HIV/AIDS (although New Zealand's document draws an unfortunate contrast between the Old Testament God and Christianity). To date, these bodies have not addressed some other important issues, e.g., the magnitude of funding for HIV/AIDS research and therapy or issues raised by the experimental use of new therapeutic agents.

VIII. GENETIC ENGINEERING

Little has been published on this subject by the churches in the Anglican Communion. With the recent advent of gene therapy, additional discussion may be forthcoming.

One harbinger may be Resolution A095, adopted by ECUSA at the 1991 General Convention. The resolution finds "no theological or ethical objection" to (1) diagnostic or therapeutic "medicinal materials" produced through genetic manipulation or (2) gene therapy, provided these interventions are intended to prevent or alleviate human suffering. The resolution calls for equitable access to the benefits of the new technologies, regardless of financial status. It finds "unacceptable" the use of genetic screening of "adults, newborns and the unborn" to permit discrimination in employment or insurance ([24], p. 251).

IX. CONCLUSIONS

The constitutive bodies of the Anglican Communion have attempted to respond to issues perceived by their members as significant. Several of the churches in the industrialized world have addressed similar families of problems. The most helpful statements tend to be the products of commissioned authors or small working parties – even if those groups can only record their disagreement. The profile that emerges is support for a series of reasonable middle-of-the-road positions, quite consistent with the Communion's intellectual roots: a broad definition of health; some differentiation of views on the various new technologies for reproduction; support for abortion rights, but abortion as a "tragic" choice; disapproval of both prolonging and hastening dying; calls for universal access to health care, and compassion for HIV/AIDS patients. Some of these positions require the member churches to stand against powerful forces in their cultures.

While these documents reveal some significant cross-fertilization among member churches, increased conversation might well be helpful to all parties. The Anglican Communion is unlikely to attempt to develop a massive, coherent teaching magisterium on all questions of biomedical ethics. Part of the genius of Anglicanism is its flexibility and tolerance for divergent views. The autonomy of national churches, and of judicatories within them, requires each group to work through a problem for itself. The federal character of the Communion is compatible with some strategies of information sharing, however. At a minimum, improved communication would help leaders of the member churches as they analyze and develop responses to biomedical issues.

Indiana University
Bloomington, Indiana, U.S.A.

ACKNOWLEDGMENTS

We want to thank The Rev. Mary J. Mail for her invaluable assistance in the research and writing of this essay. This essay could not have been completed without the cooperation of the following persons: William R. Atkin, Reader at Law, Victoria University of Wellington; The Most Reverend Dr. P. F. Carnley, Archbishop of Perth; Phyllis Creighton, Anglican Church of Canada; Karen Evans, Librarian, Resource Center, Anglican Church of Canada; The Reverend Dr. John Morgan, University of Queensland; and David Skidmore, Secretary, the Board for Social Responsibility, Church of England. We acknowledge with deep gratitude their gifts of time and effort.

We also wish to thank Jo Mutch and Gordon Light, Anglican Church of Canada; Colin Honey, Kingswood Center for Applied Ethics, Crawley, Western Australia; Alastair V. Campbell, Bioethics Research Centre, University of Otago, New Zealand; and Tom Ross, Acting General Secretary, The Church of England National Council for Social Aid.

Indiana University
Bloomington, Indiana, U.S.A.

BIBLIOGRAPHY

1. Anglican Church of Canada: 1980, "Official Statements: GS/1980 June/Act 41", Church House Library (mimeo).
2. Anglican Church of New Zealand: 1984, "In Vitro Fertilisation", n.p.
3. Archbishop of Canterbury's Commission on Urban Priority Areas: 1985, *Faith in the City*, Church House Publishing, London.
4. Baycroft, John, ed.: 1990, *Whose Child Is This? Ethical, Legal, Social, and Theological Dangers of "Surrogate Motherhood"*, Anglican Book Center, Toronto.
5. Blacker, Russell: 1992, "Euthanasia – Part I", *Crucible* (January-March 1992), pp. 15-24, and "Euthanasia – Part II", *Crucible* (April-June 1992), pp. 74-85.
6. Board for Social Responsibility, Church of England: 1975, *On Dying Well: An Anglican Contribution to the Debate on Euthanasia*, Church Information Office, London.
7. Board for Social Responsibility, Church of England: 1982, press release, n.p.
8. Board for Social Responsibility, Church of England: 1985, *Personal Origins: The Report of a Working Party on Human Fertilisation and Embryology of the Board for Social Responsibility*, Church Information Office, London.
9. Board for Social Responsibility, Church of England: 1986, *Not Just for the Poor: Christian Perspectives on the Welfare State*, Church House Publishing, London.
10. Board for Social Responsibility, Church of England: 1989, "Working for Patients" (mimeo), Board for Social Responsibility, London.
11. Board for Social Responsibility, Church of England: 1992, *Community Care and Mental Health*, General Synod of the Church of England, London.
12. Carnley, P. F.: 1984, "When Does Human Life Begin"?, *Anglican Messenger*, October 1984, p. 4.
13. Carnley, P.F.: 1991, "The Sinister Side of the Human Reproductive Technology Bill", *Anglican Messenger*, February 1991 (reprint, unpaged).
14. Carnley, P.F.: 1991, untitled reprint, *Anglican Messenger*, May 1991 (unpaged).
15. Carter, James H.: 1991, "Optimum Health and Wellness: A Holistic Approach", in Sjoerd L. Bonting, ed., "Health Concerns: Report and Background Material Prepared by the Standing Commission on Health of the Episcopal Church" (mimeo), San Francisco, Calif.
16. Church Assembly Board for Social Responsibility, The: 1965, *Abortion: An Ethical Discussion*, Church Information Office, London.
17. Creighton, Phyllis: 1977, *Artificial Insemination by Donor: A Study of Ethics, Medicine, and Law in Our Technological Society*, Anglican Book Center, Toronto.
18. Creighton, Phyllis: 1992, "Interim Report on the Disposition of Frozen

Human Embryos" (mimeo), Toronto.

19. Hawes, Arthur: 1990, "Mental Health in Society", *Crucible* (July-September 1990), 116-121.

20. Heyward, Oliver: 1984, "The Ethics of IVF: Where the Debate Is", in [27].

21. Joint Commission on AIDS, The: 1991, "Report of the Commission", in *The Blue Book: Reports of the Committees, Commissions, Boards, and Agencies of the General Convention of the Episcopal Church, 1991*, Episcopal Church Center, New York.

22. Journal of the General Convention of the Protestant Episcopal Church in the United States of America, 1973: 1973, Episcopal Church Center, New York.

23. Journal of the General Convention of the Protestant Episcopal Church in the United States of America, 1988: 1988, Episcopal Church Center, New York.

24. Journal of the General Convention of the Protestant Episcopal Church in the United States of America, 1991: 1992, Episcopal Church Center, New York.

25. Morgan, John: 1991, "Euthanasia and Death in Contemporary Debate", *Church Scene* (February 7, 1991), pp. 5-6.

26. National Council for Social Aid [Church of England]: 1989, *Responding to AIDS*, National Council for Social Aid, London.

27. Nichols, Alan, and Hogan, Trevor, eds.: 1984, *Making Babies: The Test Tube and Christian Ethics*, Acorn Press, Canberra.

28. *Planned Parenthood of Southeastern Pennsylvania v. Casey*, 60 USLW 4795 (1992).

29. Provincial Public and Social Affairs Committee of the Anglican Church [of New Zealand]: n.d., "Submissions to the Justice and Law Reform Committee on the Status of Children Amendment Bill 1986".

30. Provincial Public and Social Affairs Committee, Anglican Church of New Zealand: n.d., "Surrogate Motherhood: A Christian Perspective" (mimeo).

31. Provincial Public and Social Affairs Committee of the Anglican Church [of New Zealand]: 1987, "AIDS" (mimeo).

32. Public Affairs Unit of the Social Responsibility Commission of the Anglican Church [of New Zealand], The: 1989, "Submissions to the Justice and Law Reform Committee on the Crimes Bill 1989", n.p.

33. Robinson, Lillian: 1991, "Infertility and Reproductive Technology", in Sjoerd L. Bonting, ed., "Health Concerns: Report and Background Material Prepared by the Standing Commission on Health of the Episcopal Church", mimeo, San Francisco, Calif.

34. *Roe v. Wade*, 410 U.S. 113 (1973).

35. *Rust v. Sullivan*, 59 USLW 4451 (1991).

36. Scott, David A.: 1992, "Changing Teachings on Abortion", in Timothy F.

Sedgwick and Philip Turner, eds., *The Crisis in Moral Teaching in the Episcopal Church*, Morehouse Publishing, Harrisburg, Pa.

37. Smith, David H.: 1986, *Health and Medicine in the Anglican Tradition: Conscience, Community and Compromise*, Crossroad, New York.

38. Smith, David H., and Granbois, Judith A.: 1992, "Assisted Reproduction", in Timothy F. Sedgwick and Philip Turner, eds., *The Crisis in Moral Teaching in the Episcopal Church*, Morehouse Publishing, Harrisburg, Pa.

39. Social Responsibility Commission, Anglican Church of New Zealand: 1989, "Submissions to the Social Services Committee on the Contraception, Sterilisation and Abortion Amendment Bill 1989", Wellington.

40. Standing Commission on Health, The: 1991, "Report of the Commission", in *The Blue Book: Reports of the Committees, Commissions, Boards, and Agencies of the General Convention of the Episcopal Church, 1991*, Episcopal Church Center, New York.

41. Standing Commission on Human Affairs and Health, The: 1982, "Report of the Standing Commission on Human Affairs and Health", in *The Blue Book: Reports of the Committees, Commissions, Boards, and Agencies of the General Convention of the Episcopal Church, 1982*, Episcopal Church Center, New York.

42. Standing Commission on Human Affairs and Health, The: 1988, "Report of the Standing Commission on Human Affairs and Health", in *The Blue Book: Reports of the Committees, Commissions, Boards, and Agencies of the General Convention of the Episcopal Church, 1988*, Episcopal Church Center, New York.

43. Task Force on Abortion, Anglican Church of Canada: 1989, *Abortion in a New Perspective*, Anglican Book Centre, Toronto.

44. "Unofficial Journal of the Thirty-third General Synod": 1992, Anglican Church of Canada, Toronto (mimeo).

45. Walters, William, A.W.: 1984, "IVF Technology and Its Major Ethical Implications", in [27].

46. *Webster v. Reproductive Services*, 492 U.S. 490 (1989).

47. Whytehead, Lawrence, and Chidwick, Paul, eds.: 1980, *Dying: Considerations Concerning the Passage from Death to Life*, Anglican Book Center, Toronto.

STANLEY SAMUEL HARAKAS

EASTERN ORTHODOX BIOETHICS

This survey of Eastern Orthodox bioethical writings for the period 1990-1992
will begin some supplementary bibliographical material that has come to the
attention of the author since the publication of the first bibliography two years
ago ([24], pp. 85-101). That material will be followed by bibliographical entries
for the 1990-1992 period. During this period, books consisting of collections
of articles by various authors and at least one significant journal edition on a
single theme have been published. Many authors have also dealt with multiple
topics in articles.

This has made it difficult to categorize themes. To have used a strict topical
plan for this survey would have fragmentized coherent works. I have therefore
chosen to treat multiple-author single works as wholes, while selecting
dominant themes from other works to provide general headings. The reader,
however, should understand that during this period, the Orthodox have
produced works that, in the main, are cross-disciplinary in character.
Unfortunately, this means that those seeking information on a particular topic
may have to approach the material from the biographical list of specific articles
and by reading large parts of this article to find their subjects of interest. Consequently, this chapter should be seen as providing an overview that emphasizes
an interdisciplinary and inclusive approach rather than a strict topical approach,
although topics such as contraception, abortion, organ transplantation, sexuality,
and death and dying are discussed and highlighted.

I. ADDITIONAL BACKGROUND BIBLIOGRAPHY

Nicholas E. Metsopoulos, Professor of Ethics and Dogmatics at the University
of Athens School of Theology, published a number of volumes during the past
decade dealing with the methodology of Eastern Orthodox ethics and some
works dealing, directly or indirectly, with bioethical issues. In 1983, Professor
Metsopoulos published two important works on methodology. The first was
Following the Truth [28], in which he addresses fundamental issues of Orthodox
Christian ethical methodology. This work is the text of a talk given by Prof.
Metsopoulos at a meeting of the Panhellenic Union of Theologians March 26,
1983 and is based on John 2:4. He develops his theme in seven points, calling
as an essential fifth point for the correct fulfillment of the requirement to
"follow the truth" as an expression of the Orthodox Christian ethos. He
argues that there have developed two dangerous tendencies in Orthodox

B. Andrew Lustig (Sr. Ed.), Bioethics Yearbook: Volume 3, 117-131.
©1993 Kluwer Academic Publishers.

thought regarding the living of the Christian life. "The one tends to present Christian ethical teaching as a collection of rules and commands, in a most Western scholastic manner, which people are called to follow in life in order to be good Christians" ([28], p. 9). Metsopoulos rejects the idea that rules are "despotic commands, to which the human being is called to obey, as a simple slave of the one who gives the command" ([28], p. 12).

The second view, "apparently in reaction to the first, tends to deny the very existence of Christian ethics and the Christian ethical commands and to lead to a full subjectivity. Everything for the Christian, many say, is freedom and love" ([28], p. 10). Metsopoulos counters that "[F]reedom in Christ indicates a voluntary conformity with the will of God" ([28], p. 10), within the context of regeneration in Christ and new life in Christ. Thus, "[T]he commands of God are ... His paternal guidelines (hypodeixeis)"; they are brotherly counsels (protropai) that give specificity and content to the new life in Christ ([28], p. 12).

This debate is of importance for bioethical concerns, of course, since without the existence of an organized body of knowledge and an appropriate methodology for Orthodox Christian ethics, nothing could be said authoritatively on bioethical questions from the Eastern Orthodox point of view.

Metsopoulos takes up several issues of importance in his 1983 work *Topics of Orthodox Ethical Theology* [29], a volume designed for use by students of theology at the University of Athens. In the first several sections, he returns to the topic of the place of ethics in Orthodox Christian theological teaching and the Christian life, rooting ethics in the soteriological experience of the Christian faith ([29], pp. 15-50). In the second part of the book, he discusses particular topics, among them concern for the body and care of life ([29], pp. 126-133). In the third part, entitled "Life and Death in the Life in Christ", Metsopoulos focuses primarily on theological and ethical themes, but also discusses physical death ([29], pp. 174-182). The final section deals with killing in self-defense, the death penalty, indirect involuntary killing, suicide, self-sacrifice, euthanasia and organ transplantation from deceased donors ([29], pp. 193-207). Each of these topics is dealt with in a brief manner consistent with the basic ethical principles developed earlier in the volume.

In a 1989 volume dealing with the commands of God and their place in Orthodox Christian ethics, Professor Metsopoulos contributes to the discussion of the place of commands or moral laws in Orthodox theology today. This debate has been initiated by theologians who have begun using existentialist categories to interpret Orthodox theology and certain dimensions of the Orthodox ethos. In their writings, they have condemned and rejected the idea that ethics can have a place in the Orthodox way of thinking. In response to this intellectual trend in present-day Greece and elsewhere Metsopoulos has written several works in which he makes brief efforts to affirm the opposite view, *viz*, that there is important place for commandments in the Christian tradition and the Christian life.

Metsopoulous develops those views more fully in his subsequent work, *The Commands of God: Existence, Basic Characteristics, Fulfillment, and Content of the Divine Commands* [30]. There he roots his understanding in Scriptures and in the patristic tradition, where the "existence, basic characteristics, fulfillment, and content of the divine commands" are clearly articulated. He counters the view that the moral commands are primarily heteronomous impositions upon free human existence, arguing instead that the moral commands indicate how a person should conform to that which truly serves his or her welfare ([30], p. 6). This fully documented 216-page work presents biblical and patristic evidence in an ordered treatment of the subject. While not dealing directly with bioethical topics, Metsopoulos does discuss particular topics related to marriage and family, death, healing, medicine, diet, drugs, sexuality, the body, and the natural world.

A. *Contraception and Abortion*

The question of when ensoulment occurs is discussed by Nicholas P. Basileiades in a 64-page booklet published in 1986, and designed for a popular readership, entitled *When is the Human Embryo "Ensouled"? The "Zero" Time of Human Life* [2]. Basileiades holds the position, on the basis of biblical, patristic, doctrinal, liturgical and scientific evidence, that conception means that both body and soul are brought into being simultaneously. He concludes the study with a strong argument against abortion. Since the embryo is understood to be a psychosomatic unity in the womb, its destruction is in fact the killing of a human being.

B. *Organ Transplantation and Death*

In a 1987 speech to diocesan physicians and health care workers, entitled "Organ Transplants From a Christian Perspective" [35], the Metropolitan of Demetrias, C. Paraskevaides, bases his comments on two principles: human intrinsic value as created in the divine image and the Christian moral norm of agape-love. He notes that earlier views based their ethical approach primarily on the first principle, tending to see organ transplants only as violations of the integrity of the body. The opposition to organ transplants is supported in part by several canons of the early church that express opposition to self-mutilation. However, Paraskevaides places these canons in context to show that their intent was to reject dualistic approaches to life and inappropriate motives. In the case of organ donation, the canons do not apply. Rather, considerations of donor, recipient, and their mutual relationship cast a totally different light on contemporary organ transplantation. While generally expressing support for the practice of organ donation on the basis of Christian love, Paraskevaides notes certain ethical concerns raised by the procurement of organs from those about to die and those who have just died. He discusses measures designed to encourage the expression of free choice by both donors and recipients. He also raises questions about current brain death criteria and recommends that further diagnostic steps be taken to verify death. Finally, Paraskevaides affirms the sanctity of the human body and respect for it, even in death, as religious values. With these caveats in place, he expresses cautious support for organ donation.

Heikki Makkonen of the Orthodox Church of Finland has written a study of the traditions related to death in the lives of Orthodox Christians in a period marked by war. In his 1989 volume, *Death in the Orthodox Tradition* [25], Makkonen traces the survival rate of Orthodox death-related beliefs and practices in a Finnish Orthodox region that had to be abandoned by the Finnish Orthodox when it was ceded to the Soviet Union. Some of these Orthodox Finns moved to two cities, one traditionally Orthodox, the other in a region with a dominant Lutheran population. The author examines the traditions on death in the informants' birthplace and the survival of those traditions from 1930-1985 in the two cities. The 283-page volume begins by outlining Orthodox teaching about death based on doctrinal teaching, catechetical material, and the relevant liturgical texts. According to the study, the Orthodox who moved into dominantly Lutheran areas suffered erosions of practice, while those in the traditionally Orthodox city maintained their traditions on death more successfully. Makkonen summarizes as follows:

[T]he traditional way of handing on the traditions linked with death to the future generations in the homes and at school has become more difficult . . . However, there have not been any significant changes in the basic understanding of faith. The traditional Orthodox understanding of death and resurrection, the faith in the immortality of the soul and in eternal life have been preserved in the midst of the great upheaval ([25], p. 281).

However, some customs related to death have been given up, probably because of an unwillingness to be "different" in predominantly Lutheran environments.

II. 1990-1992 PERIOD

A. *General Approaches*

Physician Edward B. Anderson raises the issue of a distinct medical ethic for Eastern Orthodox Christianity in his 1992 article, "Is There an Orthodox Medical Ethic"? [1]. Anderson argues that such an ethic does not exist, holding that there are no overarching principles of medical ethics in Eastern Orthodoxy. Instead, Anderson points to such Orthodox themes in the ascetic tradition as sin, almsgiving, the body/spirit relationship, and the goal of the salvation of the soul. He discusses some bioethical questions in order to show that no specific bioethical principles exist in the Orthodox tradition and holds that "the answers to medical ethical problems that each Orthodox Christian may encounter in his lifetime will best be answered in the courses of his own spiritual labor" ([1], p. 17).

Stanley S. Harakas, in his volume, *Living the Faith: The "Praxis" of Eastern Orthodox Ethics* [14], takes a broader approach to Orthodox theological ethics. In the first chapter, Harakas seeks to show that Orthodox ethics draws on the whole of the Orthodox theological, liturgical, ascetic, canonical, and historical tradition in addressing ethical issues, including bioethical issues. He addresses numerous topics related to bioethics throughout the volume, including ethical relations to the self and the body ([14], ch. 4), the maintenance of life ([14], ch. 5), and the family ([14], ch. 8). In Chapter Four, which discusses the body, Harakas develops major sections on "Obligations to the Body", "The Health of the Body", "Clothing", "Housing", "The Purity of the Body", and "The Responsibility for Life". "The Responsibility for Life" discusses, among other topics, suicide, indirect suicide, self-sacrifice, sickness, healing, and death.

Under the section entitled "Bioethical Concerns" in Chapter Four, Harakas describes an Eastern Orthodox method for bioethics. He follows this with a section on "The Protection of Life", including short discussions of the allocation of scarce medical resources, human experimentation, abortion, organ transplants, mental health issues, aging, suffering, death, dying and euthanasia. In a section entitled "The Transmission of Life", Harakas briefly addresses questions of sexual behavior from an Orthodox Christian ethical perspective: contraception, population control, artificial insemination, in vitro fertilization, surrogate motherhood, egg grafts, sterilization, and genetic counseling and screening. He emphasizes as the common denominator the high regard for human life as a composite of spirit and body in the Eastern Orthodox faith tradition.

B. *Illness and the Patient as Person*

The January 1991 issue of *Aktines* (the monthly periodical published by the Union of Christian Scholars and Scientists in Greece) was devoted to the topic of "The Patient as a Person". In the introduction to the issue, "Responding to the Patient As A Person"[27], George Merikas, a physician and member of the Academy of Athens, stresses a wholistic approach to human life terms, i.e., one that sees the patient not only as the locus of illness but as a unity composed of spirit and body.

In the same issue [18], a short article by T. Ketseas entitled "The Spiritual Purposefulness of Illness According to the New Testament" was based on an examination of several New Testament passages, including John 9:1-4 and 2 Corinthians 12. The author, in holding that "illness helps each person put his or her life in order", sees illness from a spiritual perspective as an occasion for the care of the soul. From a societal perspective, illness is seen as an impetus for the cultivation of social values such as mutual concern and love.

In the second article, Demetrios Oraiopoulos discusses the question of

"Technology and Humanistic Medicine" [34]. He argues that technological advances have created a chasm between patient and physician. He urges that the physician strive to take the experience of the patient seriously in offering both a diagnosis and a therapeutic plan. In the third article of this *Aktines* issue, A. S. Koutselinas addresses the question of "Medical Responsibility and the Human Being" [20] from the perspective of a rational rather than a religious ethic. He emphasizes the principles of autonomy, justice, beneficence, and equality. As a deontological principle, Koutselinas stresses the duty of healing, and as a teleological principle, he offers a form of utilitarianism. As a solution to the questions raised by issues of medical responsibility, he calls for the development of *kanones* (codes) with ethical, social and scientific content.

Professor George Daikos, addresses "The Quality of Medicine and the Quality of Life" in the fourth article [10]. Daikos describes the potential for conflict between medical technology and the requirements of person-centered care. This conflict produces a "climate" that is not always conducive to concern for the patient's quality of life overall; rather, quality of life tends to be identified with the technological quality of medical care. Daikos charges that by substituting a "dry technocratic professionalism" ([10], p. 190], for the Hippocratic conviction of the sanctity of life, medicine fails to support the fuller meaning of quality of life for both for patient and physician. He quotes historian and theologian Demetrios Constantelos, who recommends that one serve the patient as if one were serving God, thus restoring medicine to a religious and theological matrix.

Basilike A. Lanara, a Professor of Nursing, has published in Greece a volume entitled *Heroism as a Nursing Value: A Philosophical Perspective*. The fifth article in the *Aktines* special issue, entitled "The Patient as a Suffering Person" [23], is based on the ideas he presented in that book. Lanara notes that sharing in the pain of the suffering person is itself a painful experience. Thus, such sharing is often avoided by nurses and physicians who objectify the patient and "place" the patient in an exclusively technological context. Lanara argues that if the health care professional struggles to respond to his or her questions about the meaning of illness and pain, it becomes possible to renew the deposit of personal faith in God. That renewed faith can then assist the health care professional in treating the hospitalized patient as a person. Michalis T. Melingkos, a cardiologist, emphasizes theological and philosophical perspectives in the sixth article, entitled "From Psychosomatic Medicine to the Medicine of the Person" [26]. Melingkos's thesis is that medicine has moved from the treatment of illness to the treatment of the patient as a psychosomatic unity to the recognition that the patient is a person who should be understood to existing in communion with others and with the larger environment, including the transcendent spiritual environment. "The human being is a biopsychosocial and spiritual being. The human being lives as an individual in an organized community, and has a powerful relationship with the natural and spiritual worlds which form his environment" ([26], p. 202). Drawing on the work of Paul Tournier, Melingkos argues that, since "the medicine of the person is a spiritual-psychosomatic medicine", the only fully effective medicine is "a medicine of the person" ([26], p. 205). Within this perspective, the physician and other health care professionals "offer a human service entrusted to them by God" ([26], p. 207).

In the final article of the special issue, Demetrios Constantelos, an historian, traces the meaning of "person" from the thought of ancient Greece through the Byzantine Hellenic-Christian tradition [8]. Constantelos finds strong continuities between the earlier and later periods and sums up the theme of the *Aktines* volume by reaffirming the theological underpinnings of the concept of personhood. He concludes that the dignity and significance of the person finds ultimate support in one's relationship with God. In that context, medicine also finds its fitting and appropriate orientation.

C. *The Contemporary Moral Climate for Bioethics*

Bishop Herman (Joseph Swaiko), of the Orthodox Church of America and St. Tikhon's Seminary in South Canaan, Pennsylvania, published an article in 1991 entitled "AIDS, Addictions, Abortion: The Deadly Power of Sin" [16], in which he argues for the interconnectedness of these phenomena in contemporary life. He concludes that, although exceptions exist, AIDS, the various addictions, and the practice of abortion are, in the main, connected with human sinfulness. In the transcription of a talk entitled "The Crisis in Morality" [15], Stanley S. Harakas also seeks to provide a background for dominant contemporary moral thinking that has contributed to the breakdown of traditional ethical values in the western world. The talk, originally addressed to the faculty and students of St. Tikhon's Theological Seminary in S. Canaan, Pennsylvania, and published in 1992, deals with many issues, a number of which are bioethical in character. Harakas argues for a "sin connection" among many issues and traces the roots of new attitudes to the wide acceptance, even within religious traditions, of an extreme existentialist philosophical stance. Harakas judges this view to be one-sided and ultimately out of touch with the theological and pastoral tradition of the Church.

D. *Reproductive Issues*

Writing in 1991 in the diocesan periodical, *Alive in Christ*, seminary professor and priest John Kowalczyk discussed the "Disregarding of the Sanctity of Life" [21]. He writes, "The cataclysmic result of the abandonment of the Christian ethic is the rejection of the doctrine that all human life is sacred, being created in the image and likeness of God and the subsequent loss of the protection, by law, of that life" ([21], p. 24). He presents, as illustrations of his thesis, changes in public life over the past several decades on topics such as abortion, infanticide, euthanasia, assisted suicide, sexual perversions and violence, and the "death of the family". He focuses particular attention on the issue of assisted suicide, provoked by the activities of Dr. Jack Kevorkian. Kowalczyk distinguishes between active and passive, as well as voluntary and involuntary, euthanasia. He judges that there changes in public thinking are attributable to a shift from biblical perspectives to humanistic rationalism, thus resulting in the increase of moral evil in society.

Alexander M. Stavropoulos, a member of the faculty of the University of Athens, Greece, discussed persons who become parents of a child that is not conceived through normal marital relations in an article, entitled "Substitutionary Parenthood" [43]. The article focuses on the interpersonal relations of substitute parents and the child(ren) who have come into their care, and encourages individuals involved in such situations to adopt a child-oriented perspective.

E. *Contraception/Abortion*

Metropolitan Chrysostomos (Zapheires) of Peristerion, Greece, had published in the periodical *Theologia* a series of articles on abortion, occasioned by the debate over the legalization of abortion in Greece. The content of these articles was discussed at length in Volume One of the *Bioethics Yearbook* ([24], pp. 93-96). These articles, slightly revised, were subsequently published in a 360-page volume, *Abortions and the Orthodox Church: Theses and Antitheses* [45].

Basilio Petra, a Roman Catholic scholar in Italy, has specialized in the field of Eastern Orthodox Ethics. He published a volume in 1991, *Between Heaven and Earth* [38], which provided Italian readers with an introduction to Eastern Orthodox ethics. The first part of the 284-page volume deals with several theoretical issues, including the relationship between theology and ethics, the relationship of the canons and ethics, and the connections between ethics and the practice of *economia*. The second part discusses several issues of practical ethics, all having bioethical themes, and chosen because of their controversial nature within the Orthodox tradition. Petra's treatment is both descriptive and analytical. The controversial nature of Orthodox teaching on contraception is treated in the first two chapters of Part Two under the general heading, "A Theology in Difficulty". The first chapter discusses the 1937 Encyclical of the Church of Greece, which expressed disapproval of contraception, and the role of Seraphim Papacostas in its writing. The second chapter on contraception discusses the teachings of various Orthodox theologians on the topic. Chapter Three of Part Two traces the contemporary discussion within Orthodox Christian ethics on the issue of abortion and summarizes various approaches to the issue in light of the Orthodox concept of "involuntary sin" ([38], Part Two, Ch. 3, Sec. 6).

F. *Suicide*

Elias Boulgarakes, professor at the Theological School of Athens, published a volume in 1992, *Suicide and Ecclesiastical Burial* [3], on the question of whether persons who commit suicide can receive church burial. The accepted practice in the Orthodox Church, based on canon law, is that suicide is self-murder, thus not allowing time for repentance and confession before death. A church funeral has been denied to suicides unless it can be certified by a psychiatrist or physician that the person was emotionally ill. However, Boulgarakes recommends that the church adopt a more lenient position.

G. *Aging, Sickness and Dying*

In their book, *On the Issues of Aging, Sickness and Dying* [17], two Orthodox priests, Andrew Jarmus and Stephan Jarmus, a father and son team, have co-authored an 84-page book of pastoral and ethical significance. The authors, who are clergy of the Ukrainian Orthodox Church in Canada, originally wrote the chapters as part of their clinical pastoral programs. Their focus, consequently, is on pastoral concerns but their discussion contains much of bioethical significance.

Andrew Jarmus begins the work by discussing "Some Issues in the Care for the Elderly" ([17], pp. 11-20). He focuses on the isolation and marginalization experienced by the elderly, both at home and in institutional settings. In the second and longest chapter of the book, Stephen Jarmus considers "The Problem of Illness and Death: A Discussion" ([17], pp. 21-42). The first sections are an effort to understand the world of the ill person under three headings: "Illness and the Psychological State of the Sick Person", "The Spiritual Needs of the Sick Person", and "The Sick Person and the Family". The balance of the chapter deals with issues related to dying and death: "The Dying Process and the Person's Reaction To It", "The Effect of Terminal Illness on the Behaviour of the Person", "The Family in the State of Anticipating Bereavement", and "The Problem of Unresolved Grief".

The third chapter deals with "Concepts of Death and Attitudes Towards It". The volume ends with additional observations, including reflections on the impact of death on children, a touching case study of a dying man, and a final theological assessment of death.

H. *Marriage and Issues of Sexuality*

William Basil Zion, a priest of the Orthodox Church and chair of the Department of Religion at Queen's College in Kingston, Canada, has written a major work on marriage from an Eastern Orthodox Perspective, *Eros and Transformation: Sexuality and Marriage, An Eastern Orthodox Perspective* [46]. In the first five chapters, Zion examines the biblical, patristic, and liturgical tradition on marriage, as well as various contemporary Orthodox theological approaches to marriage. Among contemporary views, he distinguishes Greek approaches to marriage, understood as incarnationally expressive in personalist and sacramental terms, from Russian views, rooted in a love-mysticism that has sophiological dimensions. He then discusses divorce in Chapters Six and Seven by tracing the historical development of the Orthodox position. That historical discussion allows Zion to affirm the permanency of marriage, but also to provide a rational for divorce and remarriage in the Church.

Chapters Seven through Nine deal with contraception, masturbation, and homosexuality. Zion recognizes the controversial arguments within Orthodox moral reflection on contraception. After surveying the literature, he opts for a limited use of contraception within marriage. In the eighth chapter's discussion of masturbation, Zion treats the topic in a sophisticated way, judging that the circumstances and context of the act have significant impact on its appropriateness or inappropriateness in a particular situation. He carefully distinguishes its moral status in varied vocations and circumstances of life, showing how these may impact on the moral assessment of the act. He holds that, "[I]n an Orthodox moral theology, masturbation must be seen as a complex phenomenon, often sinful, but not necessarily destroying a graceful union with God" ([46], p. 5). The chapter is a useful "case study" in doing Orthodox ethics.

Zion discusses homosexuality in the ninth chapter. Early negative judgments on homosexual activity are distinguished from "psychological homosexuality". Zion supports the traditional disapproval of homosexual acts because they cannot express the kind of love envisaged by sacramentally expressed life. Nevertheless, in the spirit of Christian compassion, he rejects a harsh judgmental approach toward homosexuals.

Zion's last chapter urges the Church to adopt a positive approach to human sexuality as a potential vehicle for living the God-like life.

III. BIOETHICS IN AN INTERDISCIPLINARY MATRIX

John T. Chirban edited two books in 1991, with essentially the same content, under the titles, *Health and Faith: Medical, Psychological and Religious Dimensions* [5] and *Healing: Orthodox Christian Perspectives in Medicine, Psychology, and Religion* [6]. Both contain papers presented at a national conference of the Orthodox Christian Association of Medicine, Psychology and Religion (O.C.A.M.P.R.), but the former is augmented by additional material. References below are made to the first volume, but in the second, the editor emphasizes the interdisciplinary character of healing in his introductory keynote paper. The rest of the papers deal with the relationship of healing to science and faith, genetic engineering, depression, AIDS, and miracles. The interdisciplinary approach to health is discussed by John Chirban ("Healing and Spirituality" [7]), Demetrios J. Constantelos ("The Interface of Medicine and Religion" [9]), and Bishop Nicholas, primate of the Carpatho-Russian Orthodox Church in the U.S.A. ("Science and Morality: When Technology and Ethics Meet" [32]).

The section on genetic engineering contains two papers, one by scientist Peter H. Diamandis, the other by theologian John Breck. Diamandis's "Genetic Engineering: Scientific Perspective" [12] is a description of genetic engineering and technology in language that is comprehensible to the layperson. He discusses the possible implications of genetic engineering on religious thought, and asks the provocative questions, "What more is the human being than a very complicated assemblage of the proper atoms? What and where is the spirit or the soul"? ([12], p. 48). In anticipating the potential for good and evil arising from genetic engineering, Diamandis recommends the "drawing of the line". However, he cautions against those who would "blindly demand a stop to this research", even though he admits that "genetic and molecular engineering may in fact not have any limitations other than those imposed by the laws of nature" ([12], p. 49).

In his article, "Genetic Engineering: Religious Perspectives" [4], Fr. John Breck expresses strong reservations. Because he considers genetic engineering "inherently dangerous", his concern is also one of limits. He distinguishes between the therapeutic use of the technology and "innovational eugenics", approving the first while rejecting the second as applied to human beings. Breck makes several practical proposals for monitoring and fostering the discussion from an Orthodox Christian perspective.

The next section discusses depression. The three papers in this section ([11]; [19]; [22]) discuss specific bioethical issues such as suicide, but in general treat depression from the therapeutic perspective.

Part Four of the volume is entitled "AIDS and Cancer: The Role of the Helping Professionals", with the two diseases treated separately ([6], pp. 76-114). The personal account and reflection of cancer patient Georgia Photopoulos, "Experiences in Cancer: Bridging the Gap Between Patients and Professionals" [39] is the only paper on cancer. In addition to the articulating personal experiences that are of great help in understanding the experience of cancer patients, the author asks challenging questions of caregivers regarding their relationships with cancer patients.

The remaining four articles in Part Four of the volume focus on AIDS. Physician George J. Pazin, in his "Human Immunodeficiency Virus [HIV] Infections and Acquired Immunodeficiency Syndrome [AIDS]: Impact on Lifestyles in the Twenty-first Century" [37], discusses the changes that need to occur in sexual relations, in light of AIDS. He calls for a cautionary and non-promiscuous pattern of behavior, but also recommends fundamental changes in attitudes toward sexual values. Peter Poulos discusses relationships with AIDS patients in "Psycho-Social Issues in Caring for Persons with AIDS: A Theological Perspective" [41]. His paper is a theologically based appeal for caring and sensitivity on the part of caregivers, family and friends. Fr. Milton

B. Efthimiou, in "AIDS: Is It A Moral Crisis"? [13], discusses the attitudes and reactions arising from the AIDS epidemic in social relations. He answers his title's question in the negative: "Although there is a relationship between sickness and man's sinful condition, sickness cannot be considered a punishment that man suffers for his personal sins". On the other hand, while calling for compassion and love in dealing with AIDS patients, he also affirms that ". . . no one should falsely promise solutions that would lead people to doubt that monogamy and self-control not only make moral sense but medical sense as well" ([13], p. 97).

The final article on AIDS in this volume, is a report by a special interdisciplinary committee sponsored by O.C.A.M.R. [33]. Among the topics covered, it discusses the reception of Holy Communion and AIDS according to Orthodox practice, premarital screening for AIDS, and education about how to avoid HIV infection.

The last part of the book is devoted to the topic of "Miracles and Technology". Theoharis C. Theoharides introduces miracles as phenomena that generate wonder in his paper, "Miracles and Technology: A Medical Perspective" [44].   The late Fr. John Meyendorff, in an article entitled "Miracles: Medical, Psychological and Religious Reflections" [31] stresses two points: (1) the fallen condition of the world means that any action that moves the world's condition closer to its purpose as created by God may be understood as miraculous; and (2) those efforts which, in part, contribute to such restoration, whether through medicine or acts of faith, deserve the name "miracle". He says, "If we really believe that the world as it is now is not the world that God wanted it to be – that it is a corrupt, fallen world – then miracles and healings can be thought of as partial restorations of how God wants the world to be" ([31], p. 124).

In an article entitled "God, Miracles and Quantum Mechanics" [42], Constantine Sarantidis argues that the reluctance of moderns to accept miracles, as understood by the early Church, is based on an outdated idea of physics. Newtonian mechanistic physics has been replaced by quantum physics, which affirms a fundamental indeterminacy of subatomic matter. He suggests that

Christians need not be embarrassed by miracles. Instead of seeing miracles as God overturning or interfering with the course of nature, we can more positively see them as ordering events-restoring and creating order and wholeness where it is lacking or has been damaged ([42], p. 132).

The book concludes with an article by nurse Karen Piligian on the topic, "Therapeutic Touch: Using Your Hands for Help or Healing" [40]. After outlining some recent scientific literature on the topic that supports the practice of therapeutic touch, she describes her own positive experience with the practice.

IV. CONCLUSION

This bibliographical review of writings among the Eastern Orthodox during the 1990-1992 period has focused on the interrelations of bioethics and other aspects of human experience. The literature avoids the tendency to isolate the discipline of bioethics from broader concerns. This arises in part from an overall Eastern Orthodox perspective that sees all of life as under the care of God, but also because of the fundamental Trinitarian cast to Orthodox theology, which stands before the mystery of life and the mystery of Triune God, in the knowledge that the reduction of the meaning of any part to itself alone is ultimately a distortion and a falsehood.

Holy Cross Greek Orthodox School of Theology
Brookline, Massachusetts, U.S.A.

BIBLIOGRAPHY

1. Anderson, E. B.: 1992 "Is There an Orthodox Medical Ethic"? *Epiphany*, Vol. 12, No. 2, pp. 13-17.
2. Basileiades, N. P.: 1986, *Pote "Empsychoutai" to Anthropino Embryo: E Ora "Meden" tes Anthropines Zoes* (Greek, "When is the Human Embryo "Ensouled"? The "Zero" Time of Human Life"), The Brotherhood of Theologians "O Soter", Athens.
3. Boulgarakes, E.: 1992, *Autoktonia kai Ekklesiastike Taphe*, (Greek, "Suicide and Ecclesiastical Burial"), Armos Publications, Athens.
4. Breck, J.: 1991, "Genetic Engineering: Religious Perspectives", in [6].
5. Chirban, J. T., ed. 1991, *Healing: Orthodox Christian Perspectives in Medicine, Psychology and Religion*, Holy Cross Orthodox Press, Brookline, Massachusetts.
6. Chirban, J.T., ed., 1991: *Health and Faith: Medical, Psychological and Religious Dimensions*, University Press of America, Lanham, Maryland, pp. 51-55.
7. Chirban, J.T., "Healing and Spirituality", in [6], pp. 3-11.
8. Constantelos, D. J.: 1991 "The Meaning of the Person in the Ancient Greek and Helleno-Christian Tradition" (Greek, *He Ennoia tou Prosopou sten Archaia Hellenike kai HellenoChristianike Paradose*), *Aktines*, No. 522, pp. 208-222.
9. Constantelos, D. J.: 1991 "The Interface of Medicine and Religion", in [6], pp. 13-24.
10. Daikos, G.: 1991, "The Quality of Medicine and the Quality of Life" (Greek, *He Poiotes tes Iaktrikes kai he Poiotes tes Zoes*), *Aktines*, No. 522, pp. 185-191.

11. Demakis, J.: 1991, "Depression: Medical Perspective", in [6], pp. 61-66.
12. Diamandis, P. H.: 1991, "Genetic Engineering: Scientific Perspective", in [6], pp. 43-50.
13. Efthimiou, M. B.: 1991, "AIDS: Is It A Moral Crisis"?, in [6], pp. 93-97.
14. Harakas, S.S.: 1992, *Living the Faith: The Praxis of Eastern Orthodox Ethics*. Light and Life Publishing Co., Minneapolis, MN.
15. Harakas, S.S.: "The Crisis in Morality", *Alive in Christ*, Vol. VIII, No. 1, Spring, 1992, pp. 44-49.
16. Herman, Bishop (Joseph Swaiko): 1991, "AIDS, Addictions, Abortion: The Deadly Power of Sin", *Alive in Christ*, Vol VII, No. 2, Summer, p. 1 ff.
17. Jarmus S. and Jarmus A.: 1989, *On the Issues of Aging, Sickness and Dying*, The Ecclesia Publishing Co., Winnipeg.
18. Ketseas, T.: 1991,"The Spiritual Purposefulness of Illness According to the New Testament" (Greek, *"He Pneumatike Skopimotes tes Nosou Kata ten Kainen Diatheken"*) *Aktines*, Jan., no. 517, pp. 15-17.
19. Kokonis, N.D.: 1991, "Depression: Psychological Perspective", in [6], pp. 67-70.
20. Koutselines, A. S.: 1991, "Medical Responsibility and the Human Being" (Greek, *"Iatrike Euthune kai ho Anthropos"*), *Aktines*, No. 522, pp. 177-184.
21. Kowalczyk, J: 1991, "Disregarding the Sanctity of Life", *Alive in Christ*, Vol VII, No. 3, Winter, pp. 24-25.
22. Krommydas, N.: 1991, "Depression: Religious Perspective", in [6], pp. 71-74.
23. Lanara, B.A.: 1991, "The Patient as a Suffering Person" (Greek, *"Ho Asthenes os Paschon Prosopon"*), *Aktines*, No. 522, pp. 192-199.
24. Lustig, B.A. *et al.*, eds. *Theological Developments in Bioethics: 1988-1990, Bioethics Yearbook: Volume 1*: 1991, Kluwer Academic Publishers, Dordrect.
25. Makkonen, H.: 1989, *Kuolema Orthodoksisessa Perinteessa* (Finnish, *Death in the Orthodox Tradition*), University of Joensuu Publications in Theology, Joensuu.
26. Melingkos, M.T.: 1991, "From Psychosomatic Medicine to the Medicine of the Person" (Greek, *"Apo ten Psychosomatike Iatrike sten Iatrike tou Prosopou"*) *Aktines*, No. 522, pp. 200-207.
27. Merikas, G.: 1991, "Responding to the Patient as a Person" (Greek, *"He Antimetopise tou Asthenous os Prosopon"*), *Aktines*, No. 522, pp. 163-170.
28. Metsopoulos, N. E.: 1983, *Peripateein en Aletheia*, (Greek, *Following the Truth*), Athens.
29. Metsopoulos, E. N.: 1983, *Themata Orthodoxou Ethikes Theologias A'* (Greek, *Topics of Orthodox Ethical Theology*, 1), Publications of the

University of Athens, Athens.

30. Metsopoulos, N. E.: 1989, *Ai Entolai tou Theou: Yparxis, Basikoi Characteres, Epitelesis kai Periechomenon ton Theion Entolon*, (Greek, *The Commands of God: Existence, Basic Characteristics, Fulfillment and Content of the Divine Commands*),n.p., Athens.

31. Meyendorff, J.: "Miracles: Medical, Psychological and Religious Reflections", in [6], pp. 121-125

32. Nicholas, Bishop, "Science and Morality: When Technology and Ethics Meet", in [6], pp. 25-39.

33. O.C.A.M.P.R.: "Interdisciplinary Report on AIDS: Special Committee", in [6], pp. 99-103.

34. Oraiopoulos, D.: 1991, "Technology and Humanistic Medicine" (Greek, *"Techonologia kai Anthropistike Iatrike"*), *Aktines*, No. 522, pp. 171-176.

35. Paraskevaides, C.: 1987, *Oi Metamoscheuseis apo Christianike Apopse* (Greek, *Organ Transplants From a Christian Perspective*), Volos, Greece.

36. Paraskevaides, C.: 1992, *Engephalikos e Kardiakos Thanatos? Symbole sten Exeliktike Poreia ton Metamoscheuseon* (Greek, *Brain or Heart Death?: A Contribution to the Developing Procedures Regarding Organ Transplants*), Athens.

37. Pazin, G. J.: 1991, "Human Immunodeficiency Virus [HIV] Infections and Acquired Immunodeficiency Syndrome [AIDS]: Impact on Lifestyles in the Twenty-first Century", in [6], pp. 77-82.

38. Petra, B.: 1991, *Tra Cielo e Terra: Introduzione Alla Teologia Morale Ortodossa Contemporanea*, (Italian, *Between Heaven and Earth: An Introduction Concerning Contemporary Orthodox Moral Theology*), Edizioni Dehoniane, Bologna.

39. Photopoulos, G.: 1991, "Experiences in Cancer: Bridging the Gap Between Patients and Professionals", in [6], pp. 105-114.

40. Piligian, K.: "Therapeutic Touch: Using Your Hands for Help or Heal", in [6], pp. 135-142.

41. Poulos, P.: 1991, "Psycho-Social Issues in Caring for Persons with AIDS: A Theological Perspective", in [6], pp. 83-91.

42. Sarantidis, C.: 1991, "God Miracles and Quantum Mechanics", in [6], pp. 127-133.

43. Stavropoulos, A.M.: 1992, *Anapleromatike Gonikoteta kai Alla Keimena* (*Greek, Substitutionary Parenthood and Other Texts*), n.p., Athens.

44. Theoharides, T. C.: 1991, "Miracles and Technology", in [6], pp. 117-120.

45. Zapheires, C.: 1991, *Ai Ambloseis kai e Orthodoxos Ekklesia: Theseis kai Antitheseis*, (Greek, *Abortions and the Orthodox Church: Theses and Antitheses*), n.p., Athens.

46. Zion, W. B.: 1992, *Eros and Transformation: Sexuality and Marriage, An Eastern Orthodox Perspective*, University Press of America, Lanham, Maryland.

HASSAN HATHOUT AND B. ANDREW LUSTIG

BIOETHICAL DEVELOPMENTS
IN ISLAM

I. INTRODUCTION

Islam is the third of the monotheistic Abrahamic religions following Judaism
and Christianity, both of which Islam recognizes and whose moral code Islam
shares. Islam, however, has also developed a comprehensive system, the
Shari'a, that covers all aspects of individual and collective human life. The
primary sources of the Shari'a are the Quran (to Muslims, God's very words)
and the traditional teachings and deeds (Sunna) of the Prophet Muhammad.
Issues not specifically mentioned in these two sources are ruled on by
"analogy" (i.e., intelligent reasoning matching new issues with issues judged
by the Quran or Tradition) and the unanimous consensus of Muslim scholars.
When an issue is clearly settled by the Quran or Tradition, the verdict is final,
for "It is not fitting for a believer, man or woman, when a matter has been
decided by Allah (Arabic word for God) and His messenger, to have any
option about their decision. Anyone who disobeys Allah and His messenger
is indeed clearly on a wrong path" (Quran 33:36). However, the major part
of Islamic jurisprudence is the product of human thinking responding to new
events in new times and places. In its response, Islamic jurisprudence always
heeds the five objectives of the Shari'a: the protection of faith, of life, of mind,
of ownership, and of offspring. A basic premise in Islam is that everything is
lawful unless it is otherwise specified by the Quran and Tradition or unless it
conflicts with the objectives of the Shari'a.

II. EUTHANASIA

In response to emerging and incessant efforts to legalize euthanasia in the
United States and in Holland, the Islamic Center of Southern California at Los
Angeles issued a position paper on the subject that reiterates the Islamic stand
universally held by the various juridical schools and expressed by modern
religious conferences [7]. The paper develops a number of conceptual and
practical aspects of the Islamic response to issues of euthanasia and assisted
suicide. The following subsections trace the central elements of that discussion.

B. Andrew Lustig (Sr. Ed.), Bioethics Yearbook: Volume 3, 133-147.
©1993 Kluwer Academic Publishers.

A. *The Sanctity of Human Life*

The sanctity of human life is a basic value as decreed by God even before the times of Moses, Jesus, and Muhammad. Commenting on the killing of Abel by his brother Cain, God says in the Quran: "On that account, We ordained for the Children of Israel that if anyone slew a person – unless it be for murder or spreading mischief in the land – it would be as if he slew the whole people. And if anyone saved a life, it would be as if he saved the life of the whole people" (Quran 5:32). The Quran also says: "Take not life which Allah made sacred otherwise than in the course of justice" (Quran 6:151 and 17:33). The Shari'a detailed the conditions under which the taking of life is permissible, whether in war or in peace, and specifies rigorous prerequisites and precautions to prevent lax application of these exceptions.

B. *Is There a Right to Suicide?*

Islam does not recognize a right to suicide. Since human beings did not create themselves, they do not own their lives. Rather, they are entrusted with them and charged to safeguard them according to Allah's purposes. God is the owner and giver of life and His rights in giving and taking life are not to be violated.

In Islam, attempting to kill oneself is both a crime and a grave sin. The Quran says: "Do not kill (or destroy) yourselves . . . for verily Allah has been to you most merciful" (Quran 4:29). To warn against suicide, the Prophet Muhammad said: Whoever kills himself with an iron instrument will be carrying it forever in hell. Whoever takes poison and kills himself will forever keep sipping that poison in hell. Whoever jumps off a mountain and kills himself will forever keep falling down in the depths of hell (narrated by Bukhari and Muslim).

C. *The Concept of Mercy Killing*

The Shari'a listed and specified the indications for taking life (i.e., the exceptions to the general rule of sanctity of human life). Those exceptions do not include, nor make allowance for, any notion of mercy killing. Human life is an intrinsic value to be respected unconditionally, irrespective of other circumstances. The concept of a life not worth living does not exist in Islam.

Taking life to escape suffering is not acceptable in Islam. Prophet Muhammad taught: "There was a man in older times who had an infliction that taxed his patience, so he took a knife, cut his wrist and bled to death. Upon this God said: My subject hastened his end . . . I deny him paradise" (narrated by Bukhari). During one of the military campaigns, one of the Muslims was killed. The companions of the Prophet praised his gallantry and efficiency in fighting, but to their surprise, the Prophet commented, ""His lot is hell". Upon inquiry, the companions learned that the man, after being seriously injured, "supported the handle of his sword on the ground and plunged his chest on its tip, [thus] committing suicide" (narrated by Bukhari and Muslim).

The Islamic Code of Medical Ethics, which was endorsed by the First International Conference on Islamic Medicine renders the following judgment:

Mercy killing – like suicide – finds no support except in the atheistic way of thinking that believes that our life on this earth is followed by void . . . The claim of killing for painful hopeless illness is also refuted, for there is no human pain that cannot be largely conquered by medication or by suitable neurosurgery [10].

There is another more positive aspect to pain and suffering, for patience and endurance are highly regarded and highly rewarded values in Islam. Thus, the Quran teaches that "[t]hose who patiently persevere will truly receive a reward without measure" (Quran 39:10). Or again, "bear in patience whatever [ill] may befall you: this, behold, is something to set one's heart upon" (Quran 31:17). The Prophet Muhammad taught that "when the believer is afflicted with pain – even that of a prick of a thorn or more – God forgives his sins and his wrongdoing is discarded as a tree sheds off its leaves" (narrated by Bukhari and Muslim). When means of preventing or alleviating pain fall short, this spiritual dimension can be very effectively invoked to support the patient who believes that accepting and standing unavoidable pain will be to his/her credit in the hereafter.

III. ISSUES IN CLINICAL MEDICINE

A. *The Financial Costs of Care*

There is no disagreement that the financial costs of maintaining the incurably ill and the senile is a growing concern. Consequently, one increasingly hears the argument that there is, in some instances, not merely the "right to die" but the "duty to die". According to this argument, when the human body has outlived its productive span or when its maintenance poses an unacceptable burden on society at large, it should be disposed of rather than allowing it to deteriorate gradually.

Such logic is completely alien to Islam. Core values always take priority over issues of cost. Care for the weak, old, and helpless is a value for which people should willingly sacrifice time, effort, and money. Such care begins, naturally, with one's own parents, and is a duty enjoined by the Quran:

Your Lord decreed that you worship none but Him, and that you be kind to your parents. Whether one or both of them attain old age in your life, say not to them a word of contempt but address them in terms of honor. And lower to them the wing of humility out of compassion, and say: My Lord, bestow on them Your mercy even as they cherished me in childhood (Quran 17:24-25).

Because such care is a virtue ordained and rewarded by God in this world and the next, believers do not view it as a debit but as an investment. When individual means can no longer cover the costs of needed care, according to Islam that care becomes the collective responsibility of society.

B. *The Legitimacy of Effective Pain Relief*

In an Islamic setting, the question of euthanasia does not arise, because it is deemed in all cases to be religiously unlawful. The patient should receive compassion and every possible psychological support from family and friends. The doctor is a crucial partner in providing such support and is the specific provider of effective therapeutic measures for the relief of pain. A dilemma may arise when the dosage of analgesic necessary to alleviate pain also runs the risk of hastening the patient's death. From the religious point of view, what is critical here is the doctor's intention: is it his intention to kill or to alleviate pain? To be sure, intention is beyond verification by the law, but it does not escape the ever watchful eye of God who, as the Quran states, "knows the treachery of the eyes, and all that hearts conceal" (Quran 40:19). In a practical vein, therefore, the Islamic Code of Medical Ethics makes the following recommendations:

In his/her defense of life, however, the doctor is well advised to realize his limit and not transgress it. If it is scientifically certain that life cannot be restored, then it is futile to diligently keep on the vegetative state of the patient by heroic means of animation or preserve the patient by deep freezing or other artificial methods. It is the process of life that the doctor aims to maintain and not the process of dying. In any case, the doctor shall not take a positive measure to terminate the patient's life [6].

C. *The Distinction between Medical Treatment and Ordinary Care*

The seeking of medical treatment for illness is mandatory in Islam, according to two sayings of the prophet: "Seek treatment, subjects of God, for to every illness God has made a cure", and "Your body has a right on you". However, when treatment no longer holds promise, it ceases to be mandatory. This judgment applies to surgical and pharmaceutical measures, as well as (according to the majority of scholars) to artificial means of life support. Ordinary needs of life, i.e., basic care, are regarded differently; they are viewed as the right of every living person and therefore not categorized as "treatment". The latter include food, drink, and ordinary nursing care, and are not to be withheld as long as the patient lives.

D. *The Legitimacy of Brain-Death Criteria*

An interesting development here, as noted in Volume One of the *Bioethics Yearbook*, is the acceptance by Islamic scholars of total brain death as a measurement that a person has withdrawn from life even if artificially animated. Certain rulings, based on analogy to an old juridical rule called "the movement of the slain" therefore become applicable to the "brain-dead" patient. Those rulings allow for the removal of artificial life support and the legitimacy of procuring organs for transplantation ([5], pp. 112-113).

IV. NEW REPRODUCTIVE TECHNOLOGIES AND PRACTICES

A. *The Status of Marriage in Islam*

Islam prescribes that the joining of a man and a woman to form a family should be a sacred bond documented and legitimized by the marriage contract. Marriage serves two ends: (1) the physical and spiritual union of two halves into one whole, and (2) the begetting of children whose rights are to be protected – including the right to know their proper lineage, the right to receive nurture and care, and the right to receive their legitimate inheritance.

B. *Theological Aspects of Fertility Control Methods*

In Islam, marriage is the only legitimate context for sexual union and reproduction. The status of birth control within marriage, however, has been the subject of ongoing scholarly debate within the tradition. At the First International Conference on "Bioethics in Human Reproduction Research in the Muslim World", Dr. Mohammed Raafat Osman carefully analyzed the theological aspects of fertility control within marriage [9]. Osman offers a wide-ranging and careful discussion of different scholarly opinions on various methods of birth control, including coitus interruptus, the use of condoms, diaphragms, cervical caps, spermicides, and contraceptive pills. With regard to withdrawal, Osman concludes that the preponderance of Islamic opinion allows coitus interruptus "on the basis of clear-cut Ahadith and that the arguments opposing it cannot be validated" ([9], p. 83). Although withdrawal "to alleviate burdens", including burdens "ensuing from too many children and insufficient means to care for them", may seem to "run counter to trust in God, we cannot state that withdrawal is forbidden by Shari'a" ([9], p. 84).

Osman concludes that the use of condoms, diaphragms, and cervical caps is licit in the tradition, since, "[i]f the preponderant opinion is in favor of withdrawal, [these methods are] allowed by analogy" ([9], p. 87). With regard to the use of spermicides, however, Osman cites evidence from the Regional Arab Federation for Fertility Care that "the chemical components of these medicines [are] detrimental to the health of women when absorbed" into the body ([9], p. 89). Consequently, he concludes that the use of spermicides is not permitted:

From the viewpoint of Shari'a, this contraceptive method cannot be allowed[,] considering that any method detrimental to the health of the individual is prohibited, as explained by the Prophet, peace be upon him, who said: "Inflict no harm on yourself nor on others" ([9], p. 89).

By the same token, since contraceptive pills "may in some cases be harmful to women, causing liver trouble and other problems", Osman concludes that "they cannot be allowed by Shari'a unless it is medically proved that they do not harm women" ([9], p. 90).

Finally. Osman emphasizes that in circumstances when family planning methods are chosen, Islam "dictates that a woman should be treated by a physician", because "a woman's body or part thereof should not be bared before a male physician, except in pressing and urgent cases" ([9], p. 85).

V. FEMALE CIRCUMCISION

In an address to the First International Conference on "Bioethics in Human reproduction Research in the Muslim World", Dr. Hamid Rushwan, an official of the World Health Organization, provided medical details about various types of female circumcision and discussed the origins of and the rationale given for the practice [10].

According to Rushwan, female circumcision is generally performed on young girls, usually seven or eight years old, although some African tribes perform it on infants and other societies on young adult women. In many cases, the procedures is done under "poor hygienic conditions" and without anaesthesia. Female circumcision is differentiated into four types, according to degree of severity. The least drastic first type, analogous to male circumcision, "consists of cutting the clitoral prepuce circumferentially to remove it". The second type "involves removing the glans clitoris or even the entire clitoris", and sometimes part or all of the labia minora. The third type, called infibulation or "pharaonic circumcision", "involves removing not only the clitoris but also labia minora, the raw edges of the wounds are then sewn together leaving only a tiny opening for urination and menstruation". The fourth type, rarely performed, is called introcision, and "involves enlarging the vaginal opening by cutting the perineum" ([10], p. 65), usually to reverse undue tightening.

Although the exact origins of the practice are unknown, both Herodotus, who visited Egypt in the mid-5th century B.C.E., and the Greek geographer Strabo "reported the practice of this custom in ancient Egypt" ([10], p. 67) Herodotus also noted that the ritual was practiced by Phoenicians, Hittites, and Ethiopians as well as Egyptians ([10], p. 67). Today the practice survives in "large areas of Africa among a variety of tribes" and has also been reported in Malaysia and Indonesia ([10], p. 68).

According to Rushwan, there is no "clear reference in the Holy Quran [or] in the confirmed traditions (*Hadith*) of the Prophet Mohammed" ([10], p. 69). Thus the "confusion which may have arisen with regard to religious interpretation is probably due to generalization from male circumcision [which is religiously commanded] to the female" ([10], p. 69).

Rushwan concludes that there is no specific religious basis for female circumcision. Since the practice is performed on young children prior to the age of consent and inflicts "harm which might amount to loss of life", he therefore urges the following: (1) professionals under the health care system should be educated against the practice and [should] act as important advocates for its elimination; (2) strict measures must be taken to stop the practice being performed by those health workers, especially doctors and midwives; and (3) professional organizations must set strong measures to prevent the practice within their respective professions ([10], p. 70). The practice is not performed in the vast majority of Muslim nations, and it certainly antedates Islam.

VI. RESEARCH ON HUMAN SUBJECTS

A. *International Guidelines*

On the occasion of the symposium held under this title at Geneva, Switzerland, February 5-7, 1992, co-sponsored by CIOMS (Council for International Organizations of Medical Sciences) and WHO (World Health Organization), Dr. Hassan Hathout offered the following basic Islamic perspectives regarding research on human subjects.

Because medicine is necessary for life, its establishment is a religious mandate. By juridical rule, whatever is necessary to uphold a necessity becomes itself a necessity; thus, since research is necessary for the progress of medicine it becomes juridically mandatory. This mandate for research also includes research on human subjects, so long as the latter does not conflict with the protection and promotion of basic human rights spelled out by the Sharia. The Islamic Code of Medical Ethics includes the following items:

There is no censorship in Islam on scientific research, be it academic to reveal the tradition of God in His creation, or applied aiming at solving a particular problem.

Freedom of scientific research shall not entail the subjugation of Man, telling him, harming or subjecting him to definite or probable harm, withholding his therapeutic needs, defrauding him or exploiting his material need.

The methodology of scientific research and the application resultant thereof, shall not entail the commission of sin prohibited by Islam such as fornication and adultery, confounding genealogy, deformity or tampering with the essence of human personality, its freedom and eligibility to bear responsibility [6].

Over a decade has passed since that Code was promulgated and the ethics of research on human subjects becomes ever more dynamic and complex. It is, therefore, difficult to formulate international guidelines capable of transcending cultural, economic, and political barriers. The achievements of CIOMS and WHO have been salutary, but sensitive areas remain to be sorted out.

1. The Persistence of Cultural Differences.

Cultural differences persist between nations and regions; thus one should be sensitive to the limits of generalizing from a Western model. Nonetheless, this caution should not be made the pretext for excusing lax international or interregional research safeguards or for accepting a double standard in the research use of human subjects.

In a 1991 paper entitled "Epidemiology and Ethics", K.S. Khan of Pakistan described some researchers in developing countries as agents of the First World who operate in the Third. In Khan's judgment, they appear to identify more with their first world peers than with their own nationals, and seem more concerned with gaining research results than in protecting the interests of their subjects [8]. Khan asserts that so-called "consent" is often documented by procuring signatures or thumb prints without an iota of genuine explanation. Such a sham is a travesty of honesty and of Islamic law, for the latter stipulates that a contract is not valid unless it is fully understood and freely consented.

With regard to medical research funded by the West, the picture grows even more confused. Western slogans about the inherent equality of all human beings are often belied by actual patterns of medical research. According to Khan, drugs and procedures that have been banned in their countries of origin have been exported to the Third World. In light of that problem, Dr. Mahmoud Fathalla, Director of the WHO Special Program of Research Development and Research Training in Human Reproduction, has offered a number of recommendations on international research protocols. Two of his recommendations are especially noteworthy. First,

It is unjustifiable to do clinical trials on therapies that are unlikely to become available to people in the country or community. For example, drugs that are likely to be non-affordable or non-marketable should not be tested in a given population. This applies in particular to industrial and international research ([3], p. 176).

This principle concords with a basic requirement of distributive justice, which dictates that "it is not appropriate that volunteers from only one sector of the society should carry the burden of research. [Rather], volunteers should be drawn equally from among groups who can potentially benefit later on from the outcome of the research" ([3], p. 177).

Second, as a practical corollary to the first principle, Fathalla recommends that local personnel should be utilized as much as possible and that ethically conducted epidemiological or field study "should leave something behind in the community in which it was conducted" ([3], p. 178).

2. Ethical Guidelines for Human Reproduction Research at Al-Azhar University

At the First International Conference on "Bioethics in Human Reproduction Research in the Muslim World", Dr. Abdel Fattah El Sheikh, the Rector of Al-Azhar University, noted that "[e]thical guidelines are governed by cultural and religious values" ([2], p. 307). Thus, guidelines for research on human reproduction must take account of and seek to protect the significance of the family in the Muslim world, even as they serve to enhance medical progress in research on human reproduction.

The specific guidelines for research on human reproduction at Al-Azhar University are as follows:

1. [T]he research should widen the scope of medical knowledge and comply with the needs and priorities of the society in which it is undertaken;
2. Results from the research cannot be obtained from the animals on which experiments are conducted;
3. [T]he researcher should endeavor to arrive at the targeted results making as few experiments as possible on research subjects, and ensure that research subjects shall be exposed to the least possible risk or inconvenience . . .;
4. [T]he researcher should be qualified, knowledgeable of the research topic, and experienced in research methods and scientific analysis. He will use his knowledge and expertise to protect research subjects against any risk;
5. [S]cientific references and experimental studies relevant to the research have been reviewed to identify as far as possible the risk to which research subjects might be exposed;
6. [R]esearch subjects are informed of the research objectives and of the consequences of their participation, in particular of any risk or inconvenience to which they may be exposed;
7. [R]esearch subjects have clearly and explicitly signified their consent. If the consent of a guardian is required, in one form or another, it should be ascertained that the rights of research subjects have not been forfeited.
8. [A]ll precautions have been taken to ensure the confidentiality of information obtained by the researcher and . . . this information shall not be used at any time to the detriment of the research subject ([2], pp. 307-308).

In order to implement these guidelines effectively, El Sheikh recommends that a specially constituted committee should review "the protocol of research both scientifically and ethically" ([2], p. 308). The committee should include among its members "those who represent different specializations and not only scientists of human reproduction". Its membership, therefore, "should include physicians, theologians, lawyers, social scientists, nursing staff, and also a member of the society where the research will be conducted to represent the research subjects' views" ([2], p. 308).

3. *Ethics in Research on Pregnant Mothers*

Dr. Mohammed M. Fayad, Professor of Obstetrics and Gynecology at Cairo University School of Medicine reported on the ethics of research on pregnant mothers at the First International Conference on "Bioethics in Human Reproduction Research in the Muslim World" [4]. The rate of maternal and perinatal mortality is very high in developing countries, with more than a half million each year dying from complications of pregnancy and childbirth. In order to gain new knowledge about the mechanism of diseases associated with pregnancy and to assess and apply "new tools of modern technology for the well-being of mother and child", Fayad urges that research on pregnant mothers be continued because animal models, while important as preliminary research, often cannot be straightforwardly applied to humans without specific research on human subjects ([4], p. 57).

Fayad expresses caution in evaluating the ethics of such research, because pregnancy is a "special case which entails two individuals at the same time, the mother and the fetus" ([4], p. 57). Because Islam respects and protects human life as sacred, even in its intrauterine phase, both pregnant women and their fetuses must be safeguarded; thus research on pregnant women is permissible only if it "does not entail any risk for mother or child" ([4], p. 62). Fayad therefore sets forth the following guidelines for research on pregnant women:

1. The deliberate exposure of a fetus to the uncertain consequences of an experimental intervention unrelated to the pregnancy is unacceptable.
2. Any woman who is or is likely to become pregnant would be excluded from clinical study especially in drug trials.
3. A pregnant woman should, in no circumstances, be the subject of non-therapeutic research that carries any possibility of risk to fetus or neonate.
4. Therapeutic research on pregnant women is permissible only with a view to improve the health of mother without prejudice to [the] fetus.
5. Research on pregnant mothers is permissible if it aims to enhance the viability of [the] fetus or aid its healthy development. ([4], p. 59).

Finally, Fayad reaffirms the importance of the provisions of the Second Helsinki Declaration of Ethics that call for a multi-disciplinary advisory committee to assess both the "scientific and ethical aspects" of all such proposed research. ([4], p. 60).

VII. ETHICS IN RESEARCH INVOLVING ANIMAL SUBJECTS

In an address to the First International Conference on "Bioethics in Human Reproduction Research in the Muslim World", Dr. Mohamed T. El-Khayyal noted that, at about the same time codes of ethics were introduced to regulate human experimentation, there also arose "widespread national movements to impose legislation for the prevention of cruelty to animals" ([2], p. 184). According to El-Khayyal, although there is general acknowledgement "that animals are indispensable for the advancement of science", there is also increasing criticism raised "against their indiscriminate use or against subjecting them to undue pain and stress" ([2], p. 184). He suggests, as a context for further reflections, that we address this question with a spirit of respect for the status of animals in the order of God's creation:

> Everyone dealing with animal testing should be well aware of the fact that animals are not just neutral objects created by God simply as a means of publishing new research work for the sake of promotion, but rather that animals think [sic] and feel, they see and hear, they eat and drink, and therefore, they bear in many ways resemblance to man ... We, the more powerful and better privileged, owe them at least this moral obligation: if we have to make use of them to subserve our own needs, let us then do so with kindness and understanding, without exposing them to any undue stress or pain ([2], p. 189).

El-Khayyal recommends that alternative methods to animal testing should be encouraged with a view to limiting the number of animals used in research and to limiting their suffering ([2], p. 185). Such methods include the use of various mediums (isolated organs, tissue sections and cultures, isolated cells and tissue cultures, incubated hen's eggs, microorganisms, etc.) as well as biochemical analysis and computer simulation. Nonetheless, El-Khayyal cautions against concluding that animal testing can be replaced by such alternatives, because of several inherent limitations, especially that "an intact organism is mandatory to understand properly the overall picture of [a given] drug's action" and that "disease conditions [often] cannot be reproduced in vitro" ([2], pp. 187-188).

As a practical recommendation, El-Khayyal reaffirms the importance of institutional review boards to ensure implementation of the Helsinki Guidelines. In addition, he recommends that a "national committee (or perhaps a subcommittee from the Egyptian Society of Pharmacology and Experimental Therapeutics) should be formed" to evaluate and supervise the use of animals in research ([2], p. 188).

VIII. GENETIC ENGINEERING

The attitude that Islam has taken toward science has always been a positive one. Not only has there never been confrontation between them, but the pursuit of knowledge is a religious duty for every Muslim. In Islamic juridical terminology, the equivalent of the term "scientific research" is called "the revealing of God's tradition in His Creation" and is part of man's duty as God's trustee of the earth. Because Islam has no institutional clergy, there has been no censorship of research during the era of Islamic civilization. Muslim and non-Muslim scientists have experienced no impediments to their scientific efforts, which helped Europe to emerge from the Dark Ages into the Renaissance.

With regard, then, to genetic engineering, Islam would place no obstacles upon genetic research. However, five Islamic governing rules are relevant to assessing the applications of genetic research. The first rule elaborates the five goals of Islamic jurisprudence, which are specified as the preservation and protection of self (i.e., life), of mind, of faith, of ownership, and of offspring. The second rule reminds Muslims of God's gift to humanity as expressed in the passage from the Quran, "[A]nd He has made subservient to you as from Himself all that is in the heavens, and on earth" (45:13). That passage has been interpreted by exegetes as giving man the mandate to make conscious use of the nature that surrounds him and, it would seem, the nature within him. These two rules, taken together, grant the human race a free hand to harness and manipulate nature in ways that ensure the fulfillment of the five specified goals of Islamic jurisprudence.

However, this does not mean that there are no constraints upon research or its applications. A third rule, in the form of one verse from the Quran about "changing God's creation", is germane to a discussion of appropriate limits to be placed on genetic engineering. The Quranic version of the story of Adam and Eve reports that Satan tempted both to eat from the forbidden tree, that they both sinned by disobeying God, that they both repented, and that they both were forgiven. They were then entrusted with the noble mission of populating the earth, and the human race was charged to act as God's vice-regent. When Satan saw events turn in man's favor, he asked God for a second chance to put Adam's progeny to the test. God granted Satan's request but said He would provide them with the guidance needed to immunize them against Satan's temptations, except for those who willfully reject God's guidance in favor of Satan's wiles. In an expression of his plans to lead mankind astray, the Quran quotes the rebellious Satan addressing God about the human race: "Verily of thy servants I shall most certainly take my due share, and shall lead them astray, and fill them with vain desires. And I shall command them so that they cut off the ears of cattle [in idolatrous sacrifice], and I shall command them and they will *change God's creation*" (authors' emphasis). The passage then continues: "But all who take Satan rather than God for their master do indeed, most clearly, lose all. He [Satan] holds out promises to them and fills them with vain desires, yet whatever Satan promises them is but meant to delude the mind". (4:119). The expression "changing God's creation" in answer to Satan's lures has commanded attention and generated debate over the centuries. Genetic engineering might appear to be an obvious example of succumbing to Satan's temptation to "change God's creation". However, it is the consensus of Islamic scholars that this verse from the Quran should not be construed a ban on genetic engineering, for if applied broadly, it might also ban many forms of therapeutic surgery (including appendectomy, tonsillectomy, cholecystectomy and others) that are life-saving and life-promoting even though they entail a change in God's creation.

Since neither the Quran nor the Sunna make mention of genetic engineering, the juridical rule is based on legitimate reasoning, i.e, reasoning that does not conflict with the spirit of Islam or the five goals of Islamic jurisprudence. The text of this fourth guiding rule is the following: "Wherever the welfare exists, there stands the statute of God". The feasible conclusion, therefore, is that there are no restrictions on genetic research, but that the biotechnological applications of such research should be individually allowed through juridical sanctions that ensure their use for the benefit of humanity.

Finally, the fifth rule is the juridical dictum, "Harm and harming are not of Islam". Applications fostering human life, health, and welfare are not only permissible but are acts of commendable charity that will be rewarded by God. Dangerous applications, exemplified by concerns in the 1970's about the military exploitation of biological warfare, are obviously objectionable. So are exotic applications, doing things solely because they can be done or merely to satisfy curiosity, or applications motivated by desires and inclinations that are prohibited by Islam. In all cases, rigorous precautions should be taken to guard against unforeseen or untoward complications.

It is not possible here to discuss the applications of genetic engineering in detail, but a few of them should be mentioned here. One application which is to be commended is gene therapy done to correct genetic errors. This therapy is the equivalent of organ transplantation at the molecular level, although its application to the germ line will clearly require additional evaluation. More problematic will be the application of similar eugenic techniques to genes to alter behavioral or personality traits. To date, however, there has been little specific discussion in Islam of the potential and the perils of eugenic applications.

The ethics of genetic engineering, however, involves more than issues of research goals and appropriate applications, for competition among centers and laboratories has increased secrecy and suspicion. In such a climate, issues of competition evoke secrecy and the market directs research. The issue of accessibility and equity in the distribution of benefits are serious concerns of justice. Thus the contemporary marriage between science and industry promises blessings even as it prompts caution. Genius has the right to be amply rewarded, but also a duty to be graciously discharged, with a delicate balance between that right and that duty. It is no accident that "balance" is mentioned thirteen times in the Quran. As scientists decipher creation, they should be mindful of the Creator; as the Quran says, "Amongst His worshippers, the learned heed Him most".

In view of all this, it is perhaps time for an Ethical Code on Genetics to be prospectively written, before we are overtaken by the rapidly accelerating pace of the genetics revolution. All parties concerned should contribute to the formulation of the Code, which, even if it is not legally binding, should be carefully crafted to provide clear moral guidance.

Islamic Center of Southern California
Los Angeles, California, U.S.A.

Center for Ethics, Medicine, and Public Issues
Houston, Texas, U.S.A.

BIBLIOGRAPHY

1. El-Khayyal, M., 1992: "Ethics in Research [on] Animal Subjects", in [11], pp. 183-189.
2. El-Sheikh, A.F., 1992: "Establishment of Ethical Committee on Scientific Research [at Al-Azhar University", in [11], pp. 306-308.
3. Fathalla, M., 1992: "Ethics in Medical Research", in [11], pp. 173-182.
4. Fayad, M., 1992: "Ethics in Research on Pregnant Mothers", in [11], pp. 56-63.
5. Hathout, H., 1991: "Islamic Concepts and Bioethics", in B.A. Lustig (sr. ed.), *Theological Developments in Bioethics 1988-1990*, Kluwer Academic Publishers, Dordrecht, pp. 103, 117.
6. International Organization of Islamic Medicine (later: International Organization of Medical Sciences – IOMS), 1980: "Islamic Code of Medical Ethics", IOMS Publishers, Kuwait, pp 79-80.
7. Islamic Center of Southern California, 1991: "Position Paper on Euthanasia" (manuscript).
8. Khan K.S., 1991: "Epidemiology and Ethics: The Perspective of the Third World", in Bankowski, Z., Bryant, J.H., and Last J.M. (eds.)., *Ethics and Epidemiology: International Guidelines*, Geneva, CIOMS, pp. 70-75
9. Osman, M.R., 1992: "Theological Aspects of Fertility Control Methods", in [11], pp. 78-92.
10. Rushwan, H., 1992: "Female Circumcision, An Ethical Concern", in [11], pp. 64-70.
11. Serour, G.I. (ed.), 1992: *Proceedings of the First International Conference on "Bioethics in Human Reproduction Research in the Muslim World"*, International Islamic Center for Population Studies and Research, Al-Azhar University, Cairo, Egypt.

PAUL NELSON

LUTHERAN PERSPECTIVES ON BIOETHICS

I. INTRODUCTION

A. *Lutheran Moral Theology*

The reform movement (eventually denominated "Lutheran") within "the one holy catholic and apostolic church" was, among other things, an attempt to reconceive the Christian moral life. Indeed ethics was very near the heart of the Lutheran reformers' dispute with Rome. It could hardly have been otherwise since, semi-Pelagian theology and a merit-centered piety had become, by the dawn of the 16th century, thoroughly entrenched in the pervasive corruption of the institutional church. To protest the abuses and to begin to set things right necessarily involved rethinking fundamental religious and moral issues.

Summoned to explain themselves before an imperial diet in 1530, the Lutheran reformers offered what has become known as the *Augsburg Confession*, a text universally regarded among Lutherans as a valid and authoritative interpretation of the faith of the Church Catholic. "It is taught among us" they wrote "that we cannot obtain forgiveness of sin and righteousness before God by our own merits, works, or satisfactions, but that we receive forgiveness of sin and become righteous before God by grace, for Christ's sake, through faith". Aware that their understanding of "justification" was considered in some quarters to be antinomian, they hastened to explain its implications for "sanctification" or "the new obedience". "It is also taught among us that such faith should produce good fruits and good works and that we must do all such good works as God commanded, but we should do them for God's sake and not place our trust in them as if thereby to merit favor before God" ([46], pp. 30-31).

Along with this change in the motivation for the moral life came a radical secularization of the content of good works. For example, Martin Luther – himself an Augustinian monk – denounced with characteristic vigor the folly of imagining the mortifications of monastic asceticism or the practice of pilgrimages to be divinely ordained good works. "God has commanded that a man should care for his wife and children, perform the duties of a husband, and serve and help his neighbor". Squandering a considerable sum on a

B. Andrew Lustig (Sr. Ed.), Bioethics Yearbook: Volume 3, 149-184.
©1993 Kluwer Academic Publishers.

pilgrimage to Rome while permitting family and neighbors "to suffer want back home" was "disobedience and contempt of the divine commandment" ([23], p. 59). The needs of ones' neighbors, understood comprehensively and in very down-to-earth terms, determined the content of moral obligation.

[The Christian] "should be guided in all his works by this thought and contemplate this one thing alone, that he may serve and benefit others in all that he does, considering nothing except the need and advantage of his neighbor . . . This is a truly Christian life. Here faith is truly active through love [Gal. 5:6], that is, it finds expression in works of the freest service, cheerfully and lovingly done, with which a man willingly serves another without hope of reward; and for himself he is satisfied with the fullness and wealth of his faith"([23], p. 302).

Thus the material and psycho-social dimensions of human welfare became the focus of moral attention. Moral duties emerged from family, social, vocational, and political relationships, "stations" in life that could become schools for virtue.

A consequence of the secularization of morality within the Lutheran confessional perspective is the tradition's reliance on reason. According to a standard account, Lutheran Christians "do not discover what is to be done by special revelation, or by deduction from Scripture, or by 'praying about it' and obeying the next impulse from within. [They] discover what is to be done by rational consideration of the situation and of the neighbor's possibilities in it" ([12], p. 149). This opens the way to moral discourse with other traditions and is conducive to common agreement. As Luther once said, "Better to be ruled by a wise Turk than a foolish Christian"!

In Scandinavia today, many Lutheran ethicists write from a humanistic perspective that is not distinctly or uniquely Christian. Only in Norway does one frequently encounter arguments specifically grounded in the Bible or Christian tradition. Elsewhere predominant approaches to ethics are Kantian or influenced by Jurgen Habermas' "discourse ethics". Many ethicists continue in the tradition of the Danish theologian Knud Løgstrup who denied the possibility of a specifically Christian ethic, preferring instead to base ethics on the ontological structure of human relationships (see *Bioethics Yearbook* Vol. I, pp. 120-122). Teleology within certain deontological limits is widespread among Scandinavian theological ethicists. Recently there has emerged, particularly in Denmark, interest in combining Christian and humanistic perspectives. Sometimes this blending is cast in terms of a "narrative ethic" which seeks to enrich secular ethics by recovering its deep roots in Jewish and Christian traditions ([29], pp. 320-321). This development bears a family resemblance to "post-liberal" theological ethics in the United States.

According to the Danish theological ethicist Viggo Mortensen, the church has four resources to contribute to the plenary discussion of bioethics. The Christian conceptions of human nature and the world offer an alternative to materialistic views and provide a firm grounding for claims about human dignity. Second, biblical perspectives on human action may offer guidance for handling certain problems. The love commandment and the ethical arguments of the theological tradition are a third resource. Finally, depicted in the biblical narrative of Jesus is an exemplary life of compassion freely given in service to others ([29], p. 322).

These Christian resources complement humanistic perspectives. A 1989 Norwegian Church Council report, "More Than Genes", found universal acknowledgment of human dignity and integrity in such documents as the 1931 Guidelines of the German Interior Ministry, the Helsinki Declarations of 1964/75/83, and the 1982 American "Guidelines for Biomedical Research Involving Human Subjects" ([29], p. 319). Thus, there is a clear basis for agreement and common endeavor in bioethics and human rights more generally.

Although one may speak of "the secularization of morality" within the Lutheran tradition as a whole and particularly among the Scandinavian humanistic ethicists, one should not overlook the fact that there are theological reasons internal to the tradition that orient Lutherans along these lines. It is a stance grounded in a "doctrine of creation" elaborated from the first article of the Nicene Creed: "I believe in God, the Father Almighty, maker of heaven and earth". The natural sense of justice shared by Christian and Turk alike reflects the fact that God is the creator and sustainer of all. "When Gentiles who do not possess the law carry out its precepts by the light of nature", according to St. Paul, "they display the effect of the law inscribed on their hearts" (Romans 2:14). Thus, there are biblical and other theological warrants for the identification of a generically human ethic with Christian love of neighbor.

Yet, the Lutheran tradition has seldom failed to appreciate the degree to which the goodness of God's creation is deformed by human sin. As an Evangelical Lutheran Church in America Social Statement observes: "Sin is both a condition of alienation from God and the acts that issue from this condition. Human judgments, actions, organizations, and practices are marked by a distortion of God's will and purposes for life" ([43], p. 3). The universal and all-pervasive character of this distortion has sometimes been employed as a rationalization for moral laxity, sloth, or even nihilism. At its best, however, it has served to cultivate a salutary awareness of moral ambiguity and to hedge against legalism.

The sober recognition that we are less than perfect people living in a far from perfect world, along with the conviction that we are, nevertheless, forgiven sinners are the two benchmarks of a Lutheran moral vision. The former precludes self-righteousness and underlies the sense that often we can do little else but choose between greater and lesser evils. The latter makes choice and action possible despite the attendant ambiguities. According to the Social Statement quoted above, "We are empowered so that we might do what is effective in serving the needs of the neighbor" ([43], p. 3). Not bound by any rigid legalism, Christians are free to be resourceful and pragmatic in the service of their neighbors, especially those who are most vulnerable.

A colorful illustration of this Lutheran emphasis on Christian freedom is Luther's dubious advice to confessors presented with difficult cases of conscience. Suppose, for example, a woman had unknowingly married a man suffering chronic impotence and later was "desirous of having children or [was] unable to remain continent". In the absence of today's reproductive technologies, it might seem that she had only two choices, both of them unhappy; suffer or jeopardize her eternal destiny. Were the man unwilling to submit to a divorce, Luther suggested that the woman might have intercourse with his brother or some other willing surrogate. Any child so conceived should be ascribed to the husband and supported as his heir. If the husband refused to consent to these arrangements, Luther "would counsel her to contract a marriage with another and flee to a distant unknown place". In Luther's mind, it was a situation of necessity requiring a "judgment of charity". Desiring "to bring to [his] afflicted brethren in this captivity what little comfort [he] can", Luther asked, "What other counsel could be given" ([23], pp. 233-235)?

In such circumstances, moral rules may have to yield to a natural sense of justice. Prudent moral agents understand this and will act accordingly in their professional or public roles no less than in their personal lives. For example, Luther observed, "No state is governed successfully by means of laws. If the ruler is wise, he will govern better by a natural sense of justice than by laws. If he is not wise, he will foster nothing through legislation, since he will not know what use to make of the laws nor how to adapt them to the case at hand". Good and wise rulers "will themselves be the very best of laws, and will judge every variety of case with a lively sense of equity" ([23], p. 226). What Luther demanded of 16th century princes is now required of all men and women in contemporary Lutheran social teaching. A recent Evangelical Lutheran Church in America document acknowledged that Christians must face complex bioethical decisions "in all their ambiguity, knowing they are responsible ultimately to God, whose grace comforts, forgives, and frees [them] in [their] dilemma" ([28], p. 1). (Further discussion of Lutheran theological ethics may be found in *Bioethics Yearbook Vol. I*, pp. 119-122).

B. *The Lutheran Churches*

Lutheran churches are "evangelical" and "confessional"; evangelical in the sense that they are grounded in and normed by God's reconciling love, and confessional in that they accept certain statements of belief as being authoritative. All Lutheran churches "confess" the three great ecumenical creeds (the Apostles', Nicene, and Athanasian), the *Augsburg Confession*, and Luther's *Small Catechism*. The Evangelical Lutheran Churches of Denmark, Norway, and Iceland accept only these but the Evangelical Lutheran Churches of Sweden, Finland, Germany, and the United States embrace as well all the other confessional documents collected in *The Book of Concord*. However, in other respects the latter churches are by no means alike. For example, the churches of Sweden and Finland retain the tradition of Apostolic Succession while the others do not. The Lutheran Church – Missouri Synod in the United States subscribes to the quite unLutheran notion of biblical literalism and allows considerable congregational autonomy, while the Lutheran churches of Scandinavia are highly secularized, centralized, tax supported, national churches to which more than 90% of their populations nominally belong. In Finland and Sweden, the church has a constitutional right to make recommendations to the government regarding matters to be discussed below, yet in Denmark, by law, no one may speak in the name of the church. A few Lutheran church bodies in the United States and elsewhere are fiercely protective of their Lutheran confessional identity, while after the Second World War, the German regional Lutheran churches joined with Reformed and United churches to form the federated Protestant Church in Germany.

Lutheran churches address bioethics in a variety of ways. Study materials prepared by staff or church members with relevant expertise writing as individuals or as committees are distributed to foster reflection and discussion throughout the churches. These may also be produced by inter-church organizations such as the Lutheran Council in the United States of America or the Lutheran World Federation. More authoritative are documents such as Social Statements whose teachings constitute official policy of the church. Staff members and others who may speak in the church's name are expected adhere to the positions taken. Occasionally, Lutheran churches address judicial, legislative, or other governmental bodies expressing their views on issues in law and public policy. In the case of the Evangelical Lutheran Church in America, these representations must have a clear basis in official Social Statements. No less important, but often overlooked, are the ways in which the church regularly attends to bioethics in its preaching, pastoral care and counseling, and administration of hospitals, nursing homes and other social service agencies.

In Sweden and elsewhere in Scandinavia, there is a tradition of appointing commissions to advise Parliament and the government on complex controversial matters of public policy. "Underlying this tradition is a strong belief in rational approaches to problems, in planning, and piecemeal social engineering [as well as] . . . a willingness to compromise" ([13], p. 17). Typically, a commission dealing with bioethical issues would include one or two theologians and possibly others able to represent Christian perspectives in the commission's deliberations. Their eventual report is circulated among government agencies and non-governmental organizations including the churches. The Church of Sweden's Research Department organizes a task force to study the issues and make a recommendation to the General Synod, the church's highest decision-making body, which determines the church's official response to the commission proposal. While the Parliament is free to ignore the church's advice, its views are usually given serious consideration.

Finally, it should be recognized that, as might be expected in the tradition of Luther and the Reformation principles of *sola fide* (faith alone) and *sola scriptura* (scripture alone), the churches do not understand themselves to have a magisterium or formal teaching office *per se* whose judgments should bind the consciences of individual Lutheran Christians. A large majority of Lutherans would ignore them in any case. For example, according to the recent European Values Study, "fewer than half of all . . . Germans and Scandinavians expressed confidence in their church", and only 11% of Danish and Swedish respondents "felt the church provided adequate answers to the problems of family life" ([38], p. 962). A more positive warrant for ecclesiastical modesty concerning the status of its pronouncements can be found in Luther's paradoxical dicta (following St. Paul): "A Christian is a perfectly free lord of all, subject to none. A Christian is a perfectly dutiful servant of all, subject to all" ([23], p. 277). At its best, Lutheran social teaching in bioethics aspires to exemplify Christian freedom in the service of human welfare.

C. *Lutheran Perspectives on Bioethics*

The first volume in the *Bioethics Yearbook* series focused exclusively on North American Lutheran perspectives. The present report will expand its coverage to include European Lutheran views. It will also discuss new developments in the United States, such as the Evangelical Lutheran Church in America's *amicus curiae* brief in the celebrated Cruzan Supreme Court case, its recent Social Statement on Abortion, and its new Message on Social Issues concerning "End of Life Decisions". While Lutheran churches in the United States began to address bioethical issues (in the early 1960's) ten or fifteen years before their counterparts on the Continent, since the late 1970's the Europeans have engaged them as well.

Language, distance, and the occasional nature of much of the material tend to inhibit American cognizance of European social teachings. Fortunately, two recent German publications have significantly diminished the difficulty. Hartwig von Schubert's *Evangelische Ethik und Biotechnologie* ([36]) surveys debates on a number of bioethics issues in Austria, Switzerland, and Germany. The comprehensiveness of the presentation is evidenced by his compilation of a 54-page bibliography of primarily German sources. A second volume edited by Jurgen Hübner and von Schubert, *Biotechnologie und evangelische Ethik: die internationale Diskussion* ([14]), includes chapters on theological discussions of bioethics in France, Switzerland, the United Kingdom, Canada, the United States, The Netherlands, and the Scandinavian countries. Since it is not possible to duplicate here the voluminous references to primary sources found in these books, I wish to call them to the attention of *Bioethics Yearbook* readers. Also, I am happily obligated to acknowledge my "absolute dependence" on Kees van Kooten Niekerk's invaluable survey of the Scandinavian literature in the second volume ([29] in [14]). It may be assumed that my characterizations of theological bioethics in that part of the world are borrowed from him unless otherwise indicated.

Swedish church involvement in bioethics began in 1975 when the Swedish Ecumenical Council distributed a translation of a text published by The Hastings Center in the United States. This was the first in an ongoing series of Council publications. In 1978, 1981, and 1983 the Nordic Council of Churches organized conferences in Finland, Sweden, and Norway on ethical aspects of genetic engineering. A prominent voice in Swedish bioethics is Holsten Fagerberg, a Lutheran theologian at the University of Uppsala, who served as a consultant and member of government bioethics commissions. He has published widely and edited two books in 1980 and 1984: *Foster, familj, samhalle, Fosterdiagnostikens innesord och etik* (Fetus, Family, Society: The Meaning and Ethics of Prenatal Diagnostics) and *Medicinsk etik och manniskosyn* (Medical Ethics and the View of Man) The former represents the work of a committee of physicians and theologians convened by the Conference of Bishops and the latter is a mainstay of medical and nursing school reading lists ([21], p. 31).

In Norway the first bioethics publication was issued by a Christian physicians' organization in 1980. Two years later, the Norwegian Bishops' Conference offered a report, "Ethical Viewpoints on Genetic Counseling and Prenatal Diagnosis". The Norwegian biblical scholar and theologian Jacob Jervell has served as a member of the ethics committee of the Council for Medical Research and participated in many official discussions on bioethics and public policy.

The Danish scene is quite different in that by law no one may speak on behalf of the church as an institution or corporate entity. It is, as the Danes readily insist, a "people's church" and officials, clergy or theologians may speak only as individuals. Danish theologians and philosophers interested in bioethics founded in 1980 the Forum for Theology and Natural Science and have served on government ethics councils considering matters such as the legal regulation of work in human genetics and artificial reproduction.

Bioethics came to Germany relatively late. In 1986 the first bioethics centers opened in Bocchum, Tübingen, and Hanover. The same year, the Akademie fur Ethik in der Medizin was organized and launched the journal *Ethik in der Medizin*. However, in several quarters bioethics has not been well received. Many Germans have deep apprehensions about this new discipline. For many, the very term "bioethics" has unwelcome connotations of instrumental rationality, utilitarian calculation, and biotechnological capitalism. At a deeper level, talk of genetic screening and manipulation or quality of life and euthanasia revives horrific memories of Nazi atrocities. This accounts in some measure for the passion of the "antibioethics movement" which in 1989 furiously protested the visit to Germany of the prominent utilitarian bioethicist Peter Singer. Some of his invitations were withdrawn, an entire conference was canceled, and where he was allowed to speak, his lectures were coercively disrupted. According to one account of what has become known as "the Singer affair", hostility toward the discipline is widespread within German universities. "Now an interest in Anglo-American bioethics might jeopardize an academic career" ([34], p. 22).

The same authors report that the German medical, scientific, and political establishments are content with traditional conceptions of the ethics of science or the medical profession. Moreover, they accept "the smoothly functioning representative role of the churches and their theologians" and are loathe "to disturb this with a possible pluralism in moral theories" which would result from the admission of bioethics ([34], p. 24). However traumatic secular bioethics has been, for at least two decades the German churches have actively fostered discussion of bioethical issues. The Evangelical Church in Germany and the Conference of Catholic Bishops have published material individually and on one occasion jointly. The regional Protestant churches, religious communities, and local parishes have sponsored educational events, and bioethical topics are sometimes addressed in the religious instruction that takes place in the public schools. In addition, religious institutions like the Protestant and Catholic Academies and the Institute for Interdisciplinary Research of the Evangelische Studiengemeinschaft in Heidelberg have sponsored conferences and working groups ([35], sec. 2.5.4.1).

Both in Scandinavia and in Germany, the Lutheran churches have made very significant contributions to bioethical reflection. Some of their concerns and positions will be described below. The degree to which they have often worked cooperatively with each other, with free churches, and sometimes with the Roman Catholic Church is remarkable, particularly in comparison with the paucity of such efforts in the United States. Perhaps it is the secularity of their societies that induces them to work together. In such contexts, their differences may pale in relation to their common convictions and their witness to a largely indifferent society.

For instance, in 1989 the German [Catholic] Bishops' Conference and the Council of the Protestant Church in Germany adopted a joint declaration on the protection of life. The working party that produced the document understood that "differences between the Catholic and Protestant sides on the question of an effective protection of prenatal life could not be overlooked" ([11], p. 3). But neither were those differences to be overemphasized so as to obscure "a very high degree of unanimity" on other issues and even on many aspects of abortion. Moreover, the text was embraced by all of the member and guest churches of the Council of Christian Churches. These include the Greek Orthodox Metropoly, Baptist Union, United Methodist Church, Old Catholic Church, Mennonites, Moravian Church, Syrian-Orthodox Church, Old Reformed Church of Lower Saxony, Free Evangelical Church, Quakers, Independent Lutheran Church, Christlicher Gemeinschaftsverband Mulheim/Ruhr Gmb H, and the Salvation Army. "In view of the degree and timing of their co-operation, these churches' acceptance of the declaration should be understood as signifying general agreement and not as applying to every single statement in the text" ([11], p. 3). Even with this qualification, the document represents an impressive display of ecumenicity.

II. NEW REPRODUCTIVE TECHNOLOGIES

German reflection on the new reproductive technologies can not ignore the sobering historical experience of Nazi eugenics and *Rassenhygiene*. Lutheran and other Protestant ethicists are wary of the possibility that the burgeoning applications of biotechnology may foster "a biologistic view of life" that erodes proper respect for human dignity. Knowledge of the human genome and the ability to initiate life in vitro may offer a powerful if not irresistible temptation to confuse the creature with the creator. Varying degrees of confidence or skepticism about society's ability to enjoy the benefits of biotechnology without succumbing to its risks are found among Protestant ethicists ([37], p. 9; [18]; [26]). Of course, some of the new practices seem more dangerous than others.

Homologous artificial insemination (AIH) is unobjectionable, but heterologous artificial insemination (AID) and surrogate motherhood are generally rejected. Critics often fear that such practices may generate destructive tensions in the couple's relationship and that they instrumentalize the donor, surrogate, and child. Moreover the child may be deprived of knowledge of his or her genetic origin, something that is rightfully his or hers. Those who do accept AID reject donor anonymity and insist that medically assisted procreation not be commercialized ([37], p. 22).

The permissibility of *in vitro* fertilization (IVF) is more controversial in Protestant circles. That it is artificial or unnatural is not the issue as it would be on a physicalist interpretation of natural law. Human will and artifice may legitimately exercise control over natural processes, as Protestant acceptance of contraception demonstrates. What is troubling about IVF in the eyes of some Protestants is the "danger that it promotes an ideology of unlimited possibility" ([37], p. 21). This does not necessarily mean that these parties are absolutely opposed to IVF. Compassion for the childless often precludes a total rejection of the practice, notwithstanding reservations about overemphasizing the importance of procreation for a couple, particularly for the woman. Furthermore, according to Hartwig von Schubert, "the physical unity of parents and children" is highly esteemed among Lutherans ([37], p. 20). Since IVF makes this possible and does not seem to pose any risk for the prospective child, it can not be said to violate some fundamental parental duty. Should the admittedly real ideological danger noted above be placed as an insurmountable obstacle in the path of childless couples? Many Lutherans would think not.

Another issue posed by IVF concerns the treatment of embryos. In 1987 both the Roman Catholic and Protestant churches issued statements counseling against the use of IVF ("Donum Vitae" and "zur Achtung vor dem Leben"). Their joint declaration of 1989, "God Loves All That Lives: Challenges and Tasks for the Protection of Life", states that the dignity of prenatal life is equally valid *in vitro* as *in vivo* ([11], p. 41). Therefore, one should not create embryos that will not be implanted, use them as a means to others' ends as in non-therapeutic research, or place them at risk of damage or destruction by experimentation or freezing.

Even the smallest movement in the direction of allowing research which makes use of embryos as "expendable" crosses an essential boundary. It is a question here of the protection of supreme values, in the last resort of the reverence for human dignity and every person's right to life, which are anchored in articles 1 and 2 of the constitution ([11], p. 41).

The churches called for legal protection of embryos by various means including the penal code.

Nevertheless, the Embryo Protection Act of 1991 defined human life as beginning only at the *end* of the fertilization process (twenty-four hours). The effect of this stipulation is to allow time for pre-implantation diagnosis and to eliminate the "spare embryo" problem, since zygotes not to be used may be discarded during the first twenty-four hours. To date, the churches have not addressed this discrepancy with their earlier counsel ([37], p. 26).

The "ideology of unlimited possibility" is not confined to procreative matters. Human genetics is a fertile field for excessive ambition. Protestant ethicists point to the dangers of positive eugenics. "Social medicine" or strategic approaches to the population as a whole (rather than the relief of individual patients' pain and suffering) is seen as an "essentially authoritarian . . . biologistic ideology" ([37], p. 13). Attempts to restrict genetic diversity or "improve" physical states are as misguided as they are dangerous.

Some forms of genetic manipulation, however, are perfectly acceptable. "Somatic genetic therapy is regarded to be one of the various means of substitutive medicine and should be pursued in accordance with the usual standards of riskful medical experimentation" ([37], p. 18). But manipulation of human germ cells is another matter. Protestant ethicists are aware of the great benefits that individuals and their potential offspring might derive from the alteration of germ cells, but it is not endorsed because, "the development of such therapy would imply extensive and destructive experiments with human embryos" ([37], p. 16).

There is Protestant support for genetic screening so long as informed consent is guaranteed and safeguards against discrimination are in place. Reservations about genetic screening and prenatal diagnosis pertain to the possible assumption that abortion would routinely follow the discovery of defects. Many see abortion on fetal indication as an "irresolvable conflict'; "either we kill the fetus or we accept the enormously painful future for all persons concerned" ([37], p. 17). If justice is to be done to the seriousness of the moral claims on all sides in such tragic situations, recourse to abortion can not be automatic or specified in advance according to some catalogue of indications ([37], p. 18).

Scandinavian theologians and churches have given new reproductive technologies an extraordinary amount of attention. The starting point for these discussions is the fact that the desire to have children is a great good and involuntary childlessness is often experienced as a painful loss. At the same time, they recognize that childlessness is not a disease. The wish for a child, intense as it may be, ought not be confused with having a right to a child ([29], p. 348). Some authors are troubled by the subsumption of procreation by Western technological culture, and there are feminists who regard the technologization of procreation (particularly IVF) as a form of male conquest that undermines the value of traditional female nurture. Others fear that infertile couples will feel themselves under acute psychological pressure to employ these methods and thereby be deprived of the opportunity to accept and adapt to their situation ([29], p. 358).

These concerns must be taken into account in any adequate moral assessment, though they are not in themselves decisive. Ultimately, the legitimacy of medically assisted procreation depends on whether or not the welfare of the desired child is kept centrally in view ([29], p. 348). Some procedures will meet this test; others may not. Even when procedures are judged to be morally legitimate, theological opinion does not support public financing of medically assisted reproduction. There is widespread feeling that public funds are better allocated to caring for existing children in need and to preventing infertility in the first place ([29], p. 358).

While there are no serious objections to AIH, AID has many critics. In 1983 a Swedish state commission recommended that AID be restricted to married women or to women living in a stable heterosexual relationship of a marital character. The commission expressed the opinion that having both a mother and father in the home was vital to childhood development ([19], p. 78). Thus the limitation was consistent with the best interest of the child-to-be. They also suggested that insemination be conducted in a public hospital and only with the consent of the husband or partner. The sperm donor must be identifiable in a registry for seventy years so that the child may eventually have access to this information. These recommendations were enacted into law in 1985, the first such legislation in Western Europe ([6], p. 346). A few theologians find AID problematic because of the intrusion of a third party into the marital relationship. Most, however, find it unobjectionable in principle and acceptable within the legal restrictions.

The same commission issued a second set of recommendations concerning IVF. As with AID, it should be available only to women cohabiting with a male partner whose consent is required, and the procedure should be performed in a general hospital. In addition, the egg may be implanted only in the woman from whom it was recovered. It must be fertilized with the semen of the husband or cohabitant. The commission believed that allowing egg or sperm donation in conjunction with IVF would undermine a humanistic view of human nature. As before, the commission recommendations eventually became law ([20], p. 315; [6], p, 346).

In their 1989 report, "More Than Genes", a Norwegian Church Council working group acknowledged that they had not been able to reach a consensus on IVF. Among the concerns expressed were:

(1)   that IVF was developed by illegitimate research;
(2)   that it might be premature to accept or reject IVF as a remedy for childlessness;
(3)   that the work required to establish its acceptability would itself be unacceptable; and
(4)   the fact that IVF involves embryo research can not be used against IVF without further argument ([29], p. 353).

Similar concerns underlie the Danish law that forbids experimentation with fertilized eggs *in vitro* except in an established IVF procedure to achieve pregnancy. "Thus a form of medical treatment is accepted, but attempts to improve its methods are prohibited" ([47] p. 153). Here the law represents a compromise between conflicting moral values.

Scandinavian discussions often link IVF to embryo research, itself a highly controversial issue. Some of the more biblically oriented theologians (particularly in Norway) hold that embryos are entitled to full protection and may not be used a means to others' ends, laudable as those may be, lest the human dignity of the embryos be denied. Other theologians, while granting the embryo's human dignity, are nonetheless prepared to accept some forms of experimentation if they serve human interests that are so vital as to override the embryo's right to life. The prevention of miscarriages and birth defects or the development of therapies for fetuses and premature infants might qualify by this standard. In 1985 the Swedish Ecumenical Council (which includes the Church of Sweden), the Swedish Christian Youth Council, and the Catholic Episcopate declared that life may be sacrificed only for the highest purposes and therefore advocated a general prohibition of embryo research except during the first fourteen days when it is vital for the betterment of human life; there is no other way to obtain the necessary knowledge; and both the egg and semen donors have given their informed consent. The Free churches of Sweden concurred with the general prohibition but rejected the possibility that there might be any legitimate exceptions ([29], pp. 360-361).

This ecumenical position was taken in response to the 1984 report of a Swedish state genetic ethics commission that recommended allowing research during the first 14 days. In 1991 a law was implemented restricting embryo research to the exceptional circumstances described by the Ecumenical Council: a fourteen day limit, donor consent, and vital research results otherwise unobtainable, with the additional stipulation that the embryo not be implanted but destroyed at the end of allowed period ([29], pp. 345, 361, 364).

Only in Norway has there been theological objection to the "unnaturalness" of IVF. Most Scandinavian theologians are more concerned with the freezing or discarding of embryos and the risks of prematurity or multiple births ([29], p. 351). Many are also troubled by the fact that IVF places a heavy burden (discomfort, dehumanization, inconvenience, and emotional and financial investment) on women already burdened by childlessness, while it offers only a limited prospect for a successful outcome.

Opposition to surrogate motherhood, however, is almost universal and without exception. Indeed, it is illegal. Scandinavian theologians regard it as an unnatural form of reproduction that severs the connection between biological and social parenting. It may also create conflict between the surrogate and the social parents if both or neither want the child once it is born. (The later possibility may arise in the event of parental separation or a birth defect or handicap.) The surrogate may find it psychologically difficult to give up the child, whatever she may have thought before insemination. Finally, theologians object to any commercialization of procreation. Children should not be treated as if they were merchandise or transferable property. Even the two theologians who would be prepared to allow surrogacy in the interest of respecting the autonomy of the parties do so only on the condition that it not become a commercial transaction ([29], pp. 355, 357).

Another topic of theological and ecclesiastical interest in recent years is genetic manipulation. Biblically oriented theologians reject positive eugenics because human nature as created and willed by God rests upon a genetic foundation. Modifications aimed at making "better" humans would usurp the authority of the divine creation and efface the distinction between the creature and creator. More humanistic theologians make the same judgment, but on the grounds that positive eugenics compromises human genetic integrity and dignity ([29], p. 346). Theologians of both schools observe that positive eugenic initiatives would presuppose too much knowledge of what constitutes "health" and "sickness" now and in the future, and overlook the complex interaction between genes and environment ([29], pp. 344, 346).

At the same time, these theologians are not opposed to negative eugenics in the form of somatic cell gene therapy. This intervention is not significantly different in principle from other experimental therapies and should be governed by the usual ethical requirements for medical experimentation, principally informed consent. Germ cell therapy, on the other hand, is subject to the same indictment the churches made of positive eugenics. It poses a risk to human genetic integrity, makes reckless assumptions about what is desirable, and cannot be perfected without illegitimate experimentation. In response to the government's genetic ethics commission, the Swedish Ecumenical Council noted in 1985 that the line between gene therapy and positive eugenics modification is so fine and likely to be transgressed that germ cell therapy ought to be prohibited ([29], p. 293).

Two related developments are worthy of mention in this connection. The Swedish Ecumenical Council in 1991 rejected the use of fetal tissue in medical research. In 1992 the General Synod of the Church of Sweden mandated a study of genetic engineering and patent law which is now under way.

As was noted above, Scandinavian societies value autonomy very highly. This is the basis for their legal arrangements concerning abortion. The advent of genetic screening and counseling prompted theologians and churches to ask whether parental autonomy should be absolute when a child-to-be's life is at stake. As defenders of human dignity, they had to ask whether society has a duty to protect unborn life from discrimination on the basis of a defect or handicap ([29], p. 338). These questions generated considerable public and parliamentary controversy in Norway where, according to one observer, "it takes very little to arouse suspicion of 'genetic manipulation,'" of "tinkering with human nature, life itself or what God has created" ([3], p. 331).

In 1989 the Norwegian Church Council sharply criticized prenatal screening and counseling because its intention, according to the Council, "is the extermination of the sick and not help for a family in need" ([29], p. 339). To routinely counsel screening on certain indications was seen as not-so-subtle encouragement of recourse to abortion. The church suspected that genetics counselors were inclined to favor abortion and insufficiently non-directive in their dealings with clients ([29], p. 342).

Many theologians throughout Scandinavia concur with the Church of Norway that acceptance of abortion on fetal indication is a dangerous flirtation with the idea that some lives are "unworthy". However, most would disagree emphatically with the Norwegian church's surprising allowance of selective abortion when the continuation of the pregnancy would place an unbearable burden on the family ([29], p. 340). In this judgment the Church of Norway stands alone. Yet it is very Lutheran to feel responsible for addressing the needs of family and society and to be willing, on occasion, to override the usual moral rules in order to meet those needs.

Religious opposition to prenatal diagnosis has also been reported in Denmark, especially in rural areas ([47], p. 144). In 1990 the Danish government's Ethics Council reported that its members did not agree on whether parents should have an absolute right to know the results of prenatal testing. They were agreed, however, that only the most serious conditions or diseases could justify selective abortion. A minority of the Council (among them the two theologians) suggested that society should establish precise boundaries, because in the future an increasing number of conditions will be diagnosable in utero ([29], p. 340).

Generally, Scandinavian theologians (with perhaps a single exception) accept the practice of prenatal diagnosis. However, they call for further attention to questions such as:

(1) What are the goals and consequences of prenatal diagnosis?
(2) Whether and when does a positive diagnosis justify abortion?
(3) Who should decide about diagnosis - parents, doctor, and/or society?
(4) What is the extent of and relation between the freedom of counselors and clients?

While no theologian would consider Down Syndrome a sufficient justification for abortion, there is less agreement on other diagnoses.

In Sweden these questions have been examined and re-examined since 1980, when an ecumenical panel of experts created by the Bishops' Conference of the Church of Sweden concluded that prenatal diagnosis could be accepted in principle because in most cases it preserves human life, paves the way for future treatment, and allows the fetus to be seen and treated as a patient. The panel did call for restrictions "because one aim is to abort defective fetuses" ([6], p. 347).

In reply to the Swedish National Board of Health and Welfare's 1982 Report on Prenatal Diagnosis, the Archbishop of the Church of Sweden and the Council of Free Churches "supported those aspects of medical genetics which emphasize research on treatment, and not only diagnosis of fetal defects". Expressing concern about the impact of prenatal diagnosis on social attitudes toward the handicapped and society's willingness to provide adequate support for their medical and educational needs, the Lutheran and Catholic monthly magazines followed up with a series of articles on the Christian view of the human person, emphasizing "the humanistic view that value is not contingent upon bodily constitution" ([6], p. 348).

The Swedish Ecumenical Council in 1985 accepted anencephalus and in some cases spina bifida, but never Down Syndrome, as conditions justifying abortion. When this organization returned to these issues in 1990, in response to the 1989 report of a government commission on prenatal diagnosis and late abortion, it approved withholding information about the sex of the fetus because sex is not a disease and such knowledge could be used to discriminate unfairly. The Council suggested that withholding this information could be justified as an extension of confidentiality between the physician and the fetal patient. For Scandinavian Lutherans, selective abortion is acceptable only in the context of social regulations that limit autonomy, and only as a last resort.

III. ABORTION

A. *European Developments*

Among Scandinavian theologians, abortion is generally considered a moral evil because it terminates a human life ([29], p. 331). In the circumstances of a fallen world, abortion may sometimes be necessary as the lesser of two evils, but its fundamental character should not be obscured. While abortion is readily available throughout Scandinavia, recent developments in genetic counseling and prenatal diagnosis and therapy have prompted second thoughts about the status of the fetus. However, individual autonomy remains highly esteemed as a moral value, and there has been no significant popular support for more restrictive legislation.

Since 1973 Danish women have had the right to induced abortion before the twelfth week of pregnancy. The law requires that information be provided about the procedure, its risks and consequences, and on services available should the woman choose to continue the pregnancy, but the decision is considered to be purely private and no reason is required. After the twelfth week, in the interest of avoiding complications, permission must be obtained. It is readily given in cases of rape, incest, risk to the woman's health, fetal abnormality, or for social reasons. The law has wide public support, although it has been criticized by the Roman Catholic bishop and some bishops of the Danish Evangelical Lutheran Church. Opposition to abortion is a key plank in the platform of the Christian Democratic Party which represents approximately 2.5% of the voters. Its efforts to change the current law have been unsuccessful ([4], p. 153).

Norwegian law is quite similar: "free" abortion through the twelfth week and for one of several indications thereafter. As time goes on, the reasons offered must be stronger, particularly after the eighteenth week. At viability, only a threat to the woman's life is deemed a sufficient indication ([5], p. 333). Earlier it was noted that Norwegian theological ethicists are more biblically oriented than their Nordic neighbors. This is but one manifestation of the fact that "the general cultural and specifically moral heritage that flows from Lutheran tradition [here in one of its most pietistic forms] is more influential and perceptible in Norway . . . than in other Scandinavian countries", especially in the nursing and medical professions. The membership of the Norwegian Association of Christian Physicians is 7-8% of all Norwegian doctors. The Christian People's Party wins 10% of the electorate and there is a politically powerful fundamentalist lay movement. Religious conservatives strenuously opposed the abortion law and today protest abortion following prenatal diagnosis ([5], p. 330). Thus, Lutheran perspectives are very much in play in Norwegian bioethical debates.

In Sweden, a social worker must be consulted after the twelfth week, though the decision is entirely the woman's through the eighteenth week. At that time, permission must be obtained from the National Board of Health and Welfare on the basis of "special reasons". Abortion after the twenty-second week (viability) is very rare ([6], p. 349). This legal framework represents the popular consensus. What anti-abortion sentiment exists is directed toward abortion on fetal indication ([21], p. 320). Some religious moralists fear that routine recourse to abortion after prenatal diagnosis will undermine the meaning of human dignity.

Among the many challenges faced by the newly reunified Germany is that of determining the legal status of abortion. In the former German Democratic Republic, abortion was a woman's private decision until the twelfth week; abortion after that time required the approval of a medical panel ([49], sect. 2.7.4.4). Across the border in the Federal Republic, abortion has been legally prohibited since 1976. Nevertheless it is possible to secure an abortion exempt from legal penalty under the following conditions:

(1) The woman must declare that it is her free will to abort;

(2) A physician must confirm the indication;

(3) A social counselor or physician must advise her about the social support available should she elect to continue the pregnancy;

(4) The procedure must be performed by a gynecologist other than the doctor who confirmed the indication.

Until the twelfth week, psychosocial, ethical or criminal (pregnancy resulting from rape or incest) indications are sufficient. Eugenic reasons are legitimate indications until the twenty-second week, and medical reasons (threat to the woman's life) are an exempting condition at any time ([35], sect. 2.5.1.5). Generally, it is not difficult to obtain an exemption, though some areas (e.g., Bavaria) are less liberal than others. Despite the formal legal differences – a term model in the East and an indications policy in the West – the practical effect of the laws is not much different except in the most conservative regions.

Abortion legislation adopted for the new Germany will require consultation at any stage of the pregnancy. Some Social Democrats regard this as a significant compromise of women's right to self-determination. The law is currently under review by the courts. If it is not approved, the present law of the Federal Republic will remain in force. In either case, the result would seem to be at odds with the protection afforded zygotes and embryos (after 24 hours) by the 1991 Protection of Embryos Act.

The Council of the Protestant Church in Germany, and the German [Catholic] Bishop's Conference agreed in 1989 that "according to God's will termination of pregnancy should not occur". The commandment against killing was understood to apply to "the killing of an unborn child". Even in conflict situations where the woman's life is at risk and abortion is indicated on medical grounds, there remains "a burden on the conscience" ([11], p. 43). Since a woman's right to self-determination "reaches its limit when it infringes on another's right to life . . . [it] cannot justify the disposing of the life which is developing in her". At the same time the churches observed,

If a pregnant woman does not see herself in the position of being able to accept the life which is taking shape within her, then her decision, although it is contrary to God's commandment, must not be condemned sweepingly and a priori as arbitrary domination over human life. The reasons and circumstances which lead to such a step are rather a challenge to dialogue, to sympathy, and to active help ([11], p. 44).

While understanding themselves "as advocates of the life and human dignity also of the unborn child", the churches are obligated "to stand by all those with counsel and help who have fallen into a situation of distress" ([11], p. 44).

In fact, the churches provide services that satisfy, though they surpass, the legal requirement of preabortion counseling. The Council declaration devoted considerable attention to the style of the churches' counseling. Counseling should offer acceptance and comprehensive support while seeking, if possible, to involve the women's partner and family. Commitment to respect for the unborn and to the woman places the church in a difficult position. The Council recognized that nothing can "relieve the woman of her decision" and that ultimately she may "not see herself in a position of being able to accept he child's life". Yet the Council insisted that the certification that counseling had occurred not be taken for granted. The church expected to have "a serious conversation" that did not simply proceed on the assumption "that mitigating circumstances [that qualify the woman for an exemption under the penal code] are in fact present" ([11], p. 45).

To their credit, the churches took a very comprehensive view of the problems of abortion. Needs for family planning, affordable housing, flexible work hours, child care, family leave, household assistance, financial support, education, and debt and re-employment counseling have to be addressed by the church as well as by the state in order to remove obstacles standing in the way of accepting unborn life. The churches discussed psychological issues such as emotional dependence and self-respect as well as attitudes and values concerning sex, marriage and family.

Regarding the treatment of abortion in the penal code, the churches stated:

The [C]atholic church has always declared that she cannot and will not come to terms with the present legal state of affairs . . . Sections 218ff. of the penal code book should not be declared sacrosanct . . . The Protestant Church in Germany has made it clear . . . that current penal law regulations concerning the termination of pregnancy are not completely satisfactory, but that a better protection of prenatal life can be expected rather from a development of conscience and a growth of awareness as well as from socio-political measures and that it is therefore not working for any change in the current legal position ([11], p. 53-54).

Although they were differently disposed toward the present law, the churches were agreed that "the regulations currently in force are not sufficiently guarded against misuse in practice" and, in any case, legal justification was not equivalent to moral justification ([11], p. 54). Specifically, they objected to the leniency with which the indication of special distress is confirmed. They urged that a higher threshold be required: e.g., the exhaustion of possibilities for alleviating the distress. The churches also recommended mandatory training in psychosocial counseling for persons authorized to conduct the requisite session. Finally, they objected to the current practice of allowing the counseling and the decision about the exempting indication to be conducted by the same person on the same occasion. "A separate counseling session would provide better conditions for the arguments in favor of carrying on with the pregnancy to be expressed" ([11], pp. 54-55).

B. *U.S. Developments*

In 1973 the United States Supreme Court determined that women have a constitutional right, free from state intrusion, to seek (though not necessarily to secure, if they are unable to pay for it) an abortion in the first trimester of pregnancy. Since this was seen as a matter of liberty or privacy, no reasons needed to be given and no public authorization was required. At the same time, the court indicated that during the second trimester, individual states could regulate the practice of abortion to protect the woman's health. At viability (which the court located in the third trimester), the state began to have a legitimate interest in the protection of fetal life and could go so far as to ban abortion except in cases where the woman's life or health (psychological as well as physical) was at risk.

Ever since, there has been intense controversy and much litigation concerning abortion. Opponents, non-religious as well as religious, have rejected the Supreme Court's attempted resolution of the issue and advocated legislation to ban or restrict abortion. Some states and municipalities have sought to require informed consent, parental or spousal notification, and/or a waiting period. Such requirements and bans on public funding of abortion have been challenged in the courts. In 1992 the United State's Supreme Court upheld what it called the "essence" of the controversial right to abortion while permitting states to regulate abortion in ways that do not place a "substantial obstacle in the path of a woman seeking an abortion before the fetus attains viability". The court rejected regulations that have the purpose or effect of imposing an "undue burden" on the woman. The meaning and limits of this decision will doubtless be tested by further legislation and litigation.

At the second biennial Church-wide Assembly of the Evangelical Lutheran Church in America in September 1991, a Social Statement on Abortion was adopted by a more than two-thirds majority. The challenge faced by the church in reconciling the discrepant positions of its two principal predecessor church bodies was described in *Bioethics Yearbook* Vol. I (pp. 129-134). The new ten page Statement was debated for six hours over two days. Forty-eight procedural votes were taken as the delegates considered more than sixty amendments ([1], pp. 20-21). The arduous parliamentary maneuvering demonstrated that serious differences of opinion concerning abortion were no less prevalent in the church than in American society as a whole.

Committed to both "the life of the woman and the developing life in her womb", the Statement tried to transcend the familiar rhetoric of "pro-life" and "pro-choice" and the assertion of clashing claims to absolute rights. On the central question of the status of the fetus, the Statement indicated that, "human life in all phases of its development is God-given and, therefore, has intrinsic value, worth and dignity . . . [which] human beings are called to respect and care for" ([43], pp. 2-3). Thus, "the strong Christian presumption is to preserve and protect life. Abortion ought to be an option only of last resort" ([43], pp. 3-4). Although the Statement spoke of "sin", it did so only in general terms without focusing exclusively on abortion.

"Because of the Christian presumption to preserve and protect life", the Statement announced, "this church, in most circumstances, encourages women with unintended pregnancies to continue the pregnancy" ([43], p. 6). At the same time, it recognized that "there can be sound reasons for ending a pregnancy through induced abortion" ([43], p. 6). The Statement identified three such reasons: a "clear threat to the physical life" of the woman; involuntary or non-voluntary intercourse – the latter interpreted to include "situations in which women are so dominated and oppressed that they have no choice regarding sexual intercourse and little access to contraceptives"; and "extreme fetal abnormality, which will result in severe suffering and very early death of an infant" ([43], p. 7). The significant moral issues attendant to abortion at any stage of fetal development become more serious as time goes on. Expressing opposition to post-viability abortion, except perhaps in rare cases of threat to life or newly discovered extreme abnormality, the statement urged that "if a pregnancy needs to be interrupted after this point, every reasonable and necessary effort should be made to support this life, unless there are lethal fetal abnormalities indicating that the prospective newborn will die very soon" ([43], p. 7).

The text originally proposed to the Assembly went on to observe that there was no agreement in the church concerning other circumstances, if any, in which abortion might be morally responsible. However in the interest of highlighting the church's consensus on the basic norm, the delegates deleted this reference to possible further exceptions. Certainly, that choice was politically prudent, since it foreclosed the possibility of conservative and liberal amendments attempting to specify instances of impermissible and permissible abortions. Such a debate would have been highly divisive and might well have undermined the hard-won support for the Statement as a whole.

Nevertheless, that course left readers to wonder about the church's attitude toward abortion in circumstances of social distress. The Statement was very thorough in deploring the diverse social, economic, and sexual ills that may lead a woman to consider abortion her best or only option. It called for "a realistic assessment of what will be necessary to bear, nuture and provide for children over the long-term and what resources are available". Moreover, it conceded that due to a variety of difficult circumstances in which women find themselves, "What is determined to be a morally responsible decision in one situation may not be in another" ([43], p. 6). Detractors from both ends of the spectrum of convictions about abortion have pointed to an imbalance or disjunction between the Statement's analysis of putative reasons for abortion and its explicit moral judgments ([4], p. 9). As one critic put it, "The Statement draws 'pro-life' conclusions on the basis of an essentially 'pro-choice' rationale" ([45], p. 12).

Disappointed as the champions of relentless consistency may be, the Statement is doubtless a reflection of the "mixed feelings" many Lutherans continue to have about abortion. Were the Statement to have been more single-minded in either direction, it probably would not have been adopted. The process by which Social Statements are produced is, after all, political, and church politics, no less than any other kind, necessarily involves compromise.

Turning to the public policy implications of the church's views, the Statement sought to reduce the need for recourse to abortion. Prevention of unintended pregnancies by means of sex and parenting education programs and by making safe, effective contraception and voluntary sterilization available to all was a priority concern. The church also advocated increased social "support for life after birth". Health care, housing, guaranteed income support, child care, flexible working hours, maternity and paternity leaves, equalization of women's and men's incomes, vigorous enforcement of parental financial responsibility, and child abuse prevention were identified as needing greater attention in both the public and private sectors.

Acknowledging that "government has a legitimate role in regulating abortion", the statement indicated that regulation should aim at "the preservation and enhancement of life [without] unduly encumbering or endangering the lives of women" ([43], p. 9). Therefore the church opposed:

- the total lack of regulation of abortion;
- legislation that would outlaw abortion in all circumstances;
- laws that prevent access to information about all options available to women;
- laws that deny access to safe and affordable services for morally justifiable abortions;
- mandatory or coerced abortion or sterilization;
- laws that prevent couples from practicing contraception;
- laws that are primarily intended to harass those contemplating or deciding for an abortion.

In cases where the life of the mother is threatened, where pregnancy results from rape or incest, or where the embryo or fetus has lethal abnormalities incompatible with life, the statement concluded that, abortion prior to viability should not be prohibited by law or by lack of public funding of abortions for low-income women. On the other hand, the statement supported legislation that prohibits abortions performed after the fetus is determined to be viable, except when the mother's life is threatened or when lethal abnormalities indicate the prospective newborn will die very soon ([43], p. 10).

The Statement called for further deliberation on legal questions such as whether spousal or partner notification, parental consent for minors, and public funding for abortion (presumably in circumstances other than those envisioned above) should be required. Since important values are at stake on both sides of these issues, the church called upon its members to "participate in the public debate" and to do so "in a spirit of respect for those with whom they differ". Finally, Lutherans informed by faith and conscience were encouraged "to decide and act . . . [in all matters pertaining to abortion] in ways that are responsive to God and to the needs of the neighbor" ([43], p. 10).

At the Triennial Convention of the Lutheran Church – Missouri Synod in July 1992, more than 95% of the delegates voted for intensified efforts "to oppose abortion as immoral except as an unavoidable result of a procedure necessary to save the woman's life" ([44], p. 734).

IV. CARE OF SEVERELY HANDICAPPED NEWBORNS

The 1989 joint declaration of the Protestant Church in Germany and the German Bishops' Conference staunchly defended the "inalienable dignity" of "life that is marked by illness, handicap or death":

> In view of the crimes that were committed in Germany under such irresponsible and reprehensible slogans as "life which is not worthy of life" or "ballast existence", it still seems an urgent necessity to emphasize this. At the moment there are signs of a revival of the evil spirit which seeks to distinguish between life "which is not worthy" and life "which is worthy of living" or "valuable". Over against this we say with the utmost decisiveness: Every human being, whatever his state, whether healthy or ill, with a high or low expectation of life, whether productive or a burden on society, is and remains the "image of God". The conviction that in the final analysis it is not his own qualities but God's acceptance and calling which confer on mankind the quality of being made in God's image and thus his dignity must be held fast especially in regard to ill, handicapped, and dying life. Everything else is idolatry of the vital, the strong, and the efficient ([11], p. 29).

While the declaration does not specifically discuss severely handicapped newborns, its general observations are manifestly relevant.

Aware that even normal children can be a burden as well as a blessing, the churches observed that facing concrete challenges can lead to the surprising discovery "that one can bear greater burdens than one thought at first" ([11], p. 31). Chance occurrences and unforeseen developments must be accepted as a part of life. While the churches did not presume to offer any "generally applicable standards for assessing the limits of the extent to which burdens can reasonably be expected and borne", Christians should set the limits "as widely as possible" and plumb the extent of reasonableness "as deeply as possible" ([11], p. 32). As Christians engage in honest self-examination, they are reminded that God "can and will make good arise out of evil" and "can transform the burden into a blessing" ([11], p. 33).

Admirable as it is, this readiness to bear burdens on behalf of others does not dictate treatment decisions in every case. On the assumption that "medical treatment must always be in the genuine interest of the patient" (defined in terms of "the continuation of life in a way that is worthy of a human being"), the churches recognized that in certain circumstances treatment may be unwarranted. "If treatment does not promise any improvement, it should not be preceded with. The aim of treatment must be the prolongation of life, not the process of dying" ([11], p. 30). If applied to the most severely handicapped newborns and babies "born dying", this standard would justify withholding or withdrawing treatment in some of these cases.

V. EQUITABLE ACCESS TO HEALTH CARE

A. *European Developments*

The Lutheran churches of Scandinavia and Germany have for some time enjoyed the benefits of universal health care systems. In these countries, religious conceptions of social solidarity and shared responsibility for caring for the basic needs of others are operative in public policy. Of course, this does not mean that these systems are without problems or that the churches need have no further concern about access to health care. In their 1989 joint declaration, the Council of the Protestant Church in Germany and the German Bishops' Conference observed that shared social responsibility for health care "has led to . . . a passive attitude to one's own health and . . . too great an expectation of the help to be had from others" ([11], p. 37). The declaration called for increased personal responsibility in relation to preventive health care, diet, alcohol consumption, smoking, drugs, exercise, and life style. In light of the aging of the population and rising costs, it called for self-restraint and renewed individual responsibility for the health service system as a whole:

> Anyone who makes use of services only because he pays his contributions calls into question the fundamental principle of health insurance as a fellowship in solidarity. But it is equally certain that basic changes in the structure of the health service are necessary. But they must not be at the expense of certain sick individuals or groups such as the handicapped ([11], p. 39).

Reforms that restrict access to certain procedures already have aroused controversy and will continue to do so. For example, it is reported that in Sweden, cardiac surgery is not performed on patients over seventy years of age in Stockholm. In 1988 the Karolinska Sjukhuset, a Stockholm cancer clinic, imposed age limits on treatment for some forms of cancer. "Both the prime minister and the minister of health forcefully spoke out against the view that not everyone should be given optimal treatment, while others have argued that age limits are a poor criterion, since seventy year old people can vary greatly in physical and psychological health ([13], p. 18). It may be expected that age limits and other forms of rationing will be a subject of political debate wherever there is publically funded health care. Scarce resources, rising costs, aging populations, and taxpayer resistance assure that in the future this issue will have a prominent place on the bioethics agenda.

B. *U.S. Developments*

In continuity with the positions of its predecessor churches, the Evangelical Lutheran Church in America supports the creation of a universal health care plan. Both the promotion of human well-being and social justice require that the 37 million Americans without health insurance be afforded access to care. Moreover, the church's more than 250 social ministry organizations provide health care services throughout the United States. Rapidly rising costs and their impact on the Medicare and Medicaid reimbursement systems undermine the services those institutions can offer.

Through its Office for Governmental Affairs in Washington, D.C., the Evangelical Lutheran Church in America has joined with 14 other denominations and 30 state organizations to form the Interreligious Health Care Access Campaign. Launched in 1992, the Campaign has four basic aims for the health care system:

(1) Everyone living in the United States should have access to comprehensive health care services.
(2) Health care should be of good quality.
(3) Payments for health care should be made in a cost-effective way.
(4) Prompt and appropriate payment to the provider should be assured ([9], p. 34).

Although the Lutheran churches have advocated health care reform for many years, there is now more reason to be optimistic that such efforts might succeed.

VI. WITHDRAWING OR WITHHOLDING TREATMENT

A. *European Developments*

The Protestant and Catholic churches of Germany, in their 1989 joint declaration "God Loves All That Lives: Challenges and Tasks for the Protection of Life", held that "Even an incurably ill person, who is nothing but a burden to others, has an undiminished right to life. No doctor can give him up as a so-called 'hopeless case', as long as he is alive, and cease to afford him medical care". Echoing what they said about the handicapped (quoted above), the churches insisted that "Nobody has a right to decide about the value or lack of value of another human life – and also not about one's own" ([11], p. 66). All who live are valuable in the eyes of God, and that divine valuation is the inalienable ground of human dignity.

That is not to say, however, that medical treatment is always morally indicated. Indeed treatment can, itself, constitute disrespect.

All medical and nursing measures must be carried out with . . . respect for [the patient's] dignity. It must not be prevented that the dying person [makes] decisions affecting himself at the end of his life. That includes respecting the way the other chooses, even if one doesn't agree with it. If a terminally ill person can express himself and deliberately refuses further medical treatment, his wish is to be respected. And if he is no longer able to express himself, then the doctor should act as a good advocate in the properly understood interests of the dying and for his individual well-being. In the individual case, this principle might very well lead to the omission or discontinuance of further medical measures, if these – instead of lengthening this person's life – only lengthen his dying.

This does not mean that every wish a dying person expresses to [another], such as a doctor, must be complied with ([11], p. 66).

With regard to the administration of pain killing drugs which may shorten life, the declaration concluded, "If death is not intended to occur, but the aim of the treatment is rather to make the remaining life of the dying person more bearable, then the risk of death as side effect can be accepted". In cases where the patient is not able to express her wishes, the physician may act on "the basis of his medical knowledge that what he does is for the benefit of the patient under the given circumstances" ([11], p, 67).

B. *U.S. Developments*

In 1989 the Evangelical Lutheran Church in America submitted to the Supreme Court of the United States an *amicus curiae* brief in *Cruzan v. Director of Missouri Department of Health*. The church argued on behalf of the petitioners – parents seeking the right, free from unwarranted state intrusion, to determine the level of care appropriate for their irreversibly comatose daughter. Shortly after the automobile accident which left their daughter comatose, the parents of Nancy Cruzan authorized the surgical implantation of a feeding tube into her stomach. At that time her prognosis was uncertain, but soon thereafter she lapsed into a persistent vegetative state from which there was no possibility of recovery. Her cerebral cortex had been destroyed, although her brain stem continued to function, thus allowing her to breathe on her own. The parents eventually gave up any hope of her recovery and concluded that their daughter would not want to continue to live in this condition. They requested that the state hospital withhold any further life-support treatment, including the tubal feeding and hydration that was keeping her alive. The hospital administrator was unwilling to honor their request without a court order.

The trial court entered judgment for the parents, ruling that "[t]here is a fundamental right expressed in the Constitution as the 'right to liberty', which permits an individual to refuse or direct the withholding or withdrawal of artificial death prolonging procedures". The court was convinced, on the basis of the patient's former life-style and statements to family and friends, that she would not wish to remain in her present condition. However, on review, the Supreme Court of Missouri reversed the trial court's judgment. The majority declared that the privacy right to refuse treatment belonged only to those able to make a competent decision. They found the evidence offered at trial regarding Nancy Cruzan's wishes "inherently unreliable" and insufficient to outweigh the state's interest in preserving life, irrespective of its quality. In the absence of a living will, the majority was unwilling to grant the parents' request. The Cruzans appealed. By the time their case was argued in the United States Supreme Court, their daughter had been in a persistent vegetative state for over six years.

The brief of the Evangelical Lutheran Church in America considered the case from the perspectives of its 1982 Social Statement, "Death and Dying" and of an American Lutheran Church Task Force Report (see *Bioethics Yearbook* Vol. I, pp. 136-139). Citing those documents as well as legal precedents, the brief argued that the Missouri Supreme Court construed the constitutional right to privacy too narrowly and the state's interest too broadly. The church maintained that the presumption of parental authority is essential to [the American] tradition of individual liberty and that the right asserted by the family of Nancy Cruzan was a logical extension of prior cases regarding family privacy. Nowhere is privacy more important than in situations where families face the impending death of a loved one. The church asked the Court to consider:

that a person of faith who makes a decision to discontinue artificial hydration or nutrition should not be forbidden from doing so. We believe that for us, such a decision requires prayerful consideration of the gift of life from God, respect for the unconscious person's preferences, and hope in the resurrection over death. Continued life, ordered by state officials over family objection, should not be allowed to frustrate religious belief that accepts death as part of the created order and proclaims ultimate victory over death through the promise of the resurrection of the body. Our freedom to believe and to act on this belief is inextricably bound to the Cruzan family's struggle to do the same ([31], pp. 13-14).

With regard to the state's legitimate interest, the church argued that it should be confined to assuring a careful deliberation and fair decision on behalf of a incompetent person. The Missouri Supreme Court should have been satisfied with the trial court's finding of no bad faith on the part of the Cruzans. By sweeping aside the testimony of the patient's family and friends concerning her previously expressed wishes, "the Missouri court assumes that the state is the moral repository of individual belief concerning life and death" ([31], p. 17). Since the parents' decision could not be viewed as homicide or aiding a suicide. the court was not justified in interposing itself between Nancy Cruzan and her parents. If the state is concerned with preventing abuse of institutionalized dependent people, it should encourage rather than prevent family involvement in decision making. Absent any evidence of bad faith, who is likely to be more attentive to the interests of the institutionalized – bureaucratic regulators or loving families?

What was especially pernicious about the state's invasion of family privacy in this case was that it mandated a "continued intrusion into Nancy's body to maintain biological existence for a person who insists in the only way she is able, through her closest family, that she has had enough". The brief concluded, "When we as Christians have lived our life and our earthly bodies fail, we wish our families to be free on our behalf to repeat the words of Simeon, upon seeing the infant Jesus, 'Lord, now lettest thou thy servant depart in peace . . . , (Luke 2: 29-31)' ([31], p. 21).

The 1982 Social Statement, "Death and Dying", also served as the basis for the Evangelical Lutheran Church in America's 1992 Message on Social Issues, "End of Life Decisions". Applying the Statement's "interpretive principles" (see *Bioethics Yearbook* Vol. I, p. 136) to the issue of refusing beneficial treatment, the Message held that,

Because competent patients are the prime decision makers, they may refuse treatment recommended by health care professionals when they do not believe the benefits outweigh the risks and burdens. This is also the case for patients who are incompetent, but have identified their wishes through advance directives, living wills, and/or conversation with family or designated surrogates. Health care professionals are obligated to inform patients of medical treatment options and what in their best judgment are the potential benefits and burdens of such options. They are also obligated to obtain the consent of patients to provide treatment. Where this consent is not given, they should accept the desired limits of treatment, even when they do not agree with the decision ([28], p. 3).

Such a refusal in no way frees health care professionals "from the obligation to give basic human care and comfort throughout the dying process" ([28], p. 3).

On the central moral (if not legal) point at issue in the Cruzan case – whether artificial nutrition and hydration may ever be withheld or withdrawn – the Message set forth what may have been assumed but was not explicitly stated in the Social Statement; i.e., "artificially-administered nutrition and hydration move beyond basic [human] care to become medical treatment" ([28], p. 3). As such, they may be refused when they are "unduly burdensome" and "disproportionate to the expected benefits". That is the case "when medical judgment determines that [they] will not contribute to an improvement in the patient's underlying condition or prevent death from that condition". Nor are health care professionals "required to use all available medical treatment in all circumstances". When patients or their legal spokesperson seek to limit treatment and allow death to occur, their request should not be regarded as suicide or abandonment. "Family, friends, health care professionals, and pastor should continue to care for the person", providing "relief from suffering, physical comfort, and assurance of God's enduring love" ([28], p. 3).

VII. ACTIVE EUTHANASIA

A. *European Developments*

According to opinion polls conducted since 1985 by a pro-suicide group known as the German Society of Humane Dying, about two-thirds of Germans favor the legalization of active voluntary euthanasia ([34], p. 26). If this figure is reasonably accurate, the shadow cast by Nazi euthanasia practices must not be as long as it used to be. Nevertheless, proposals to legalize active voluntary euthanasia have been rejected by German legal and medical organizations. "Behind this resistance stood . . . physicians' insistence on traditional Western deontology that includes the Hippocratic prohibition against killing; fear of a slippery slope; and a distrust of the idea itself, with its associations of horror and taboo" ([34], p. 26).

The extreme sensitivity of the subject may help to explain Germany's reluctance to formalize procedures for the cessation of treatment. As Margaret Battin observes,

Living wills are rarely used; the durable power of attorney has only come into effect as of 1 January 1992. Do-not-resuscitate orders are rarely explicitly executed and only in exceptional cases put in written form; for the most part they are made in agreement with the family but without discussion with the patient . . . [T]here is no such thing as informed consent. In general, decisions about life – sustaining therapy are made by the physician, not the patient, and are consented to by the family ([3], p. 45).

In such a context, the churches' assertion (quoted above) that patients' wishes should be respected is more significant than it might seem to readers long accustomed to the idea of patient autonomy and comfortable with less authoritarian conceptions of the physician's role.

Another distinctive feature of the German scene is its ambivalence toward suicide, which was decriminalized as far back as 1751. Moreover, it is not illegal to assist a voluntary suicide, so long as the person is competent and informed. It is, however, the legal duty of a physician to rescue the patient. As Battin notes,

one, widely prevalent interpretation of the legal situation holds [that], although the physician is not prohibited from giving a lethal drug to a patient, once that patient has taken the drug and becomes unconscious, the physician incurs a duty to resuscitate him or her" ([3], p. 46). For obvious reasons, suicide is "a private matter, to be conducted outside the medical establishment and largely without its help ([3], p. 46).

Deep cultural values underlie these legal arrangements. Battin comments that the German language has several terms for suicide. Some of them carry the usual negative moral and pathological connotations but one, *Freitod* (literally "free death") is positive: "It is associated with voluntary individual choice and the expression of basic, strongly held personal values or ideals, especially those running counter to conventional norms, and suggesting the triumph of personal integrity in the face of threat or shame" ([3], p. 47). It is not difficult to imagine that a terminally, or even chronically, ill person in a severely debilitated condition might choose *Freitod* as an alternative to continued suffering and the indignity of the prevailing authoritarian, paternalistic style of medical practice.

All of this stands as the background to the German Protestant and Catholic churches' common witness. They began by acknowledging that "nobody has the right to pass judgment from the outside. What moves another to act and his or her possibilities of decision remain as hidden . . . as do the possible effects of an illness". They called for "a tolerance of the other person which goes beyond an understanding of his action" and does not result in any loss of respect. Attempted suicides must be, for the Christian, "only an 'accident' and a cry for help". Yet there was no equivocation in their fundamental judgment. "The person who has grasped that he does not live for himself alone cannot approve and condone suicide" ([11], p. 67).

The churches were even more adamant about "mercy killing". "Nobody could seriously consider the intentional killing of a patient against his/her wishes". But even when requested by a competent patient, "killing . . . can under no circumstances be an act of love, of compassion . . . for it destroys the basis of love". Such requests must be answered "gently, but decisively" explaining "why the desire cannot be acceded to". There must be no abandonment of the patient who asks to be killed. "A desperate person needs intensive attention in order to experience the truth that even his life is not meaningless". Of course, accompanying the dying is a most arduous service. Those who remain at their posts may find that in their own exhaustion, utter helplessness, and natural desire "not to have to stand up to this any longer", they may be tempted to entertain the self-deceptive thought that it would be best if the patient's life could be terminated "to save him [!] from further suffering" ([11], pp. 67-68).

The document indicated that physicians have additional, role-specific reasons for refusing to accommodate euthanasia requests.

If a doctor were to comply with such a request, he/she would place him/herself in a tug of war between his/her duty as a doctor to be an advocate on behalf of life and the completely different role of killing someone. If he/she were to do this out of compassion – could it be avoided that people would begin to impute other motives? That would be the end of any basis for trust between doctor and patient ([11], p. 68).

If German doctor-patient relations are as devoid of open communication and covenantal partnership as Battin describes them, it is unlikely that they could withstand the additional stresses created by the admission of active euthanasia to the menu of routine medical services.

In Sweden, as elsewhere in Scandinavia, there is general acceptance of passive euthanasia (the cessation of attempts to forestall a patient's inevitable death). There are also organizations advocating the legalization of euthanasia. To date there has been no specific legislation. According to Ingemar B. Lindahl, "[B]oth opponents and proponents have stressed the inappropriateness of legislating on euthanasia". Empirical uncertainties in prognosis and the desire to avoid "ending up in the same bureaucratic bargaining in life and death that occurs in abortion inquiries" suggest that the matter is best left "on a purely ethical level" ([20], p. 323).

B. *U.S. Developments*

Recently American voters in the states of Washington and California have defeated initiatives that would have allowed physician-assisted suicide and active direct euthanasia. Doubtless, the issue will reappear on ballots in these and other jurisdictions in the years ahead. In 1992 the two largest Lutheran church bodies in the United States reiterated their opposition to both practices. The 2.6 million member Lutheran Church-Missouri Synod did so by means of a resolution adopted at its Triennial Convention in July ([44], p. 734), while the 5.3 million member Evangelical Lutheran church in America elected to produce a Message on Social Issues entitled "End of Life Decisions". Drafted and revised throughout the summer and fall, it was officially approved by the Church Council less than a week after the California referendum.

The Message observed that "the integrity of the physician-patient relationship is rooted in trust that physicians will act to preserve the life and health of the patient". The fact that they are also obligated to relieve suffering by means of aggressive pain management (even if it hastens death) was clearly recognized. "However, the deliberate action of a physician to take the life of a patient, even when this is the patient's wish, is a different matter. As a church we affirm that 'deliberately destroying life created in the image of God is contrary to Christian conscience'"[Here the Message quoted the 1982 Social Statement "Death and Dying".] Sounding a distinctive Lutheran theme, the church acknowledged that its fundamental moral judgment may not do justice to the reality or extremity of certain cases. Without derogating from the clarity or force of its judgment, the Message "recognize[d] that responsible health care professionals struggle to choose the lesser evil in ambiguous borderline situations – for example, when pain becomes so unmanageable that life is indistinguishable from torture" ([28], p. 4).

The church opposed the legalization of "physician-assisted death which would allow . . . private killing". It expressed dispositive doubt that regulatory safeguards could assure adequate public control and warned of substantially increased potential for abuse, especially of people who are most vulnerable. Alternatively, the church suggested that "caring treatment that allows death to occur within the bounds of what is morally acceptable may reduce the appeal of physician-assisted death" ([28], p. 4). The increased use of advance directives and the availability of hospice care should diminish the perceived need for such drastic measures. Finally, the Message observed that "a more equitable health care system that more effectively responds to catastrophic illness and provides needed follow-up care should also be a priority of those concerned about end of life decisions" ([28], p. 4).

VIII. DEFINITION OF DEATH

The Catholic and Protestant churches of Germany are agreed that "the death of the brain is the sign of a person's death". According to the 1989 joint declaration, "The death of the brain in its entirety is equated with the death of the individual because it marks the end of the control of the physical and spiritual unity of the organism"([11], p. 65). The churches were content to leave to medical science the task of establishing the methods by which death is determined to have occurred.

There has been considerable debate in Scandinavia concerning the definition and criteria for death. It was not until 1987 that the Swedish Parliament passed a brain death statute (stipulating the total and irreversible loss of brain function). Critics of the new law argued that it was unnecessary because since 1973 the National Board of Health and Welfare had permitted stopping respiratory support upon determination that brain function had totally and irreversibly ceased. Proponents "pointed out that there is an obvious ethical difference between turning off the respirator because the patient has died, and – if brain related criteria are not accepted – killing the patient by turning off the respirator" ([13], p. 18). The brain death law had the advantages of eliminating the latter interpretation and allowing closure for the patient's family while preserving the possibility of obtaining usable organs for transplantation.

At about the same time, the Danish Ministry of Justice drafted a legislative proposal that would have accepted both brain and heart death as valid criteria. After a first reading in the Danish Parliament, the proposal was withdrawn. Expressing opposition to the bill was the Danish Council of Ethics, created by Parliament in 1987 to submit recommendations to the Ministry of Health. Among the Council's membership were three doctors, two theologians, two lawyers, three teachers, two writers, a pharmacist, a social worker, a nurse, a dentist, and a biologist ([33], p. 5). Of these, only the physicians and one of the lawyers, a judge who chaired the Council, favored the proposed law. According to one observer, the rest were "seemingly influenced by ultra-reactionary divines" ([30], p. 10). The Council secretary reported that the majority was not content to define death in purely scientific terms.

The Council majority held that "the everyday experience of death common to the individuals of a particular culture" should be respected. This meant that respiration, heartbeat, warmth, and normal coloration, even when artificially maintained in a brain dead patient, "continue to signify that life has not ended" ([33], p. 6). They doubted that most people and particularly the relatives would regard a body in this state as a 'corpse'.

The Council offered an alternative legislative proposal based on the following guidelines:

1. A person should be declared dead only when all brain, heart, and lung function has definitely ceased.
2. With the cessation of the brain function, the person has entered the death process.
3. The death process should not be prolonged after brain function has ceased.
4. The time of death is given by the end and not the beginning of the death process.
5. The sole purpose legitimating the extension of the death process is transplantation from beating heart donors, if the donor or his relatives have given their informed consent. The transplant procedure will end the death process but will not constitute the cause of the donor's death ([33], p. 6).

Unfortunately, this by no means resolves the problem brain death legislation seeks to correct. The Council's fifth guideline continued to "assume that a different death awaits organ donors" ([16], p. 9). Potential donors would be treated differently, which is precisely the popular apprehension that needs to be addressed. Potential donors and their families must have the assurance that those still living will not be exploited for sake of a potential recipient.

IX. ORGAN DONATION

Like their North American counterparts (see *Bioethics Yearbook* Vol. I, p. 139), the German churches have made statements encouraging postmortem organ donation as a way of "exercising the love of one's neighbor even beyond death". In no way does the practice conflict with a Christian view of the human person or proper respect for the newly dead. Nevertheless, the joint Protestant-Catholic declaration expressed some ethical concerns about donation and transplantation.

The document found that "only in rare exceptional cases" is the transplant of an organ from a living donor morally justifiable. Risk to the donor was cited as one but not the only reason for caution. Even when the practice is restricted to organs existing in pairs (e.g., kidneys), it should still be regarded as "an exceptional sacrifice". Another concern expressed concerned the psychological dynamics of coercion and dependence. The churches questioned whether, in cases of donation between relatives or friends, "the express consent of the donor always takes place voluntarily and without psychological pressure". Recipients, too, could find themselves under extreme duress because they owe their continued existence to the donor. What if rejection were interpreted as a sign of ingratitude?

With regard to cadaveric donation, the churches wanted assurance that the donor's life "is not prematurely declared to be at an end in the interest of a recipient". The document stipulated that the death of the brain "must be definitely proved [according to appropriate medical criteria] and certified by doctors qualified to do so, who must be independent of the team carrying out the transplant". In cases of emergency or where there is no record of the prospective donor's wishes, the churches regard the possibility of "presumed consent" as "a moot point" in which "the legal arrangements for the agreement of the bereaved are difficult". Finally, the document observed that "too many experiments are being made. Progress in medical science in itself is not enough to justify an organ transplant". Nor should "the mere quantitative lengthening of life" be overvalued, especially when it derives from "a refusal to accept the finiteness of human life" or tempts "a choice to benefit a certain human life at the cost of help for other human lives". The churches reject all such choices, including "when wealthy patients can 'buy' themselves an organ" ([11], pp. 64-65).

In Sweden, Catholics have expressed support for the practice of "presumed consent* but Lutherans oppose it. This is surprising in light of the high value Swedes place on social solidarity and welfare. Yet it does reflect their great respect for the sanctity of individual autonomy.

X. CONCLUSION

In accord with the purpose of the *Bioethics Yearbook* series, this chapter has concentrated on reporting the social teachings of Lutheran churches. It has not submitted them to extended critical analysis. Nor has it been possible to discuss the views of individual Lutheran bioethicists. Nevertheless, the material presented here demonstrates that Lutheran churches in the United States and Northern Europe have devoted considerable time and resources to addressing the bioethical issues confronting their societies. Although it would be difficult to identify uniquely Lutheran insights or normative commitments, it may be possible to discern in the reflection of these religious communities a common moral ethos. Sensitive to moral ambiguity, wary of legalism and self-righteousness, Lutheran bioethics aspires to promote works of mercy, love, and justice. It is pragmatic about means and prepared to work in concert with others who endeavor to ameliorate our manifold afflictions.

Wittenberg University
Springfield, Ohio, U.S.A.

ACKNOWLEDGMENTS

The author wishes to thank the following individuals for their invaluable assistance: Prof. Dr. Holsten Fagerberg (University of Uppsala), Rev. Dr. Jean Lambert (Immanuelskrykan, Stockholm), Prof. Dr. Viggo Mortensen (Lutheran World Federation, Geneva), Prof. Dr. Kees van Kooten Niekerk (University of Aarhus), Dr. Gert Nillson (Church of Sweden), Dr. John Stumme (Evangelical Lutheran Church in America) and Ms. Christine Sinnott (Wittenberg University). Travel funds were provided by the Lutheran World Federation and the Faculty Research Fund at Wittenberg University.

BIBLIOGRAPHY

1. "Abortion: 'Option Only of Last Resort": 1991, *The Lutheran* 4 (October 2), 20-21.
2. Ahlzén, R. *et al.*: 1991, *Abort, Fosterdiagnostik and Manniskovarde (Tro & Tanke,* No.7), Svenska Kyrkans Forskningsrad, Uppsala.
3. Battin, M.: 1992, "Assisted Suicide: Can We Learn from Germany"?, *The Hastings Center Report* 22 (March-April), 44-51.
4. Benne, R.: 1991, "A Reluctant 'No'", *The Lutheran* 4 (May 22), 8-9.
5. Berg, K. and Trangy, K.E.: 1989, "Ethics and Medical Genetics in Norway", in [48].
6. Bischofberger, E. *et al.*: 1989, "Ethics and Medical Genetics in Sweden", in [48].
7. Crist, J.: 1991, "A Middle Ground", *The Lutheran* 4 (May 22), 11-12.
8. Evans, M.: 1990, "Death in Denmark", *Journal of Medical Ethics* 16, 191-194.
9. "Evangelical Lutheran Church in America Participates in Health Care Campaign": 1992, *The Lutheran* 5 (March), 34.
10. Gillon, R.: 1990, "Death", *Journal of Medical Ethics* 16, 3-4.
11. "God Loves All That Lives: Challenges and Tasks for the Protection of Life" ("Gott ist ein Freund des Lebens. Herausforderungen und Aufgaben beim Schutz des Lebens"): 1989, English trans. 1991, A Joint Declaration of the Council of the Protestant Church in Germany and the German [Roman Catholic] Bishops' Conference in co-operation with the other member and guest churches of the Council of Christian Churches in the Federal Republic of Germany and Berlin (West), Gutersloher Verlagshaus Gerd Mohn, Gutersloh and Paulinus-Verlag, Trier.
12. Gritsch, E.W. and Jenson, R.W.: 1976, *Lutheranism: The Theological Movement and its Confessional Writings*, Fortress, Philadelphia.
13. Hermerén, Göran: 1988, "In Sweden, Questioning the Model of Compromise", *The Hastings Center Report* 19 (August), 17-18.
14. Hübner, J. and Schubert, H. von (eds.): 1992, *Biotechnologie und evangelische Ethik: die internationale Diskusssion*, Campus Verlag, Frankfurt am Main /New York.
15. Klein, C. and Dehsen, C. von: 1989, *Politics and Piety: The Genesis and Theology of Social Statements of The Lutheran Church in America*, Fortress, Minneapolis.
16. Lamb, D.: 1990, "Wanting It Both Ways", *Journal of Medical Ethics* 16, 8-9.
17. Lamb, D.: 1991, "Death in Denmark: A Reply", *Journal of Medical Ethics* 17, 100-101.
18. Lammers, A. and Peters, T.: 1990, "Genetics: Implications of the Human Genome Project", *The Christian Century* 107, 868-872.

19. Lindahl, B.I.B.: 1985, "Philosophy of Medicine in Scandinavia", *Theoretical Medicine* 6, 65-84.20.
20. Lindahl, B.I.B.: 1988, "Medical Ethics in Sweden", *Theoretical Medicine* 9, 309-335.
21. Lindahl, B.I.B.: 1989, "Sweden: Growing Interest in Ethics", *The Hastings Center Report* 19 (July-August), 30-31.
22. Lundblad, B.K.: 1991, "Abortion: The Lutherans' Turn", *Christianity and Crisis* 51, 382-383.
23. Luther, M.: 1988, *Three Treatises*, Fortress, Philadelphia.
24. Lutheran Church in America: 1984, *Minutes*, New York.
25. "Lutherans Say Abortion Can Be Responsible Move": 1991, *The New York Times*, September 4.
26. Meilaender, G.: 1990, "Mastering Our Gen(i)es: When Do We Say No?", *The Christian Century* 107, 872-877.
27. Meilaender, G.: 1991, *Faith and Faithfulness: Basic Themes in Christian Ethics*, University of Notre Dame Press, Notre Dame, Indiana.
28. Message on Social Issues: 1992, "End of Life Decisions", Evangelical Lutheran Church in America, Chicago.
29. Niekerk, K.: 1992, "Die Diskussion in Skandinavien" in [14].
30. Pallis, C.: 1990, "Return to Elsinore", *Journal of Medical Ethics* 16, 10-13.
31. Reece Martyn, S.D. *et al.*: 1989, "Brief Amicus Curiae of the Evangelical Lutheran Church in America in Support of the Petitioners" in *Cruzan v. Director of Missouri Department of Health and Administrator of the Missouri Rehabilitation Center at Vernon*, 110 S.Ct. 2841.
32. Rendtorff, T.: 1989, *Ethics* Vol. II, *Applications of an Ethical Theology* trans. K. Crim, Fortress Press, Minneapolis.
33. Rix, B.: "Danish Ethics Council Rejects Brain Death as the Criterion of Death", *Journal of Medical Ethics* 16, 5-7.
34. Schöne-Seifert, B. and Rippe, K.P.: 1991, "Silencing the Singer: Antibioethics in Germany", *The Hastings Center Report* 21 (November-December), 20-27.
35. Schroeder-Kurth, T.M. and Hübner, J.: 1989, "Ethics and Medical Genetics in the Federal Republic of Germany (FRG)" in [48].
36. Schubert, H. von: 1991, *Evangelische Ethik und Biotechnologie*, Campus Verlag, Frankfurt am Main/New York.
37. Schubert, H. von: 1991, "Protestant Ethics and Biotechnology: A Summary" (unpublished summary of [36]).
38. "Secularism's Persistence": 1991, *The Christian Century* 108, 962.
39. Singer, P.: 1990, "Bioethics and Academic Freedom", *Bioethics* 4, 33-44.
40. Singer, P.: 1991, "On Being Silenced in Germany", *New York Review of Books* 15 August, 36-42.
41. Social Statement: 1970, "Sex, Marriage and Family", The Lutheran Church in America, New York.
42. Social Statement: 1982, "Death and Dying", The Lutheran Church in

America, New York.

43. Social Statement: 1991, *Abortion*, The Evangelical Lutheran Church in America, Chicago.

44. Stanich, S.: 1992, *Missouri Synod Defuses A Crisis*, *The Christian Century* 109, 732-734.

45. Stuhr, W.M.: 1991, *Keep the Options Open*, *The Lutheran* 4 (May 22), 11-12.

46. Tappert, T.G. (ed.): 1959, *The Book of Concord: The Confessions of the Evangelical Lutheran Church*, Fortress, Philadelphia.

47. Terkelsen, A.J. *et al.*: 1989,*Ethics and Medical Ethics in Denmark*in [48].

48. Wertz, D.C. and Fletcher, J.C.(eds.): 1989, *Ethics and Human Genetics: A Cross Cultural Perspective*, Springer Verlag, New York, Berlin.

49. Witkowski, R. *et al.*: 1989, *Ethics and Medical Genetics in the German Democratic Republic (GDR)*in [48].

KATHLEEN NOLAN

BUDDHISM, ZEN, AND BIOETHICS

Things are not what they seem.
Nor are they otherwise.

Traditional Buddhist Saying

Because of Buddhism's central focus on transcendental enlightenment, it is
sometimes portrayed as a religion that is antithetical, or at least indifferent, to
worldly concerns, including ethics. Buddhist scholars and teachers sometimes
contribute to such misconceptions, especially in relation to the branch of
Buddhism known as Zen (Chinese, *Ch'an*; Indian, *dhyana*), which was
introduced to Americans by Zen master D.T. Suzuki in the early part of the
twentieth century as an amoral (i.e., non-moral) discipline. These
misconceptions are no doubt exaggerated by attempts to articulate the
differences between Buddhism and other religions, which often emphasize
Buddhists' reliance on direct personal experience, rather than rules or
argumentation, as the touchstone of religious and ethical truth. From this
avowedly mystical perspective, inquiry into standards of ethical conduct may
appear to be unnecessary, and an arbitrary character may appear to be
engendered in morality itself.

This is an erroneous conclusion, as modern Buddhist teachers and scholars
have begun to recognize ([65];[30];[50];[54];[99]). Early Buddhist texts clearly
stress the primacy of ethics, placing morality first among the three central
doctrines of the Buddha's teachings – sila (morality), *samadhi* (concentration),
and *prajna* (wisdom) ([83], p. 57). Morality is primary, not only because of the
dangers of practicing concentration without a thorough moral grounding, but
also because the Buddha's Middle Way, or Noble Eightfold Path, was
formulated as a "a radical critique of wishful thinking and the myriad tactics
of escapism" prevalent in his day, and, indeed, in our own ([29], p. 7). Despite
its mystical character, Buddhism is thus an extremely practical religion, a
religion of the present life and of the present moment [75]. In fact, enlightenment itself can be understood as wisdom (awakening to the true nature of
reality) expressed in the activity of compassion. Moral conduct thus forms the
foundation for all spiritual attainment ([78], p. 46), and enlightenment without
morality is not true enlightenment ([65], p. 133).

However, many Buddhist teachers have expressed considerable reluctance
towards the formulation of analytical systems in which ethics becomes an object
of inquiry independent of enlightenment itself ([32];[57]). As Zen master

B. Andrew Lustig (Sr. Ed.), Bioethics Yearbook: Volume 3, 185-216.
©1993 Kluwer Academic Publishers.

Soyen Shaku once put it, "Buddhism has nothing to do with utilitarianism or intuitionalism or hedonism or what not" ([85], p. 71). This avoidance of systematic analysis bears further exploration, not only because it is potentially quite frustrating to non-Buddhist scholars, but also because it offers important insights into Buddhist moral teachings.

EMPTINESS, ETHICS, AND ENLIGHTENMENT

One of the major themes of early Buddhist scripture was the avoidance of religious controversy and ideological debate [16]. The historical Buddha urged his followers not to become attached even to his own teachings and to avoid denigrating the views of others. Stressing the importance of each person's individual spiritual inquiry, he urged: "Do not accept anything because of report, tradition, hearsay, the handing on in the sacred texts, or as a result of logic or inference, through indulgent tolerance of views, appearance of likelihood, or as paying respect to a teacher" ([83], p. 43).

Consistent with such teachings, the Buddha himself often side-stepped contentious religious questions, either responding indirectly or reinterpreting the question in terms of internal attitudes and virtues [16]. Noting a similar tendency in the thirteenth century Zen mystic Dogen Zenji and other Buddhist teachers, Thomas Kasulis therefore argues that Buddhism establishes a virtue ethics, with a central focus on the moral person, rather than the moral act [50].

This is not an unreasonable interpretation. Buddhist texts do stress the importance of moral virtues ("perfections"), including generosity, tolerance, truthfulness, and vigor [100];[83]. Moreover, many Buddhists accept both the Noble Eightfold Path and the basic Buddhist precepts (see below) as simple, straightforward, practical guides to leading a virtuous life.

On the other hand, it might equally well be argued that reliance on the precepts gives Buddhism a strongly deontological flavor [14]. Alternatively, Buddhism could be understood in consequentialist terms, given its emphasis on *karma* (volitional actions, whether good or evil) and the importance of accepting responsibility for our actions [23]. Buddhism could also be understood as offering a narrative ethics, with its teachings couched primarily in stories, such as those found in the sutras and in Zen's famous *koans* (apparently paradoxical utterances used in meditation to cut through tangles of discursive thought and thus allow transcendental insight) [59]. Or again, based on its teachings regarding the co-origination and interpenetration of all beings, Buddhism could be portrayed as one of the earliest examples of an ethics of relationships ([42];[56].

To force Buddhist ethics into these – or other – categories, however, is to risk missing the point of the Buddha's exhortations regarding authority, even (or perhaps, especially) the authority of intellectual constructs. Categories like these manifest an inherent tendency toward dichotomization and self-reification; they can therefore separate morality into observer and observed and falsely imply that definition and description completely capture the "essence" of moral experience. By employing teaching methods that avoid this sort of hypostatization, Buddhism emphasizes its grounding in the formlessness or "emptiness" of all existence (*sunyata*).

Emptiness – the absence of an independent and abiding essence – is perhaps the most problematic concept in Buddhism; yet, it is often used as a synonym for enlightenment, and it may be said to be the "fundamental realization from which ethics and other human virtues originate" [86]; see also [42] and [56]. Frequently misunderstood as a state of blankness or vacuity [67], emptiness in a Buddhist context instead refers to an experience of reality that is direct and immediate, "empty of concepts, and therefore vivid and dynamic" ([29], p. 8]).

This seemingly paradoxical "fullness" of emptiness forms the basis for Buddhist teachings regarding the unity and interrelatedness of all being: form is no other than emptiness, emptiness no other than form. Oneness and differentiation exist simultaneously and interpenetrate perfectly in a co-dependence that is "dynamic and multiple rather than static and single" ([56], p. 248). Such wholeness is conceptually unfathomable, but it finds modern metaphors in such phenomena as holograms (in which every piece of these special laser photographs is reflected and contained by every other piece) and quantum physic's theory of nonlocal interaction (in which subatomic particles light years "apart" communicate instantaneously as part of a coordinated and indivisible universe) [95].

Anticipating these modern discoveries by nearly 2,500 years, early Mahayana Buddhists described reality in terms of the "Diamond Net of Indra", in which every particle of the universe contains and reflects all others, and in which nothing is static or fixed [19]. For Buddhists, morality is action in accord with this reality: compassion, based on a realization of emptiness, or "no-self". Again, this is not nihilistic, nor should it be understood as simple altruism; to act compassionately is to be in harmony with all beings. Compassionate activity flows naturally from the experience of enlightenment and constitutes the life of a Buddha [65].

Despite the unfamiliar terminology, this philosophical description of Buddhist ethics – in which concentration, wisdom, and morality are inextricably linked, and all are intrinsically empty, without an abiding essence – is neither totally foreign to Western thought [51] nor inherently amoral ([65], p. 144;[18], pp. 5-6). Translated into Western philosophical terms (and with a grateful nod to Heraclitus), we might say that epistemology, ontology, and ethics are inextricably linked, and that all are in flux, in a state of becoming rather than being. Noted biologist and philosopher Hans Jonas has recently made precisely such an argument, devoting special attention to the importance of this formulation for resolving the "is/ought" dichotomy that haunts most Western ethical systems [43].

THE BUDDHIST PRECEPTS

Elaborating on Buddhist ethics intellectually cannot substitute for actually manifesting compassionate activity. There is an often told story of a thirteenth century Chinese poet-statesman who asked the most renowned Buddhist monk of his time to instruct him in the essentials of Buddhist doctrine. The monk agreed and replied by reciting a version of the Three Pure Precepts: "Do no evil, do good, and purify your heart". The Chinese poet was indignant, declaring that he was interested in the highest and most fundamental teachings, not something known to every small child. The monk observed, "Known to every child but even a silvery-haired man fails to put it into practice". Abashed, the poet returned home to meditate ([85], pp. 69-70).

Indeed, simplicity is among the highest Buddhist virtues, especially in the area of morality. The correct "answer" to a moral question is generally viewed as less important than what the issue can teach the individuals involved about the nature of reality. There are no ethical dogmas and no central authority or governing body to "represent" or "speak for" Buddhism. Even the so-called Buddhist precepts (see Table 1) are generally considered guides to enlightened behavior rather than externally imposed rules of conduct.

However, the interpretation and use of the precepts serves to distinguish between the various schools of Buddhism [8]. The Theravada school (predominant in Thailand, Cambodia, Laos, and Vietnam) generally takes a more literalistic and prescriptive stance than do other schools, such as the Mahayana, out of which Zen arises, and the Vajrayana, as typified by some forms of Tantric and Tibetan Buddhism. For these latter schools, the vow to end the suffering of all beings takes precedence over any dogmatic adherence to rules ([31];[8]), and the precepts must function in accord with particular circumstances ([65], pp. 140-141;[11], p. 202;[1]).

Table 1

BASIC BUDDHIST PRECEPTS
(Mahayana Tradition)

The Three Refuges
   I take refuge in the Buddha
   I take refuge in the Dharma
   I take refuge in the Sangha
The Three Pure Precepts
   Not doing evil
   Doing good
   Actualizing good for others

The Ten Grave Precepts
1. Affirm life; do not kill
2. Be giving; do not steal
3. Honor the body; do not misuse sexuality
4. Manifest truth; do not lie
5. Proceed clearly; do not cloud the mind
6. See the perfection; do not speak of others' errors and faults
7. Realize self and other as one; do not elevate the self and blame others
8. Give generously; do not be withholding
9. Actualize harmony; do not be angry
10. Experience the intimacy of things; do not defile the Three Treasures (i.e., the Buddha, Dharma, and the Sangha)

(After Loori, Eight Gates)

The differences among the various schools of Buddhism can become quite pronounced when the precepts are called into service to deal with modern ethical and bioethical dilemmas. Buddhist morality also presents itself differently in different cultures, adapting itself to the vessel that contains it [92]. Moreover, many Buddhist authors offer their views without identifying themselves as coming from a specific culture or school of Buddhism, creating confusion about what "Buddhism" actually has to say about a given topic [44].

Within the context of the tradition, the absence of such labels and distinctions does not seem to present a major problem, perhaps because it is understood that individual Buddhists speak only from their own experience. An appreciation for diversity also follows naturally from Buddhist ontology, as well as from the historical Buddha's emphasis on tolerance and respect for the views of others. Nonetheless, as Buddhists from various schools and cultures enter the dialogues of modern bioethics, it may be useful to note the different contexts from which certain positions are or might be articulated.

I. REPRODUCTIVE TECHNOLOGY

Open your hand, it becomes a cloud;
turn it over, rain.

Zen saying

Several recent books and articles have addressed issues of sexuality and reproduction from an avowedly Buddhist perspective. Four topics raised in these materials are germane to bioethics: non-coital reproduction; sexuality (including homosexuality); contraception; and abortion.

Non-coital Reproduction

Very little has yet been written by Buddhists about the "technological" (i.e., non-coital) aspects of reproductive technologies, perhaps because Buddhists have traditionally considered all aspects of nature open to analysis, understanding, and compassionate use; in Buddhism there is nothing "mystically sacrosanct" ([33], p. 55). Buddhist monks, for example, have participated in extensive neurophysiological studies of their practice of meditation, and the Dalai Lama once remarked that if studies in neuroscience or other disciplines revealed errors in Buddhist conceptions about the nature of mind, he would gladly correct the Buddhist teachings ([33], p. 117).

Most Buddhists would presumably extend a similar attitude toward non-coital reproduction. As summarized by Shoyo Taniguchi:

As long as technology brings benefits to the couple who wishes to have a child, and as long as it does not bring pain or suffering to any parties involved, Buddhism would find no conflict in applying and using modern biotechnology. This is a basic Buddhist standpoint ([94], p. 66]).

Avoiding pain and suffering, however, is not always easily accomplished. Early Buddhist texts stress the importance of maintaining the solidarity of families and lay out duties of children to their parents and parents to their children ([83], pp. 117-119). These are primarily social duties, arising from the interconnections of the family. Children, for example, were said to owe an unconditional obligation to their mothers in particular, because of the generosity and compassion manifested in accepting the risks of pregnancy and delivery ([25], p. 71). Thus, in considering the harms that might result from such techniques as donor insemination and surrogate motherhood, it would seem necessary to take into account not only physical risks but also any confusion or pain resulting from disruption of family relationships experienced by the donors, recipients, or resulting offspring ([76];[7]).

Buddhist teachers, especially those in the Zen tradition, might also be expected to use questions about the use of non-coital reproductive techniques as an occasion to probe basic issues such as the nature of sexual impulses, the origins of procreative desires, the workings of karma, and the meaning of compassion. As discussed in the sections that follow, these issues have recently been explored in some detail.

Sexuality

Presentations of Buddhist attitudes toward sexuality can range from the puritanical and ascetic to the promiscuous and unrestrained [90]. The puritanical perspective views sexual drives as ensnaring passions, a source of grief and bondage, and a hindrance to enlightenment. On this view, sexual passion is "a negative force stirring up an unending flow of wants and needs" ([90], p. 22), a state of desire that should be suppressed or controlled in the pursuit of non-attachment. Early Buddhist monastics struggled to follow the Buddha's example of celibacy and frequently meditated on the loathsomeness of the body in an attempt to free themselves from its enticements.

Some Buddhists express the other extreme, using Tantric disciplines to redirect and transform sexual desires as an aid to enlightenment. Tantra has been commended as an approach based upon "the affirmation of life in all its forms and the validity of the phenomenal world; the innate purity of natural conditions; . . . the body as a microcosm of the universe; and the necessity of realizing the truth in this present mode of existence" ([90], p. 60). Sadly, genuine Tantra has frequently been confused with and sullied by untrained and self-serving attempts to master its profound mysteries.

Mahayana Buddhism steers a middle way between these two extremes, recognizing that human sexual urges can lead to deluded, self-centered actions, yet appreciating that these same drives can form the basis for life-giving and life-affirming intimacy ([2], pp. 37-48;[65], p. 139). Zen, in particular, has been characterized as "Tantra purified of excess" ([90], p. 85). As expressed by Zen teacher Robert Aitken Roshi:

The sexual drive is part of the human path of self-realization. With our modern, relatively permissive sexual mores, we have increased opportunity to explore our human nature through sexual relationships. At the same time, of course, there is more opportunity for self-centered people to use sex as a means for personal power. The path you choose rises from your fundamental purpose. Why are you here? ([2], p. 41).

Celibacy formed a central part of the monastic tradition in China and southeast Asia, but Japanese Buddhism embraced a married priesthood, and members of the lay Buddhist community have always been expected to attain enlightenment "within the context of ordinary existence (which, of course, includes the sexual dimension)" ([90], p. 50). Although celibacy is still an option, many American Buddhist communities have followed the Japanese example, accepting responsible sexual activity in both the lay and monastic communities.

The path of sexual responsibility presumably offers itself to all who seek to realize and manifest Buddha nature ([2], pp. 37-48). However, in the early days of Buddhism, homosexual activity was officially condemned by both the puritan and the Tantric traditions ([90], pp. 139-1400, and homosexuals were denied ordination, apparently because it was believed they could not or would not control their sexual behavior [101]. Yet the extent to which special disapprobation fell on homosexual as opposed to heterosexual drives and activities is not clear [101]. For example, the monastic rules for celibate monks (Vinaya) proscribe homosexual activity as a breach of the monastic vow, but such activities do not seem to have been singled out as especially evil or immoral: ". . . if a monk's penis enters any orifice of a human being (female, male, hermaphrodite, or eunuch), a nonhuman (demon or ghost), or an animal, even if the penetration is only the length of a sesame seed, it is grounds for expulsion (from the Order of Celibates)" ([90], p. 33).

Nor is it clear how much, if any, condemnation continues at present time. Asked for his opinion on the morality of homosexual activity, the Dalai Lama reportedly replied, "Sex is sex". Similarly, Aitken Roshi observes that Buddha nature is neither heterosexual nor homosexual, yet, at the same time, it is both heterosexual and homosexual ([2], p. 42). Thus, although Buddhist scholar and translator John Stevens suggests that acceptance of homosexuality remains controversial ([2], pp. 139-140), modern Buddhist sexual ethics seems to emphasize the integrity rather than the form of sexual activities, placing a central focus on avoiding sex that is self-serving or disregarding of others ([65], p. 139;[2], pp. 37-48;[90], pp. 140-141).

Contraception

One of the potential harms associated with sexual activity is the conception of an unwanted child. Early Tibetan Buddhists had knowledge of both temporary and permanent contraceptives, but apparently discouraged contraception as a possible interference in the workings of karma ([26] (cited in [90]). On the other hand, the necessity for birth control was always tacitly acknowledged, and various methods of contraception were regularly employed: "abstention from sex (the rhythm method), control of the male's ejaculation, and from the time of the Buddha, birth control pills" ([2], p. 139).

Some of the concerns about the use of contraceptives may have related to matters of safety. While providing abortifacients to pregnant women was forbidden under the *Vinaya* (see below), preparing fertility or contraceptive potions was apparently punished only if the woman who used the preparation died ([2], p. 35 (citing [38]). Although the early Buddhists opposed the taking of life, including prenatal life, marriage and reproduction held no privileged place within the tradition; in fact, these were generally considered secular rather than religious concerns, and there was "a decisive turning away from the [religious] sanctioning of fertility" ([58], p. 21).

These attitudes followed Buddhism as it moved into Southeast Asia, China, and Japan, and gradually evolved into a justification of contraception, so long as it was not used to promote a promiscuous life-style but rather as an aid to family planning and as a means to prevent personal, economic, or social suffering ([58], p. 116). As articulated by Shoyo Taniguchi, a modern Buddhist who writes primarily from a Theravada perspective, prevention of an unwanted pregnancy is justified because "Buddhism does not teach procreation as the essential purpose of marriage" ([94], p. 64). Indeed, intentional contraception may be seen as a form of skillful action:

. . . Here we can make use of the Buddhist theory of Cause and Effect or of Dependent Co-Arising (paticcasamuppada). The principle of this doctrine is given in a short formula of four lines: 'When this is, that is. This arising, that arises. When this is not, that is not. This ceasing, that ceases.' Simply put, it means that when the causes and conditions co-exist, there is always its effect. If the causes and conditions do not exist, there is no effect.

From this teaching, it is possible to draw the following conclusion: If one does not want to have a certain effect conditioned by certain causes, one should prevent the necessary conditions from falling together ([94], p. 64).

Modern Zen teacher John Daido Loori offers a different analysis. He focuses his inquiry on the nature of responsible and compassionate sexuality, using the third precept ("Honor the body; do not misuse sexuality") to thrust the question of what constitutes a violation back on the individuals involved ([65], p. 139). Similarly, Robert Aitken Roshi raises questions about personal vulnerability and our acceptance of cultural attitudes toward sexuality. Speaking of the risks inherent in sexual union, he implies that relying solely on contraceptives for protection is insufficient:

. . . In my view we must acknowledge that sex and fertility cannot be dissociated, whatever mechanical means we may use as birth control. Unwanted pregnancy is a painful reminder of biologically determined nature at work in our bodies; karma that cannot be evaded . . . . ([2], p. 45).

Thus, in keeping with his translation of the third precept as "no boorish sex" ([2], p. 37), Aitken Roshi identifies the most important safeguard for sexual activity to be selfless commitment – the cultivation of a life of true intimacy with another, in harmony with others.

II. ABORTION

An old Buddhist story tells of two disciples who were having an argument and sought out their teacher to resolve the matter. The first argued that wholehearted effort and strict discipline is necessary to abandon old habits and awaken to the spiritual life. "You're right", said the master. But the second disciple immediately objected, arguing that the true spiritual path is one of surrender, of letting go, and therefore cannot be obtained by effort. "You're right", said the master. A third disciple, overhearing this, remarked, "But they can't both be right, Master". To which the master replied with a smile, "And you're right, too".

This is what is most poignant about the highly charged and contentious character of the modern abortion debate: that almost every argument – pro and con – seems to emerge from the wellsprings of human sensitivity and compassion. Then, too, very few people realize how much consensus there is about some of the most fundamental issues; for example, over 70% of the U.S. population (in repeated polls over the last two decades) believe that having an abortion involves taking a human life, *and* that abortion should remain a legal option for women who feel they need it.

If Buddhism has something to contribute to the abortion debate, perhaps it is as a voice for this silenced majority, creating a space for honest inquiry into the roots of ambivalence, a place where truth can be spoken without being viewed as a betrayal of either the pro-life or the pro-choice platform. This is certainly the message of Helen Tworkov, editor of *Tricyle*, the nation's leading Buddhist periodical, in her article "Anti-abortion/Pro-choice: Taking Both Sides" [97]. As Tworkov observes, "Everything important about life is important about abortion .. ". ([97], p. 61), and ". . . dharma teachings can be used to validate either pro-choice or anti-abortion politics" ([97], p. 67). She continues:

For this very reason, abortion places American Buddhists at the crossroads of Western and Eastern perception of the individual, society, and what liberation is all about. Anyone considering abortion from Buddhist teachings -- and not from political peer pressure - is thrown back again and again on interpretation and view, on self-analysis and ambiguity. This is Buddhism at its most instructive, demanding an authentic confrontation with oneself ([97], p. 67).

Authentic confrontation begins with the realization that some Buddhists, especially those within the Theravada and Pure Land traditions, view the Buddha's teachings as much less ambiguous and open to interpretation than Tworkov suggests ([94];[32];55]).   For example, in summarizing Buddhist attitudes toward sexual ethics, John Stevens has noted that, until recent times, the Buddhist position against abortion was quite clear-cut ([90], pp. 138-139). Early Buddhist embryology was quite sophisticated, and participating in abortion was considered a violation of the first precept ("Affirm life; do not kill"), as well as the destruction of a potential Buddha ([26] (cited in 90]). Under the *Vinaya*, providing an abortifacient to a pregnant woman was clearly considered murder ([90], p. 139). More recently, Shoyo Taniguchi has given careful attention to other, "particularly Buddhistic", reasons (such as the accumulation of negative karma) for discouraging abortion as an unskillful and harmful response to an unwanted pregnancy ([94], p. 62).

Yet one of Tworkov's main points is that few Buddhists – including those who are pro-choice – would dispute these facts. As she observes:

Among my friends, one consistent difference keeps emerging: non-Buddhists argue, in sweeping socio-economic and historic terms, for pro-choice as the touchstone of women's lives. But when it comes to whether or not the fetus qualifies as life, convincing dialectics often collapse into sighs and hesitation. On the other hand, Buddhist practitioners seem to accept that abortion at any stage, unequivocally, means the taking of life ([97], p. 63).

Given that abortion means the taking of life, the central question for Buddhists, especially for those within the Mahayana and Vajrayana traditions, is "What is the most compassionate action?" For the pregnant woman herself, this means honest and intimate consideration of whether a decision to prevent birth can be made, "on balance with other elements of suffering" ([2], p. 22). To violate the first precept in this setting is no small matter, but to fail to violate it when compassion demands it also generates its own karma ([49], p. 228;[82], p. 376). One becomes heir to whatever one does ([94], p. 62).

Some Buddhists view abortion as a "necessary sorrow" ([57], p. 532), since the practice of compassion is not a practice of perfection, at least as perfection is usually understood:

... We take vows to be where the suffering is. In terms of abortion, this means staying open to the suffering of a woman faced with an unwanted pregnancy, to her lover who may or may not want the child, to the suffering of an aborted fetus, to the suffering of an unwanted baby ([97], p. 68).

As Aitken Roshi says, "Once the decision [to abort] is made, there is no blame, but rather acknowledgment that sadness pervades the whole universe. . ". ([2], p. 22).

Because Buddhist priests have, at least in recent years, expressed sympathy for parents who have chosen to abort, performing funeral services and other memorial rituals for aborted fetuses, Buddhism has been viewed as relatively "soft" on abortion [57]. However, as William LaFleur has argued, the very presence of such rituals may reinforce a sense of intimacy with the fetus and thus serve to prevent people from becoming inured to abortion ([57;[58], pp. 204-206). The *mizuko kuyo* rituals of Japanese Buddhists seem designed to express both gratitude and apology to the aborted fetus (as well as Shintoistic notions of purification and appeasement), thereby establishing a continuing relationship with the parents and relieving their burden of guilt ([57];[58];[88]).

In reinterpreting these rituals for Westerners, Aitken Roshi emphasizes the importance of maintaining compassion for all those involved and of saying farewell to this incomplete but individual and human "child unborn" ([2], pp. 21-22, pp. 175-176). At the same time, he remains always the Zen teacher, using the occasion to raise questions about these profound mysteries, life and death – the passage of waves "on the great ocean of true nature, which is not born and does not pass away" ([2], p. 175).

III. TERMINATION OF TREATMENT

When it comes –just so!
When it goes –just so!
Both coming and going occur each day.
The words I am speaking now –just so!
Death poem of Zen Priest Musho Josho, 1306

Because Buddhism offers a discipline for experiencing the joys and sorrows of life fully and unconditionally, it teaches the possibility of dying simply, clearly, and compassionately. Realizing that life and death are not two separate realities, Buddhists engage the practice of dealing with death in all its manifestations. Some Buddhists, especially those in the Tibetan tradition, emphasize the potential transformative dimensions of the process of dying, experienced through dedicating one's suffering to the benefit of others and dying without fear, without confusion, and without regret [82]. Others focus on its naturalness ([10;36]), or even deal with it playfully, as something like an art form ([37;48]).

Buddhism is a life-affirming religion precisely because it teaches that dying need not be denied, feared, or blithely ignored; instead, as the Dalai Lama observes, living and dying well become one's personal responsibility:

Naturally, most of us would like to die a peaceful death, but it is also clear that we cannot hope to die peacefully if our lives have been full of violence, or if our minds have mostly been agitated by emotions like anger, attachment, or fear. So if we wish to die well, we must learn how to live well: Hoping for a peaceful death, we must cultivate peace in our mind, and in our way of life (quoted in [82], p. ix).

Cultivating peace requires a willingness to practice non-attachment, to abandon the desire to possess and dominate ([82];[48];[62];[17]). This is the central message of dozens of books, articles, and audio and video recordings that have brought Buddhist (and other Eastern) visions of living and dying to Western audiences over the last decade. A few of these offerings deal directly with decisionmaking about medical treatment, and many offer insights, gleaned from thousands of years of working with "The Great Matter" of life and death, that can spur new thinking about how to resolve termination of treatment dilemmas and improve care for dying patients.

Healing and Dying

Buddhist teachings encourage people who are dying to take responsibility for whatever situation arises. Particularly in the Theravada tradition, this may be expressed as "accepting one's karma", that is, bearing a painful and incurable illness quietly and patiently in order to allow karma to run its course ([80];[61]. However, this does not mean that people should not try to rid themselves of illness and suffering; rather, people who are suffering (and those caring for them) should work with an illness in skillful ways, seeking a deep, wholistic healing which may manifest as recovery from a disease or injury, or as a peaceful and accepted death.

To heal is literally "to make whole", and engaging the process of dying has enormous liberating potential ([13], p. 10;[82];[62]). Meditation teacher and healing minister Stephen Levine, whose work integrates Buddhism with many other religious traditions, reports that he is frequently asked "'How do you know when to stop healing and begin to prepare for death?'" ([62], p. 203). His response illustrates the importance of practicing non-attachment in relationship to both healing and dying:

. . . In reality the opening to healing and the preparation for death are the same. When we are differentiating between healing and preparing for death we are forgetting that each are aspects of a single whole. It is all within the attitude with which one comes to life. If we don't use our symptoms as a message of our holding [i.e., attachments], then any attempt at healing which seeks to suppress that teaching slays a much deeper aspect of being. Is the healingthat affects only the body in our best interest? On the other hand, if one welcomes death as an escape, that is a rejection of life, and the same imaginary differences between life and death will occur. In either case we never touch the deathless. We never encourage the exploration of undifferentiated being out of which all healing and wisdom arise ([62], p. 203).

Similar sentiments have been expressed by Tibetan meditation master Sogyal Rinpoche:

... now more than ever before we need a fundamental change in our attitude to death and dying.

Happily, attitudes are beginning to change. The hospice movement, for example, is doing marvelous work in giving practical and emotional care. Yet practical and emotional care are not enough; people who are dying need love and care, but they also need something even more profound. They need to discover a real meaning to death, and to life. Without that, how can we give them ultimate comfort? ... ([82], p. 10).

Forgoing Treatments: Affirming Life and Accepting Death

Recognizing that the occurrence of illness, injury, and death can provide a profound stimulus for spiritual exploration and awakening, Buddhists from many different backgrounds and cultures have advocated hospice as an appropriate model of care for dying patients ([32];[62];[72];[48];[5];[80];[61]; [10]). In contrast, the positions that have been articulated concerning withholding and withdrawing medical treatment appear to be quite diverse.

For some Buddhists, respecting the first precept ("Affirm life; do not kill") means taking advantage "of whatever means of treatment and recovery are available", because human life affords a rare and irreplaceable opportunity to transcend suffering through enlightenment ([80], p. 310;[10]). Seeking and continuing treatment is therefore imperative because "there is the possibility for every disease to be cured so long as life continues" ([80], p. 310).

From this perspective, a patient who seeks death as a means to avoid a painful or drawn-out dying process short-circuits the potential for healing inherent in the experience of illness and therefore risks engendering negative karma, including what some Buddhists would understand as a painful "rebirth" ([80;[61];[48];[5];[10];[94]). Thus, if the motive is self-destruction, refusal of treatment becomes virtually indistinguishable from suicide, and both are morally unwholesome ([10;[32];[80];[61];[5];[94]). Similarly, surrogate decisions to forgo life-sustaining treatments, if motivated by self-serving aims (e.g., repugnance towards suffering and disability), are problematic because those seeking or causing the patient's death thereby generate harmful karma ([10];[32];[80];[61]).

If, however, a person does not refuse treatment for selfish reasons but instead acts compassionately (e.g., to end extreme suffering, to relieve family or friends of extreme emotional or economic burdens, or to participate more fully in the dying process), the karmic consequences will be quite different ([48], p. 129;[5];[91]). Thus, based on the particular circumstances, and especially on the intent of the decision-maker, it is possible to distinguish decisions to forgo treatment in order to engage dying as a spiritual process from similar decisions in which the intent is to commit suicide ([10];[32];[72], pp. 74-78;[48], pp. 128-134;[5];[34]).

The line between seeking versus accepting death can be quite fine. For example, in one account of the historical Buddha's teachings, several monks are expelled from the Order for encouraging a monk who was greatly distressed by a serious illness not to fear death; the monk subsequently stopped eating and died, and the monks who had offered reassurance were judged guilty of commending suicide ([72], pp. 74-75;[10], p. 209). However, faced on another occasion with a very similar case, the Buddha offered the following commentary:

'Do not commit suicide.' . . . If, however, a Bhikkhu [i.e., monk] is very much afflicted with disease and sees the Sangha [i.e., religious community] and other Bhikkhus attending upon him in his sickness put very much to trouble on account of nursing him, he thinks thus, "These people are very much put to trouble on account of me!" He then contemplates upon his life-span and finds that he is not going to live long and so he does not eat, does not clothe himself properly nor does he take any medicine, then it (i.e., suicide) may be excusable (lit. good) ([84] (quoted in [72], p. 75).

Hence, many Buddhists (especially those from the Mahayana or Vajrayana traditions) stress the importance of being willing to forgo medical or surgical interventions, either as an act of compassion or as a means to avoid distractions during the process of spiritual healing ([82];[48];[62];[36]). Tibetan meditation teacher Sogyal Rinpoche, for example, focuses on the importance of fostering peacefulness in a dying person's environment:

When a person is very close to death, I suggest that you request that the hospital staff do not disturb him or her so often, and that they stop taking tests. I'm often asked what is my attitude to death in intensive care units. I have to say that being in an intensive care unit will make a peaceful death very difficult, and hardly allow for spiritual practice at the moment of death. As the person is dying, there is no privacy: They [sic] are hooked up to monitors, and attempts to resuscitate them will be made when they stop breathing or their heart fails. There will be no chance of leaving the body undisturbed for a period of time after death, as the masters advise.

If you can, you should arrange with the doctor to be told when there is no possibility of the person recovering, and then request to have them moved to a private room, if the dying person wishes it, with the monitors disconnected . . .

Try and make certain also that while the person is actually in the final stages of dying, all injections and all invasive procedures of any kind are discontinued. These can cause anger, irritation, and pain, and for the mind of the dying person to be as calm as possible in the moments before death is . . . absolutely crucial ([82], p. 185).

IV. ACTIVE EUTHANASIA

Because of their primary focus on the intent of the decision-maker, most Buddhists writing about death and dying draw very few distinctions between decisions to forgo treatment and voluntary active euthanasia. Those who frown on decisions to forgo treatment insofar as they have any suicidal or death-seeking character generally oppose active euthanasia on the same grounds [32; 10; 80; 61]. Similarly, those who allow an exception for deciding to forgo treatment based on a compassionate intention may allow the same exception for cases of active euthanasia ([72], pp. 80-81;[63];[36]).

Some Buddhists, however, view active euthanasia as more difficult to justify than decisions to forgo treatment ([5];[48], p. 127;[77]). Chinese Buddhists, for example, may incorporate Taoist perspectives in their views on these issues, seeing termination of treatment as a form of "nonaction", in which nature simply takes its course without human intervention [77]. In contrast, active euthanasia, especially for debilitating but not immediately lethal conditions (such as Alzheimer's disease), might be seen as a more egoistic or "u-nnatural" attempt to avoid suffering ([21], pp. 107-109).

Perhaps more importantly, death via active euthanasia often involves a mode of death that most Buddhists find highly undesirable: the patient is purposely rendered unconscious ([5];[10];[61]). This kind of drug-induced unconsciousness obscures the normal process of dying and thus robs the dying patient of one of life's most potent opportunities for transcending suffering and death in enlightenment ([61];[69]). Here the precept against using drugs to cloud the mind can be invoked to affirm the Buddhist ideal of participating in one's dying, such that "it is the individual who *actively lets go*, and not medication that serves to kill the patient" ([36], p. 133). Since the precepts provide guidance for relieving suffering, some Buddhists have suggested that to grant people "release" through a painless (i.e., unconscious) death may be to confuse comfort with compassion ([98];[32];[48], p. 229). Others have noted that, given the nature of karma, it is simply "pointless to kill oneself – or aid another to do so – in order to escape" ([48], p. 135).

Thus, most Buddhists would view an unconscious death as personally undesirable; nonetheless, a few have argued in support of laws that would protect the individual's sphere of decision-making about these matters, including the choice for voluntary active euthanasia ([72], pp. 80-81;[63]). Such arguments, like those offered by Buddhists in support of legalized abortion, are not based on a desire simply to respect individual autonomy; rather, they support the notion of an ethics based on "mutuality and interdependence", in which individuals in society provide each other with the greatest possible range of opportunity for compassionate action ([72], pp. 74-81). On the other hand, the effects of legalizing active euthanasia might be harmful to some individuals, exacerbating pre-existing tensions about being abandoned or shunned during dying, especially for vulnerable populations such as the disabled and elderly

([82], pp. 375-76). Moreover, changes in the law may not actually be necessary, since the mandate to compassionate activity is not dependent on legal sanction ([36];[2]), and compassion for the dying can obviously manifest in many ways other than painless killing ([82];[62];[48]).

V. ISSUES IN PROVIDING COMFORT CARE

Buddhist authors have addressed several issues related to providing comfort care in ways that may be of interest to bioethicists; among them are three that are addressed in particularly distinctive ways: working with pain, abstaining from nourishment, and caring for patients in a persistent "coma", i.e., a persistent vegetative state (PVS).

Working with Pain

Buddhist meditation practices have frequently been offered as a complement (or an alternative) to sedative and analgesic medication regimens for dying patients ([82];[10];[62];[71];[48]). Most of these practices involve exercises such as counting the breath and simple visualizations, which encourage the release of anxiety and self-absorption in order to open to the truth of the present moment. Because they are not intrinsically related to Buddhism as a religious belief system, these and similar meditation practices are potentially available to any suffering patient; they may work particularly well with patients thought to have otherwise untreatable pain ([62], p. 119;[10];[71]).

Several Buddhist authors also emphasize the importance of having health care professionals learn to work with and accept their own pain and fear of dying ([82];[62];[10];[5];[72];[48]). Stephen Levine describes how "resistance and fear, our dread of the unpleasant" can magnify pain for ourselves and those around us: "It is like closing your hand around a burning ember. The tighter you squeeze, the deeper you are seared" ([62], p. 115). He continues:

Much of our pain is reinforced by those around us who wish us not to be in pain. Indeed, many of those who want to help – doctors, nurses, loved ones, therapists – because of their own fear of pain project resistance with such comments as, "Oh, you poor baby!" Or a wincing around the eyes that reinforces the pain of those they are treating. Those who have little room for their own pain, who find pain in no way acceptable, seldom encourage another to enter directly into their experience, to soften the resistance and holding that so intensifies suffering . . . ([62], p. 118).

Buddhist authors consistently advocate a skillful approach to pain management, encouraging the use of medications (and meditations) in doses titrated to maximize calm and lucidity ([82;[5];[61];[10];[48]):

One of the fears that we can most easily dispel is the anxiety we all have about unmitigated pain in the process of dying. I would like to think that everyone in the world could know that this is now unnecessary . . . The Buddhist masters speak of the need to die consciously with as lucid, unblurred, and serene a mental mastery as possible. Keeping pain under control without clouding the dying person's consciousness is the first prerequisite for this, and now it can be done: Everyone should be entitled to that simple help at this most demanding moment of passage ([82], pp. 180-181).

Abstaining from Eating

Buddhist literature, and especially Zen Buddhist literature, contains many stories in which individuals who were very old or ill simply stopped eating and then died. The historical Buddha apparently gave his approval to this process in circumstances where the individual "is not going to live long" and has become a burden to those providing care ([72], p. 75). Voluntary abstention from eating, or "terminal fasting" (Sanskrit, *sallekhana*) was probably a common practice in India at that time; it would normally be accompanied by other spiritual activities such as meditation or the reciting of sutras as a way of entering death calmly and alertly ([22];[12]).

In Buddhism, abstaining from eating, if not motivated by a desire to escape from life, can be accepted either as a form of self-sacrifice (self-immolation) [32], or as a natural response to terminal illness and aging – a "letting go" rather than a death-seeking action ([48], pp. 126-127;[72], p. 77). However, it is critical that the intent not be self-serving. Philip Kapleau Roshi, for example, cites with approval the case of Zen master Yamamoto, who refused to let either his living or his dying be a burden to his community:

. . . At the time of his death he was the abbot of a large and respected monastery in Japan. Having grown old – he was ninety-six at time, if I remember correctly – he was almost completely deaf and blind. No longer able to actively teach his students, he made an announcement that it was time for him to take his leave, and that he would die at the start of the new year. He then stopped eating. The monks in his temple reminded him that the New Year period was the busiest time at the temple, and that for him to die then would be most inconvenient.

"I see", he said, and he resumed eating until the early summer, when he again stopped eating and then one day toppled over and quietly slipped away ([48], p. 126).

These examples are important not only for the light they shed on the debate within bioethics as to whether "starving" invariably causes discomfort in the dying process, but also for the context they provide for respecting oral or written advance directives from Buddhists about forgoing medically supplied nutrition and hydration. Indeed, given the meaning of voluntary abstention from eating within the Buddhist tradition, recent efforts by some state legislatures to restrict competent adults from using their advance directives to refuse medically supplied nutrition and hydration may represent unconstitutional infringements on the free exercise of religion.

Caring for Individuals in a Persistent
Vegetative State

Various Buddhist sources relate death to the cessation of consciousness and the termination of natural respiration, although important "internal processes" are said to continue for some time even after death (see below – Definition of Death) ([10], pp. 204-211;[39], pp. 200-202;[82], p. 253;[72], p. 68). However, patients in a persistent vegetative state (PVS), despite their lowered, or withdrawn, state of consciousness, are considered to be alive, manifesting *prana* – "the life force" – through the presence of spontaneous respiration and other brainstem functions ([10], pp. 204-206;[39], p. 211). For some Buddhists, the presence of this interior consciousness calls for continuing a wide range of supporting treatments (including kidney dialysis, blood transfusions, and medically supplied nutrition):

Even though comatose patients are helpless with regard to their physical body, the conscious mind, which has withdrawn within, may still be working to mentally prepare the patients for death. This process of mental cultivation can continue for as long as the patient still has **prana** present in the body ... [T]herefore, despite the lack of signs of life [sic], the doctor has the responsibility to insure that the patient can continue to cultivate the mind without interrupting the **prana**, and thus avoid jeopardizing the final phase of the dying process ([10], p. 210).

Without specifying the continuation of any particular therapies, others have raised similar concerns, focusing on the potential of Western scientific medicine to take a purely mechanistic view of patients in PVS or dead by brain criteria ([28], p. 24;[81], p. 27;[41], pp. 181-182):

Fearing that ... [the current death-with-dignity movement] may not make adequate allowance for profound spiritual interchange between family members and the patient, I cannot help entertaining misgivings about [it] ... Its members insist that human dignity can no longer be maintained once consciousness has been irrecoverably lost. But, even after the level of consciousness has been lowered and life has fallen into a profound coma, interchange remains possible at the deepest levels of the mind. Under such circumstances, whether the patient can pass from life to death with dignity does not depend on connection or disconnection of a respirator or the loss or presence of consciousness. The important issue is whether the ... person is treated, not as a physical object, but as a Vessel of the Law and regarded by those around him with respectful, compassionate care and treatment ([41], pp. 210-211).

VI. ADVANCE DIRECTIVES AND SURROGATE DECISIONMAKING

Buddhists have endorsed the concept of advance directives, such as living wills and proxy statements, as a means by which individuals can clarify their intentions and communicate them to others ([82], p. 373;[36], pp. 130-140;[48], pp. 303-307;[10], p. 210;[40], p. 212). There is also support, based on such documents, or on traditional customs and cultural expectations, for respecting the wishes and opinions of the incapacitated patient's family and involving them in ongoing decisionmaking ([36];[48], pp. 303-310;[10], p. 210-211;[40], pp. 212-

215;[91], p. 21).

On the other hand, several reports of practices in Japan, China, and Southeast Asia - countries with large Buddhist populations - indicate that principles other than respect for patient autonomy motivate and shape the forms taken by surrogate decisionmaking ([53], pp. 22-23;[40], pp. 213-214; [2], pp. 51-52;[96], p. 25). Physicians from these cultures may consider it unwise or even cruel to provide full details of a patient's condition to loved ones, and would expect to bear more of the burden of decisionmaking than a pure autonomy model would dictate; they would, in turn, be held to very high standards of empathy and compassion in order to justify the family's on-going trust ([40], pp. 210-211;[53], pp. 22-23;[2], pp. 51-52). In addition, some Buddhist authors would restrict surrogates from making certain types of decisions, such as a decision to pursue involuntary euthanasia, on the grounds that no one can decide for another individual that dying will be used as a spiritual practice ([32], pp. 65-66).

Some philosophers have advanced theories about the nature of personal identity that they claim resemble Buddhist teachings ([74], p. 280); these theories have been used to call into question the assumption that the wishes of a person in good health should be respected when that "same" person becomes ill [27], p. 379]. While such claims are interesting, and the purported similarities are worthy of further investigation ([39], p. 197, footnote 5), it is worth noting the conflict and confusion that may arise from engaging abstract or conceptual "Buddhist-like" *theories* of personal identity; these are the kinds of metaphysical debates that the historical Buddha eschewed ([83], pp. 51-52).

VII. ECONOMICS AND THE DISTRIBUTION OF SCARCE RESOURCES

While recognizing each person and each person's dying process as precious, Buddhists writing about termination of treatment and care of the dying are also sensitive to the social and economic contexts in which health care is provided ([5], p. 41;[39], p. 211;[79], pp. 244-279). This is in keeping with Buddhist teachings of interdependence, in which all beings are intimately interrelated and mutually dependent, such that the action of any individual affects all others ([19];[72], pp. 73-74).

Still, the focus of Buddhist ethics has traditionally been personal rather than social morality ([83], pp. 135-149;[31], p. 328), and very little has been written about Buddhist perspectives on the social, economic, and political dimensions of health care ethics, despite calls for greater Buddhist involvement in and attention to these issues ([31];[81]). This remains an area for further inquiry, since intriguing insights may emerge from a Buddhist exploration of the ethical interface between individual and social morality ([44];[52], pp. 10-17;[2];[70]; [35];[64];[80], pp. 311-312).

VIII. ORGAN DONATION

The Perfection of Giving: ... *When one thinks, "The giving*
of the gift here gives rise to a great fruit", then give
and take is degrading, like the profit of commerce.
Ethics of Tibet, p. 135

The possibility of removing organs from an individual at the time of death in order to save the life of another (or to substantially ease the burden of a severe illness) raises interesting questions for those concerned with the care of dying patients. Buddhist authors have addressed these questions under two main categories: 1) how can and should one make a determination that death has occurred? and 2) should the dying process of one individual be disturbed in order to benefit another?

Determination of Death

Many schools of Buddhism have elaborate teachings about death and the process of dying, often centered around the concepts of karma and what is commonly called "rebirth" ([78], pp.32-34;[82];[10];[61];[48], pp. 255-300;[40]). In these teachings, the process of dying is frequently described as occurring in various stages leading up to rebirth, and respectful care of the dying and newly dead is considered essential to help assure that this rebirth will be propitious ([82], pp. 244-298;[40];[48]). These stages may be understood as the progressive dissolution of the physical and mental elements of existence: "each stage of the dissolution has its physical and psychological effect on the dying person, and is reflected by external, physical signs as well as inner experiences" ([82], p. 250).

Traditionally, Buddhists have identified the loss of consciousness and the cessation of spontaneous respiration as the most prominent external signs of death ([10], pp. 204-211;[39], pp. 200-202;[82], p. 253;[72], p. 68), but important internal processes of dissolution are believed to continue for some time after the vital signs are extinguished. A form of "inner respiration" may continue for from roughly twenty minutes ([82], p. 253) to two hours ([40], p. 227) after the cessation of breathing and heartbeat, and the life force may remain present in subtle forms for from several hours ([40], pp. 227-228) to several days ([48], pp. 164-165). Most Buddhists therefore try to avoid moving the body for several hours after death and will generally wait from one to three or more days before proceeding with burial or cremation, in order to insure that the individual's dying process remains undisturbed ([48], pp. 164-165). Chanting and other ceremonial rituals are considered appropriate during this period, and for several weeks after death ([48], p. 176).

Nothing in these traditions would forbid the medical or legal determination of death by whole brain criteria; indeed, it is tempting to correlate descriptions of the dissolution of "inner respiration" and the "departure of the life force" with the loss of brain, and particularly, brainstem function ([39];[40];[41];[10]). However, it may never be possible to say with absolute certainty exactly when the "integrating power" of the substance of life has been irretrievably lost ([40], p. 222-223). Moreover, despite the absence of an integrative force at the systemic level, some Buddhists would find evidence of the continued presence of life in the continued function of cells and organs, whether in the warmth and heartbeat of brain-dead patients maintained on life support systems or in the growth of hair and fingernails of seemingly lifeless corpses, giving evidence of continued cell division for several days after complete cardiorespiratory collapse ([32], p. 67;[40];[81]).

Thus, while recognizing the need for legally and socially binding determinations of death, Buddhists also call attention to the uncertainty inherent in determining that something that can be called "death" has occurred ([11], pp. 294-299;[48], p. 269). Categories and boundaries are useful, as a practical matter, but within Buddhist teachings, points of so-called transition--such as birth and death--are discussed with great respect for their ultimate intangibility ([78], p. 33). Some traditions, such as Zen, would also direct attention to fundamental religious questions such as "What is the nature of the self?" and "Why does Buddhism teach that 'life is the unborn and death is the unextinguished'?" ([65], p. 122).

Giving and Receiving Organs

Major debates have taken place in Japan over the proposed introduction of brain criteria for the determination of death, especially in the context of retrieving organs for transplantation ([45];[3];[47]). Although much of the opposition to the proposed standards has been attributed to perceived conflicts with Buddhist teachings, many of the issues involved seem to arise from other traditional Japanese values and beliefs. Feldman, for example, attributes the reluctance of some Japanese to donate organs to their "Buddhist ideas about reincarnation" ([28], p. 24), but concerns about survival in the afterlife and bodily reincarnation actually fit more closely with Confucian and Shinto beliefs about the unity of body and spirit than with Buddhist notions of rebirth ([41], p. 185).

However, Buddhists may indeed be extremely sensitive about the need for organs to be donated freely ([59], p. 351) and for recipients not to accept an organ out of an unseemly grasping for and attachment to life ([28];[32]). Buddhists understand a peaceful death as offering the best opportunity for spiritual awakening ([82], p. 186), and the taking of organs risks disturbing the dying process, possibly causing distraction or even pain: "This is a time of the suffering of pain of sickness and death. At such a time, not even a finger must touch (the body). The touch of a finger will seem like a blow from a great boulder . . ." ([40], p. 229).

To avoid these potential harms requires that the prospective donor make the choice to donate freely and with right intention (i.e., not for personal gain) ([32]; [82], pp. 376-377; [48], p. 169; [10], pp. 211-212). Tibetan meditation master Sogyal Rinpoche elaborates on this point in his response to a thoughtful series of questions posed by a student:

Should we donate our organs when we die? What if they have to be removed while the blood is still circulating or before the process of dying is complete? Doesn't this disturb or harm the consciousness at the moment before death?

Masters whom I have asked this question agree that organ donation is an extremely positive action, since it stems from a genuine compassionate wish to benefit others. So, as long as it is truly the wish of the dying person, it will not harm in any way the consciousness that is leaving the body. On the contrary, this final act of generosity accumulates good karma. Another master said that any suffering and pain that a person goes through in the process of giving his or her organs, and every moment of distraction, turns into a good karma ([82], p. 376).

Remarkably, this feature of generosity is so central to the Buddhist approach to the morality of organ transplantation that it even takes priority over the question of the determination of death; that is, it has been argued that – given a willing donor – a determination of death prior to organ retrieval is not truly essential ([82], pp. 376-77;[48], p. 169):

Dilgo Khyentse Rinpoche explained: 'If the person is definitely going to die within a few moments, and has expressed the wish to give his organs, and his mind is filled with compassion, it is alright for them to be removed even before the heart stops beating' ([82], pp. 376-377).

On the other hand, some Buddhists feel uncertain about the benefits to be attained by the those who *receive* the organ(s), since they may be acting selfishly ([32], p. 66), by hoping "for the death of another person in order to benefit from their organs" ([28], p. 24) or by striving to avoid death at the cost of pain to another ([40], p. 219;[48], p. 170). Some have also questioned the commercialism and self-interest that may motivate transplantation efforts ([72], pp. 115-120;[48], pp. 169-170). In light of these difficulties, one prominent Buddhist author has called for increased research into the pathology of conditions leading to the need for transplantation and maximum efforts toward developing alternative therapeutic approaches such as the artificial heart ([41], pp. 182-183).

IX. GENETICS

Nothing is wasted in a splendid reign.
                                                          Zen saying

Perhaps the earliest mention of Buddhist thought in the bioethics literature appeared in a paper dealing with genetic counseling published in the *Hastings*

Center Report in 1971 [60]. At that time, Marc Lappe first introduced the standard of compassion (that is, unselfish action, in a Buddhist sense) as a potential guiding principle for prenatal genetic counseling. Using metaphors from Buddhism and other Eastern religions, Lappe argued that relying on the standard of compassion would avoid the eugenic tendencies associated with the "Western predilection for attempting to create 'ideal situations'" ([60], p. 7). Instead, the goal of genetics from an Eastern perspective would be to minimize the impact of suffering coincident with genetic "defects" ([60], p. 8). This standard, Lappe argued, would not always lead to an easy validation of the practice of aborting fetuses with detectable genetic abnormalities, unless those abnormalities would inevitably lead to great suffering ([60], p. 8).

The attitudes expressed by Buddhists toward disability (whether genetic, congenital, or acquired) vary quite widely. Pinit Ratanakul reports that in Thailand, for example, doctors are reluctant to withhold any available treatment from impaired newborns, since such an action might reflect a repugnance of the patient's pain and suffering rather than true compassion ([81], p. 27). Similarly, the Venerable Mettanando Bhikkhu claims that "More than any other religion in the world Buddhism values life, especially human life, whatever grotesque [sic] form life may assume . . ." ([10], p. 202). He then goes on to explain the basis for this view:

The probability of being born as a human is so rare, that it has been compared to the probability of a turtle surfacing at random in the wide ocean and accidentally popping its head through the center of the only yoke floating in the ocean . . . Life is an irreplaceable opportunity to cultivate one's happiness in this lifetime and those to come ([10], p. 202-203).

In contrast, K.N. Siva Subramanian reports that in Sri Lanka neonatal mortality is generally high, and Buddhists apparently take comfort in the belief that the death of an impaired infant is the result of the workings of karma: "Quality of life rather than sanctity of life is a consideration because of a strong belief in rebirth . . .". ([91], p. 21]) In China, too, harsh conditions seem to have led to substantial support among the general public for both active and passive euthanasia of infants with very severe impairments, particularly neurological impairments [77]. Ren-Zong Qiu has argued that impaired infants in China stand in need of protection because of a cultural history of infanticide (of both female infants and "monsters", i.e., infants with severe deformities), an economy that makes raising an impaired newborn an "unbearable burden", and a political atmosphere that encourages parents to withdraw treatment from an impaired child in order to be able to have and raise a healthy one [77]. Another possible explanation of the observed and reported tendency to withdraw support from infants with impairments can be found in Taoist and Confucianist teachings emphasizing the importance of leading a meaningful life, as full members of the human community.

At the same time, both Taoist and Buddhist teachings have been used to uphold the ideals of tolerance and active acceptance of disability. For example, a famous Chinese story recounts how the Taoist sage Yu cheerfully embraced a deforming illness:

> . . . His heart was calm and his manner carefree. He limped to the well, looked at his reflection in the water and said, "My, my! How the Maker of Things is deforming me!" [His friend] Szu asked, "Does this upset you?" "Why should it?" said Yu. "If my left arm becomes a rooster, I will herald the dawn. If my right arm becomes a crossbow, I'll shoot down a bird and roast it. If my buttocks turn into wheels and my spirit into a horse, I'll go for a ride. What need will I have for a carriage? I was born when it was time to be born, and I shall die when it is time to die. If we are in peace with time and follow the order of things, neither sorrow nor joy will move us. The ancients called this 'freedom from bondage.' Those who are entangled with the appearance of things cannot free themselves. But nothing can overcome the order of nature. Why should I be upset?" ([37], p. 69).

Several reports on Japanese views of genetic issues have recently emerged ([7];[9];[68]), but again in this arena, it seems that substantial further work will be necessary in order to parse the impact of Buddhist thought from the influence of Japanese values and beliefs derived from other sources. Moreover, in many areas related to genetic technology, Japanese standards may be tracking Western or international attitudes rather than evolving in accord with any particular Japanese religious or cultural tradition [7].

As noted in relation to new reproductive technologies, Western Buddhists might be expected generally to take a favorable attitude toward genetic interventions, especially those clearly designed to respond compassionately to human suffering. For example, the Dalai Lama was once asked "If, at some future time . . . you could make by genetic engineering, with proteins and amino acids, or by engineering with chips and copper wires, an organism that had all of our good qualities and none of our bad ones, would you do it?" To which the Dalai Lama replied, "If this were possible it would be most welcome. It would save a lot of effort!" ([33], p. 35).

Buddhists for thousands of years have, in fact, chosen to put forth the effort to study and know the self – but primarily in ways other than through the sciences and technology. As Buddhist scholar Robert Thurman observes, this does not represent a failure of will or intellect, but a considered response to the direct realization of the dangers inherent in developing powers to affect the world around us which far outstrip our powers over ourselves ([33], pp. 55-57):

> In ancient India, when the Buddha established the Buddhist educational institutions, reality was approached as both outer environment and inner self, the same as in the West. The inner self, however, was chosen as the more important to understand and the more practical to control and engineer to suit human needs. This was not because of a naive belief in the irreducible human spirit or because of any sort of mysticism. Materialists were already flourishing at that time. The Buddhists themselves used materialistic reductionism in contexts where practical, especially in the development of medicine . . .

Underlying the choice of what aspect of reality, outer or inner, is more important to understand and control, is the complex of views about what reality is, what life within that reality is, what human life in particular is, what its purpose is and what its needs and prospects are. Without knowing the answers to these questions, if we just rush off and analyze aspects of the environment, modify what seems modifiable, and satisfy immediate needs without a long-term perspective, our procedure is not likely to succeed . . . ([33], p. 55).

X. OTHER ISSUES

Buddhists have devoted a great deal of attention to some topics that until recently have remained somewhat on the fringe of mainstream bioethics, especially environmental ethics ([4];[6];[15];[17];[19];[20];[24];[35];[44];[46];[70]; [73];[87];[89];[99]) and the care and use of animals by humans ([49];[66];[89]). Unfortunately, discussion of Buddhist approaches to these topics deserves a fuller treatment than the present essay will allow.

New topics also seem likely to emerge as Buddhism finds its footing in the West and begins both to challenge and respond to the myriad biomedical experiences and questions of American practitioners. Indeed, one of the major ways in which Buddhism may contribute to bioethics over the next few years is through expanding the range of topics regularly included in its discourse.

XI. CONCLUSION

The function of Buddhist ethics is to nourish and heal, manifesting wisdom in compassionate activity. In such activity, self is forgotten and the intimate harmony of the vast and infinitely interconnected universe is revealed. For Buddhists, this is a vital ethical matter – *the* vital ethical matter – because every thought, every word, every action, however small and seemingly insignificant, affects the whole. As Francis Cook says, "It is not just that 'we are all in it' together. We all *are* it, rising or falling as one living body" ([19], p. 229).

A Buddhist ethic is thus an ethic of responsibility, for oneself and for the whole phenomenal universe. Yet this is not simply "doing good", for in compassion "there is no effort involved, no sense of separation, no giver or receiver. . ." ([65], p. 22). This is the realization and actualization of selfless enlightenment:

To study the budda-way is to study the self. To study the self is to forget the self. To forget the self is to be actualized by myriad things.

Dogen Zenji, "Genjokoan" [93]

Zen Mountain Monastery
Mt. Tremper, New York

ACKNOWLEDGMENTS

Partial support for the preparation of this material was provided by the Hastings Center Project on Priorities in the Clinical Application of Human Genome Research, funded by the National Center for Human Genome Research of the National Institutes of Health # R01 HG00418-0.

Special thanks to Marna Howarth and the library staff at the Hastings Center for cheerful and efficient assistance, and to John Daido Loori (Abbot) and his students at Zen Mountain Monastery – for all their teachings. All errors of concept and interpretation are the responsibility of the author.

BIBLIOGRAPHY

1. Aitken, R.: 1991, "Interpreting the Precepts", *Buddhist Peace Fellowship Newsletter* (Spring), 23-24.
2. Aitken, R.: 1984, *The Mind of Clover*, North Point Press, San Francisco.
3. Akatsu, H.: 1990, "The Heart, the Gut, and Brain Death in Japan", 20 *Hastings Center Report* 2, 2.
4. Ames, R.T. and Callicott, J.B.: 1989, "Introduction: The Asian Traditions as a Conceptual Resource for Environmental Philosophy", in J.B. Callicott and R.T. Ames (eds.), *Nature in Asian Traditions of Thought: Essays in Environmental Philosophy*, State University of New York Press, Albany.
5. Anderson, P.: 1992, "Good Death: Mercy, Deliverance, and the Nature of Suffering", II *Tricycle* 2, 36-42.
6. Badiner, A.H. (ed.): 1990, *Dharma Gaia: A Harvest of Essays in Buddhism and Ecology*, Parallax Press, Berkeley, California.
7. Bai, K., Shirai, Y., and Ishii, M.: 1987, "In Japan, Consensus Has Limits", 17 *Hastings Center Report* 3 (Supplement), 18S-20S.
8. Barber, A.W.: 1991, in C.W. Fu and S.A. Wawrytko (eds.), *Buddhist Ethics and Modern Society: An International Symposium*, Greenwood Press, New York.
9. Bernard, J., Kajikawa, K., and Fujiki, N.: 1988, *Human Dignity and Medicine*, Excerpta Medica ICS 774.
10. Bhikkhu, V.M.: 1991, "Buddhist Ethics in the Practice of Medicine", in C.W. Fu and S.A. Wawrytko (eds.), *Buddhist Ethics and Modern Society: An International Symposium*, Greenwood Press, New York.
11. Bibel, D.J.: 1992, *Freeing the Goose in the Bottle: Discovering Zen through Science, Understanding Science through Zen*, Elie Metchnikoff Memorial Library, Oakland, California.
12. Bilimoria, P.: 1992, "The Jaina Ethic of Voluntary Death", 6 *Bioethics* 4, 331-355.
13. Birnbaum, R.: 1989, *The Healing Buddha*, Shambhala, Boston, Massachusetts.

14. Boonyoros, R.: 1991, "Buddhist Ethics in Everyday Life in Thailand: A Village Experiment", in C.W. Fu and S.A. Wawrytko (eds.), *Buddhist Ethics and Modern Society: An International Symposium*, Greenwood Press, New York.

15. Callicott, J.B. and Ames, R.T. (eds.): 1989, *Nature in Asian Traditions of Thought*, State University of New York Press, Albany, NY.

16. Chappell, D.W.: 1991, "Buddhist Responses to Religious Pluralism: What are the Ethical Issues"? in C.W. Fu and S.A. Wawrytko (eds.), *Buddhist Ethics and Modern Society: An International Symposium*, Greenwood Press, New York.

17. Chau, S.S. and Kam-Kong, F.: 1990, "Ancient Wisdom and Sustainable Development from a Chinese Perspective", in Engel, J.R. and Engel, J.G. (eds.), *Ethics of Environment and Development: Global Challenge, International Response*, The University of Arizona Press, Tucson.

18. Cook, F.D.: 1978, *How to Raise an Ox*, Center Publications, Los Angeles, California.

19. Cook, F.D.: 1989, "The Jewel Net of Indra", in J.B. Callicott and R.T. Ames (eds.), *Nature in Asian Traditions of Thought*, State University of New York Press, Albany, NY.

20. Crawford, C.: 1991, "The Buddhist Response to Health and Disease in Environmental Perspective", in C.W. Fu and S.A. Wawrytko (eds.), *Buddhist Ethics and Modern Society: An International Symposium*, Greenwood Press, New York.

21. Danto, A.C.: 1987, *Mysticism and Morality*, Columbia University Press, New York.

22. Davis, D.S.: 1990, "Old and Thin", 15 *Second Opinion* (November), 26-32.

23. De Silva, Lily, "The Scope and Contemporary Significance of the Five Precepts", in C.W. Fu and S.A. Wawrytko (eds.), *Buddhist Ethics and Modern Society: An International Symposium*, Greenwood Press, New York.

24. De Silva, P.: 1991, "Environmental Ethics: A Buddhist Perspective", in C.W. Fu and S.A. Wawrytko (eds.), *Buddhist Ethics and Modern Society: An International Symposium*, Greenwood Press, New York.

25. Dharmasiri, G.: 1989, *Fundamentals of Buddhist Ethics*, Golden Leaves Publishing Company, Antioch, CA.

26. Donden, Y.: 1980, "Embryology in Tibetan Medicine", in *Tibetan Medicine, series 1*, Library of Tibetan Works and Archives, Dharamsala, India.

27. Dresser, R.: 1986, "Life, Death, and Incompetent Patients: Conceptual Infirmities and Hidden Values in the Law", 28 Arizona Law Review 3, 373-405.

28. Feldman, E.: 1985, "Medical Ethics the Japanese Way", 15 *Hastings Center Report* 5 (October), 21-24.

29. Fields, R.: 1992, *How the Swans Came to the Lake: A Narrative History of Buddhism in America (3rd Edition)*, Shambhala, Boston, Massachusetts.

30. Fu, C.W. and Wawrytko, S.A. (eds.): 1991, *Buddhist Ethics and Modern Society: An International Symposium*, Greenwood Press, New York.

31. Fu, C.W.: 1991, "From Paramartha-satya to Samvrti-satya: An Attempt at Constructive Modernization of (Mahayana) Buddhist Ethics", in C.W. Fu and S.A. Wawrytko (eds.), *Buddhist Ethics and Modern Society: An International Symposium*, Greenwood Press, New York.

32. Fujii, M.: 1991, "Buddhism and Bioethics", *Bioethics Yearbook, Vol. 1 (Theological Developments in Bioethics: 1988-1990)*, Kluwer Academic Publishers, Dordrecht, The Netherlands.

33. Goleman, D. and Thurman, R.A.F. (eds.): 1991, *MindScience: An East-West Dialogue*, Wisdom Publications, Boston.

34. Groth-Marnot, G.: 1992, "Buddhism and Mental Health: A Comparative Analysis", in Schumaker, J.F. (ed.), *Religion and Mental Health*, Oxford University Press, New York, 270-280.

35. Heisig, J.W.: 1990:, "Toward a Principle of Sufficiency", 8 *Zen Buddhism Today: Annual Report of the Kyoto Zen Symposium* (October), 152-164.

36. Hill, T.P. and Shirley, D.: 1992, "Death in the Buddhist Tradition", in *A Good Death: Taking More Control at the End of Your Life*, Addison-Wesley Publishing Company, Inc., Reading, Massachusetts.

37. Hoffman, Y. (ed.): 1986, *Japanese Death Poems*, Charles R. Tuttle Co., Inc., Rutland, Vermont.

38. Horner, I.B.: 1982, *Book of The Discipline (6 volumes)*, Pali Text Society, London, England.

39. Ikeda, D.: 1987, "Thoughts on the Problem of Brain Death (1): from the Viewpoint of the Buddhism of Nichiren Daishonin", 26 *The Journal of Oriental Studies* 2: 193-216.

40. Ikeda, D.: 1987, "Thoughts on the Problem of Brain Death (2): from the Viewpoint of the Buddhism of Nichiren Daishonin", 27 *The Journal of Oriental Studies* 1: 203-232.

41. Ikeda, D.: 1987, "Thoughts on the Problem of Brain Death (3): from the Viewpoint of the Buddhism of Nichiren Daishonin", 27 *The Journal of Oriental Studies* 2: 151-192.

42. Inada, K.K.: 1991, "Buddhist and Western Ethics: Problematics and Possibilities", in C.W. Fu and S.A. Wawrytko (eds.), *Buddhist Ethics and Modern Society: An International Symposium*, Greenwood Press, New York.

43. Jonas, H.: 1984, *The Imperative of Responsibility: In Search of an Ethics for the Technological Age*, University of Chicago Press, Chicago.

44. Jones, K.: 1990, "Getting Out of Our Own Light", in A.H. Badiner (ed.), *Dharma Gaia: A Harvest of Essays in Buddhism and Ecology*,

Parallax Press, Berkeley, California.
45. Kajikawa, K.: 1989, "Japan: A New Field Emerges", 19 *Hastings Center Report* 4 (Supplement), 29S-30S.
46. Kajiyama, Y.: 1990, "Fundamentals of Buddhist Ethics", 8 *Zen Buddhism Today: Annual Report of the Kyoto Zen Symposium* (October), 41-60.
47. Kato, I.: 1988, *Brain Death and Organ Donation*, Japan Medical Association.
48. Kapleau, P.: 1989, *The Wheel of Life and Death*, Anchor Books, New York, New York.
49. Kapleau, P: 1981, *To Cherish All Life: A Buddhist View of Animal Slaughter and Meat Eating*, Zen Center Publications, Los Angeles.
50. Kasulis, T.P.: 1990, "Does East Asian Buddhism Have an Ethical System"? 8 *Zen Buddhism Today: Annual Report of the Kyoto Zen Symposium* (October), 41-60.
51. Kawamura, E.: 1990, "Ethics and Religion – From the Standpoint of Absolute Nothingness", 8 *Zen Buddhism Today: Annual Report of the Kyoto Zen Symposium* (October), 71-85.
52. Keyes, K.: 1987, *The Hundredth Monkey* (2nd edition), Vision Books, Coos Bay, Oregon.
53. Kimura, R.: 1986, "In Japan, Parents Participate but Doctors Decide", 16 *Hastings Center Report* (August), 22-23.
54. Kirita, K.: 1990, "Buddhism and Social Ethics", 8 *Zen Buddhism Today: Annual Report of the Kyoto Zen Symposium* (October), 1-10.
55. Klevnick, L. and Hayes, R.: 1986, "Women & Buddhism: Buddhist Views on Abortion", 6 *Spring Wind – Buddhist Cultural Forum* 1-3 (November), 166-172.
56. LaFleur, W.R.: 1978, "Buddhist Emptiness in the Ethics and Aesthetics of Watsuji Tetsuro," 14 *Religious Studies* (June), 237-250.
57. LaFleur, W.R.: 1990, "Contestation and Consensus: The Morality of Abortion in Japan", 40 *Philosophy East and West* 4 (October), 529-542.
58. LaFleur, W.R.: 1992, *Liquid Life: Abortion and Buddhism in Japan*, Princeton University Press, Princeton, NJ.
59. Lancaster, L.R., 1991, "Buddhism and the Contemporary World: The Problem of Social Action in an Urban Environment", in C.W. Fu and S.A. Wawrytko (eds.), *Buddhist Ethics and Modern Society: An International Symposium*, Greenwood Press, New York.
60. Lappe, M.: 1971, "The Genetic Counselor: Responsible to Whom"? 1 *Hastings Center Report* 2 (September), 6-11.
61. Lesco, P.A.: 1986, "Euthanasia: A Buddhist Perspective", 25 *Journal of Religion and Health* 1 (Spring), 51-57.
62. Levine, S.: 1982, *Who Dies?* Anchor Books, New York, New York.
63. Levine, S.: 1992, "No Second-Guessing: An Interview with Stephen Levine", II *Tricyle* 2, 48-50.

64. Lindbeck, V.: 1984, "Thailand: Buddhism Meets the Western Model", 14 *Hastings Center Report* (December), 24-26.

65. Loori, J.D.: 1992, *The Eight Gates of Zen: Spiritual Training at an American Zen Buddhist Monastery*, Dharma Communications, Mt. Tremper, New York.

66. Loori, J.D.: 1992, "Food: Just the Right Amount", II *Tricycle* 2 (Winter), 78-79.

67. Loy, D.: 1991, "Buddhism and Money: The Repression of Emptiness Today",in C.W. Fu and S.A. Wawrytko (eds.), *Buddhist Ethics and Modern Society: An International Symposium*, Greenwood Press, New York.

68. Macer, D.R.: 1992, *Attitudes to Genetic Engineering: Japanese and International Comparisons*, Eubios Ethics Institute, Christchurch, New Zealand.

69. MacLean, V.: 1992, "Through a Glass, Darkly", II *Tricycle* 2, 51.

70. Macy, J.: 1991, *World as Lover, World as Self*, Parallax Press, Berkeley, California.

71. Miller, O.H.: 1991, "A Sharing of Breaths", *The Quest* (Autumn), 65-69.

72. Nakasone, R.Y.: 1990, *Ethics of Enlightenment: Essays and Sermons in Search of a Buddhist Ethic*, Dharma Cloud Publishers, Fremont, California.

73. Nordstrom, L.: 1990, "Zen, Ontology, and Environmental Ethics", unpublished manuscript.

74. Parfit, D.: 1984, *Reasons and Persons*, Oxford University Press, Oxford.

75. Premasiri, P.D., 1991, "The Relevance of the Noble Eightfold Path to Contemporary Society", in C.W. Fu and S.A. Wawrytko (eds.), *Buddhist Ethics and Modern Society: An International Symposium*, Greenwood Press, New York.

76. Qiu, R.: 1989, "AID Confronts the Law in China", 19 *Hastings Center Report* 6, 3-4.

77. Qiu, R.: 1993, "Chinese Medical Ethics and Euthanasia", *Cambridge Quarterly of Healthcare Ethics* (forthcoming).

78. Rahula, W.: 1974 (2nd edition), *What the Buddha Taught*, Grove Press, New York.

79. Ratanakul, P.: 1986, *BioEthics: An Introduction to the Ethics of Medicine and the Life Sciences*, Thammasat University Printing House, Bangkok, Thailand.

80. Ratanakul, P.: 1988, "Bioethics in Thailand: The Struggle for Buddhist Solutions", *The Journal of Medicine and Philosophy* 13, 301-312.

81. Ratanakul, P.: 1990, "Thailand: Refining Cultural Values", 20 *Hastings Center Report* 2 (March/April), 25-27.

82. Rinpoche, S.: 1992, *The Tibetan Book of Living and Dying*, Harper, San Francisco, San Francisco, California.

83. Saddhatissa, H.: 1987, *Buddhist Ethics: The Path to Nirvana*, Wisdom Publications, London.
84. Sanghabhadra (Bapat, P.V. and Hirakawa A., trans.): 1970, *Samantapasadika: Shan-Chien-P'i-P'o-Sha, A Chinese Version by Sanghabbhadra of Samantapasadika*, Bhandarkar Oriental Research Institute, Poona.
85. Shaku, S. (Suzuki, D.T., trans.): 1987, "Buddhist Ethics", in *Zen for Americans*, Dorset Press, New York (original copyright 1906 by Open Court Publishing Company, Peru, Illinois).
86. Shibayama, Z.: 1974, *Zen Comments on the Mumonkan*, Harper & Row, San Francisco, California.
87. Sivaraksa, S.: 1990, "A Buddhist Perception of a Desirable Society", in Engel, J.R. and Engel, J.G. (eds.), *Ethics of Environment and Development: Global Challenge, International Response*, The University of Arizona Press, Tucson.
88. Smith, B.: 1992, "Buddhism and Abortion in Contemporary Japan: Mizuko Kuyo and the Confrontation with Death", in Cabezon, J.I. (ed.), *Buddhism, Sexuality, and Gender*, State University of New York Press, Albany.
89. Snyder, G.: 1991, "Indra's Net as Our Own", XII *Ten Directions* 1, 7-9.
90. Stevens, J.: 1990, *Lust for Enlightenment*, Shambhala Publications, Inc., Boston.
91. Subramanian, K.N.S.: 1986: "In India, Nepal, and Sri Lanka, Quality of Life Weighs Heavily", 16 *Hastings Center Report* (August), 20-22.
92. Sze-bong, T.: 1991, "The Conflict Between *Vinaya* and the Chinese Monastic Rule: The Dilemma of Disciplinarian Venerable Hung-i", in C.W. Fu and S.A. Wawrytko (eds.), *Buddhist Ethics and Modern Society: An International Symposium*, Greenwood Press, New York.
93. Tanahashi, K. (ed.): 1985, *Moon in a Dewdrop: Writings of Zen Master Dogen*, Northpoint Press, San Francisco, California.
94. Taniguchi, S.: 1990, "Bio-medical Ethics from a Buddhist Perspective", *Buddhist Digest, English Series* 26 (July), 58-70.
95. Talbot, M.: 1991, *The Holographic Universe*, HarperCollins Publishers, New York.
96. Tian-Min X.: 1990, "China: Moral Puzzles", 20 *Hastings Center Report* 2, 24-25.
97. Tworkov, H.: 1992, "Anti-abortion/Pro-choice: Taking Both Sides, I *Tricycle* 3 (Spring), 60-69.
98. Tworkov, H.: 1992, "Tender Mercies" (editorial), II *Tricycle* 2, 4.
99. Ueda, S.: 1990, "The Existence of Man--Life 'One Inch Off the Ground'" 8 *Zen Buddhism Today: Annual Report of the Kyoto Zen Symposium* (October), 165-171.
100. Wayman, A. (trans.): 1991, *Ethics of Tibet: Bodhisattva Section of Tsong-Kha-Pa's Lam Rim Chen Mo*, State University of New York Press, Albany, New York.

101. Zwilling, L.: 1992, "Homosexuality as Seen in Indian Buddhist Texts",
     in Cabezon, J.I. (ed.), *Buddhism, Sexuality, and Gender*, State Univerivery
     of New York Press, Albany.

ROBERT L. SHELTON

BIOMEDICAL ETHICS IN METHODIST TRADITIONS

John Wesley's ministry was grounded in the redemptive ministry of Christ with its focus on healing that involved spiritual, mental, emotional, and physical aspects. His concern for the health of those to whom he ministered led him to create medical services at no cost to those who were poor and in deep need, refusing no one for any reason. He saw health as going beyond a simple biological well-being to wellness of the whole person. His witness of love to those in need of healing is our model of ministry . . . ([38], p. 314).

With these words, the United Methodist Church set the framework for its 1992 resolution on "Ministries on Mental Illness", an updating of its earlier (1988) statement on "Mental Health" ([18]). The many descendants of Wesley, including those in denominations that have "Methodist" in their name, have often looked back to his work, words, and influence for moral grounding in issues of health and medicine. United Methodist historian E. Brooks Holifield provides a framework for understanding this influence:

. . . Wesley's interest in health and medicine reflected his sense of duties implicit in love. Caring for the sick, he said, helped to form and discipline love. In that sense, care for the sick became a means of grace to the visitor who cared. But to care for the sick was also to express love, and in that sense caring became a way simply of living the life of love . . . For Wesley, the notion of love was deeply embedded within the self-understanding of a community that was formed by its common journey. And in that journey, Christians cared for the sick because it was the loving thing to do ([43], p. 22).

This discussion of developments in the last two years will again focus on The United Methodist Church, with a few references to positions taken by two predominantly African-American denominations, The African Methodist Episcopal Zion Church and the Christian Methodist Episcopal Church.

I. NEW REPRODUCTIVE TECHNIQUES

Contemporary developments in facilitating fertility and reproduction are not addressed in official documents in the Methodist tradition. Inferences regarding misuse of related scientific efforts were stated before the 1990-1992 period, as were strong admonitions to both church and society to provide sound information and counseling, both medical and ethical, in family planning, fertility, and childbearing. It is likely that advances in medical science that provide assistance in fertility and conception are simply not seen as ethical issues in this denomination. As I noted in Volume One, a concern more likely to be addressed in the future will be the use of these techniques in family

B. Andrew Lustig (Sr. Ed.), Bioethics Yearbook: Volume 3, 217-241.

structures that are not of the "traditional" style, such as single adults desiring to become parents without a traditional marriage partner.

II. ABORTION

Positions regarding abortion have not changed in official statements of the Methodist tradition in the last two years. Thinking, beliefs, and concerns among members of the churches are undoubtedly as varied as that in the general population. Petitions were presented in a number of Annual Conferences of the United Methodist Church calling upon the 1992 General Conference to take a clear stance against abortion. Those efforts, however, were unsuccessful, as the Annual Conferences reiterated their support of the denomination's previous statements. Likewise, the General Conference turned back "pro-life" amendments and resolutions. The only change in documents approved by the General Conference was the addition of two sentences in the church's "Social Principles" that urge the Church to provide "nurturing ministries" both "to those persons who terminate a pregnancy" and also "to those who give birth" ([26], p. 37).

The United Methodist Church has thus continued its more than two decades of recognition that "tragic conflicts of life with life ... may justify abortion" ([26], p. 36). Although general reluctance to approve abortion is based on "belief in the sanctity of unborn human life", a concern for the well-being of the mother may lead to a conclusion that the continuance of pregnancy is not a "moral necessity" ([29], p. 126). Issues of the beginning of human life, so central in some aspects of abortion debates, are not specifically addressed in United Methodist official statements. Alluded to, and held in tension, however, are the competing interests of "unborn human life" and "fully developed personhood". If an "unacceptable pregnancy" occurs, due to "contraceptive or human failure", a "profound regard" for the former must be "weighed alongside an equally profound regard" for the latter. This balancing is particularly required, according to the resolution on "Responsible Parenthood", "when the physical, mental and emotional health of the pregnant woman and her family show reason to be seriously threatened by the new life just forming" ([29], p. 126). This resolution, originally adopted in 1976, continues to be affirmed in the 1992 Book of Resolutions.

The College of Bishops of the Christian Methodist Episcopal Church entered the arena of controversy over life's beginning in 1990 (although their church's General Conference had spoken on abortion in 1978 [7]). In a "Position Statement . . . on Abortion", the Bishops assert that abortion "... remains in its fundamental sense an intentionally induced procedure that causes a woman to miscarry in giving birth". It is critical, then, to understand what is aborted: "Life or human life?" With brief references to philosophical, biological, biblical, and theological considerations, their statement moves to the concept of "ensoulment" and distinction between "... life and life with potential". For the purposes of teaching, preaching, and counseling, they would thus put an "end point for abortion" during the second trimester of pregnancy, on the grounds that "characteristically human thinking" begins to be possible at that stage of fetal development ([8], pp. 4-5). It is particularly interesting to note the secular source cited to support this concept of human life's beginning, an article by Carl Sagan and Ann Druyan, "Is it Possible to Be Pro-Life and Pro-Choice?", in *Parade Magazine*, April 22, 1990.

Abortion as a means of birth control or gender selection are specifically rejected by both the United Methodist and the Christian Methodist Episcopal (CME) Church statements. The CME position also excludes its use for "economic purposes". The latter would advise abortion only "where pregnancy is due to rape, incest, or the fetus shows signs of extreme physical deformities or mental retardation or the mental and physical welfare and well-being of the woman is at risk" ([8], p. 5).

Especially important in the most recent statements of these two denominations is the emphasis on the pastoral function of the church regarding the issue. The CME Bishops emphasize that the "Community of Faith" should be a "Nurturing Fellowship" to the woman who must make what they insist is an "ethical decision". This "Nurturing Fellowship" must perform in such a way that a woman deciding about a pregnancy can" ... sense that the Nurturing Fellowship, her local church, loves her in spite of the decision she makes and it loves her because she acted responsibly in the matter of her pregnancy". She must be helped to consider the church's teaching and be aided by both "religious and medical" counseling. The statement concludes with affirmation of the decisional responsibility of the woman and her knowledge that "she will not be abandoned by her church" ([8], p. 5). Likewise, the several statements by United Methodists in recent years focus on a call to "all Christians to a searching and prayerful inquiry into the sorts of conditions that may warrant abortion". An abortion decision "should be made only after thoughtful and prayerful consideration by the parties involved, with medical, pastoral, and other appropriate counsel" ([26], p. 37).

The United Methodist Church, in its 1992 *Book of Resolutions*, continued to affirm its earlier actions calling for congregations and general church agencies to be involved in protecting the right to abortion in society at large, whether in local, national, or international areas. This right is addressed in the contexts of health and of the dignity and personhood of women. Churches are urged to include abortion as an option in pregnancy counseling and medical practice throughout their mission institutions, as well as to work for protection of such options in programs supported by public funding.

III. MATERNAL-FETAL CONFLICT

In general, positions of Methodist denominations have not changed regarding the conflict of life-with-life, as is noted in the above discussion on abortion.

The language of "unborn human life" being in potential conflict with "fully developed personhood" is utilized in the United Methodist documents to suggest value distinctions inherent in the struggle to balance competing claims of the fetus and the mother. The CME bishops expanded considerably on the earlier church position on abortion, with one important aspect of that expansion being an attempt to identify an "end point" for the acceptable timing of abortion. The position statement clearly implies that the interests of the fetus take priority over the interests of the mother at the time of "ensoulment", or when the beginning of "characteristically human thinking" becoming possible. The normal time for this development is assumed to be early in the second trimester, thus setting the time beyond which fetal interest should outweigh maternal interest. At the same time, the Bishops began their statement by declaring that their position is "dialectic:" "It speaks, theologically, between the claim of the rights of a woman to have control over her body and the claim of the rights of a fetus" ([8], p. 4). This "dialectical" approach proceeds through "pastoral" and "prophetic" dimensions that focus on equipping the woman to be able to make ethically mature, responsible decisions with the support of her church.

IV. CARE OF SEVERELY HANDICAPPED NEWBORNS

"All human life is the gift of God" ([30], p. 140). This theological declaration, which opens the 1992 United Methodist document on "Understanding Living and Dying as Faithful Christians", is a general reaffirmation of an earlier insistence that "Every child ... has the right to be regarded as a person and shall have the right to receive appropriate medical care and treatment" ([17], p. 309). Otherwise, no policy statements in churches of the Methodist tradition have specifically addressed this issue. As noted in Volume One, the United Methodist Church has for some time advocated rights of infants and children, as well as those with handicapping conditions, in ways that would certainly imply an obligation to provide nurturance and care for severely handicapped newborns. At the same time, the new statement on living and dying recognizes that "When a person's suffering is unbearable and irreversible or when the burdens of living outweigh the benefits for a person suffering from a terminal or fatal illness, the cessation of life may be considered a relative good" ([30], p. 142). The questions of whether a handicapped newborn has conditions of such severity as to have no opportunity for "growth and realization" are difficult ones, and the discussion that has taken place generally in medical ethics has not been addressed thus far in official Methodist policy statements, beyond laudable expectations of "considered and respectful care" to be given to all persons, regardless of age.

V. CONSENT TO TREATMENT AND EXPERIMENTATION

The 1992 "Social Principles" of The United Methodist Church reaffirmed that "those engaged in research shall use human beings only after obtaining full, rational and uncoerced consent" ([26], p. 42). The principle of consent has been a consistent theme throughout this church's policy statements about health care, especially with regard to individual autonomy and patient participation in medical treatment decisions. The role of the care-giving community in assuring that persons are sufficiently well informed to participate and give consent has often been emphasized. One recent example is found in "Understanding Living and Dying as Faithful Christians":

The right of persons to accept or reject treatment is protected in a just society by norms and procedures that involve the patient as an active participant in medical decisions. In order to safeguard the right of self-determination at a time when one may lack decision-making capacity due to dementia or unconsciousness, individuals are encouraged to designate a proxy or execute a durable power of attorney and to stipulate, in written advance directives, guidelines for their treatment in terminal illness.

All persons are endowed with the gift of freedom and are accountable to God and their covenant community for their decisions. Congregations and other church groups can play a particularly important role helping their members provide written guidance for their treatment in terminal illness and find support for implementing their own directives or those of others ([30], p. 147).

Another example, from the 1992 United Methodist General Conference, is a short statement on "Circumcision". All "involved doctors and medical institutions" are encouraged to "inform fully the parents of every newborn male concerning all the risks and benefits of circumcision prior to the giving of their consent for the procedure" ([32], p. 121).

VI. CONFIDENTIALITY

Resolutions adopted in recent years by The United Methodist Church have placed a high priority on confidentiality in medical counsel and treatment, as well as pastoral care, for a wide range of conditions and situations. Of special note is an expansion of the "Social Principles" section on genetic technology, including more stringent language regarding confidentiality. The 1988 statement had stated that "The knowledge of the chromosomes of any individual must in no case be used to his or her disadvantage. Such knowledge shall be liable to medical secrecy, to strict privacy and data protection" ([10], p. 26). The 1992 rewriting specifies:

Genetic data of individuals and their families should be kept secret and held in strict confidence unless confidentiality is waived by the individual, or by his or her family, or unless the collection and use of genetic identification data is supported by an appropriate court order ([26], p. 42).

VII. EQUITABLE ACCESS TO HEALTH CARE

The "right" to adequate health care is one of several rights reaffirmed in the 1992 edition of The United Methodist Church's Social Principles.   In connection with the Health Care Access Campaign, retired Bishop Leontine T.C. Kelly asserts, "Our driving concern is rooted in our religious understanding that everyone in the United States today has a right to health care" ([50], p. 29). These rights are to be guaranteed and protected by governments, and the church takes seriously its task to "hold governments responsible" for such protection ([26], p. 47). A significant number of policy statements in recent years have addressed access to health care in a variety of ways, as was demonstrated in Volume one. "Our basic policy position should not change" was the strong assertion, for instance, of a 1988 statement on "Supportive Policies for Families With Children". Among the policies that "we need to press for" was one that would "mandate full and complete access to health and medical care" . . . ([43], pp. 136-137). That "pressing", alluded to in no less than twenty resolutions from 1976 through 1988, is most recently expressed in the 1992 call by the church's General Conference for "Universal Access to Health Care in the United States and Related Territories". This statement begins by acknowledging that "[t]he health care system in the United States is in need of serious systemic change. We call for legislation that will provide universal access to quality health care with effective cost controls". It concludes with a challenge to "support the Interreligious Healthcare Access Campaign and its public-policy advocacy to provide access to universal health care for all" ([28], pp. 395, 398). This Campaign, in which United Methodist agencies have played an active role, participates in a national movement of concern, clearly reflected in the 1992 presidential campaign, for health care "reform".

The resolution rephrased the Campaign's "Working Principles" in calling for legislation providing a national health-care plan:

. . . that serves and is sensitive to the diversity of all people in the United States and its territories.

. . . that will provide comprehensive benefits to everyone, including preventive services, health promotion, primary and acute care, mental-health care, and extended care.

. . . with an equitable and efficient financing system drawn from the broadest possible resource base.

. . . that provides services based on equity, efficiency, and quality, with payments to providers that are equitable, cost-efficient, and easy to administer and understand.

. . . that reduces the current rapid inflation in costs through cost-containment measures.

. . . that is sensitive to the needs of persons working in the various components of the health-care system and gives special attention to not only providing for affirmative action in the recruitment, training, and employment of workers, but also for just compensation for all workers at all levels and for retraining and placement of those displaced by changes in the health-care system.

. . . that promotes effective and safe innovation and research for women and men in medical techniques, the delivery of health services, and health practices.

. . . that assesses the health impacts of environmental and occupational safety, environmental pollution, sanitation, physical fitness, and standard-of-living issues such as housing and nutrition ([28], pp. 397-398).

A final concern expressed in relation to these principles is the assurance that "persons representative of the groups most directly affected by inaccessibility to quality health care participate in all levels" of the Church's efforts to gain implementation of a national health-care policy ([28], p. 398). The inclusion of such participants is necessitated by the drastic conditions noted in this document, viz., "the poor, the aging, women, children, persons with disabilities, and persons of color are most at risk . . ." ([28], p. 396). The document from which the United Methodist resolution was developed was even more insistent about including representatives of those groups. The "Interreligious Health Care Access Campaign" includes United Methodist participation and is officially endorsed by the Women's Division of its General Board of Global Ministries. The Campaign's first "Principle" seeks a health care plan whose participation "must not be limited due to discrimination on the bases of race, income, gender, geography (urban or rural), age, disability, health status, sexual orientation, religion, country of origin or legal status" ([46], p. 1).

The CME Church has for many years advocated in its Social Creed the "provision of adequate medical care for all people" ([5], p. 5). United Methodists have likewise been global in their concern for adequate care for persons in a wide variety of circumstances. Just as the 1988 General Conference had supported the World Health Organization's "Health for All by the Year 2000", the 1992 session produced statements concerned about international blockades and embargoes that restrict access to health care and essential medical supplies ([45], p. 606), and about "strained and inaccessible" health services related to industrial and social conditions near the border between the United States and Mexico ([44], p. 645). Thus, while the most recent Methodist utterances have focused especially on health care in the United States, the church continues to insist on increasing and protecting access to care in all corners of the globe, and calls on leaders at all levels to assure such access, regardless of political or ideological views.

VIII. COST-CONTAINMENT ISSUES

The United Methodist Church, joining a growing national chorus in 1992, recognized the need to control the high costs of health care, while at the same time assuring increased access to both treatment and preventive measures. The most succinct statement is at the same time extremely general: "We seek a national health-care plan that reduces the current rapid inflation in costs through cost-containment measures" ([28], p. 397). The document describes the desired plan as one that will offer services "based on equity, efficiency and quality, with payments to providers that are equitable, cost-efficient, and easy to administer and understand" ([28], p. 397). The document's source, however, went farther in specifying what would be included: "... setting standards for the quality of medical care and guidelines for the appropriateness of medical services; regional planning and prospective budgeting for health institutions; limiting the effects of malpractice litigation; including of citizens and governments on key regulatory boards" ([46], pp. 5-6). The same "working principle" recognizes the ethical issues involved in cost containment: "However, the pursuit of cost containment should not place undue burdens on medical providers or upon those who receive services" ([46], p. 6). Thus, The United Methodist Church is aware of major societal efforts to control rising medical costs while at the same time increasing access to services. In the resolution, "Understanding Living and Dying as Faithful Christians", differences between "care" and "cure" are emphasized. The document notes the temptation to utilize expensive technology for "cure" when such effort is fruitless, despite more humane approaches to "care" in the dying process that are actually less costly. The document also recognizes the skewed priorities in program budgets and reimbursement policies for "technologically sophisticated diagnosis and treatments", even as those budgets deny or minimize payments for "less costly services that are critical for humane dying" ([30], p. 148).

The tension between efforts to maintain and improve human life, and inevitable questions about both the cost and the inappropriate use of such efforts, is properly acknowledged as a significant moral concern. Analyses of that concern, and specific suggestions for addressing it, are not found in denominational statements, but in discussion by individual ethicists, some of whom are members of this religious tradition.

IX. WITHDRAWING/WITHHOLDING CARE

We applaud medical science for efforts to prevent disease and illness and for advances in treatment that extend the meaningful life of human beings. At the same time, in the varying stages of death and life that advances in medical science have occasioned, we recognize the agonizing personal and moral decisions faced by the dying, their physicians, their families, and their friends. Therefore, we assert the right of every person to die in dignity, with loving personal care and without efforts to prolong terminal illnesses merely because the technology is available to do so ([26], p. 37).

This assertion of the "right to die in dignity" is not new for The United Methodist Church; the statement appears in the Church's "Social Principles" and in its "book of law", the *Book of Discipline*. The assertion is also supported by a passage in a 1988 resolution on "Aging in the United States of America":

... our society is called upon to respond to a basic human right of the elderly: the right to die with dignity and to have personal wishes respected concerning the number and type of life-sustaining measures that should be used to prolong life. Living wills, requests that no heroic measures be used, and other such efforts to die with dignity should be supported ([47], p. 172).

What is "new" in 1992 is the church's adoption of "Understanding Living and Dying as Faithful Christians". This document is a somewhat modified version of the common statement prepared by a United Methodist – Roman Catholic Dialogue team, "Holy Living and Holy Dying", published in 1989 and discussed in Volume One. Much of the earlier language about withholding or termination of treatment agreed to by the team of ethicists, theologians, biblical scholars, and pastoral care givers from the two church bodies was adopted in the United Methodist official resolution.

An important foundation for the ethical assertions of the United Methodist statement is stated in an affirmation regarding "The Human Condition":

Humanity is subject to disease and the inevitability of death. Death as well as life is a part of human existence. Given this relationship, we should be free from either denying or exalting death. Our propensity, however, to distrust God leads us to distort the ordered place and meaning of death. When we do, our fears and anxieties become exaggerated and we are led into despair, believing God has forsaken us.

Our human situation is further exacerbated by our sins of indifference, greed, exploitation, and violence, and by the moral failure engendered by stupidity and narrow-mindedness. As a result we have rendered our earthly environment unhealthy and produced unjust social structures perpetuating poverty and waste. This deprives much of the human family of health, robs persons of dignity, and hastens death ([30], p. 141).

A theological affirmation of Christ's transformation of suffering and death into "wholeness and life" moves from the above analysis of the human condition to a focus on "Stewardship of Life":

Life is given to us in trust: not that we "might be as gods" in absolute autonomy, but that we might exercise stewardship over life while seeking the purposes for which God made us. In this life we are called by God to develop and use the arts, sciences, technologies, and other resources within ethical limits defined by respect for human dignity, the creation of community, and the realization of love.

The care of the dying must always be informed by the principle of the loving stewardship of life. The direct, intentional termination of human life either of oneself or another generally has been treated in the history of Christian thought as contradictory to such stewardship because it is a claim to absolute dominion over human life.

Such stewardship, however, allows for the offering of one's life when a greater measure of love shall be realized through such action than otherwise would be possible, as in the case of sacrificing one's life for others or choosing martyrdom in the face of evil. When a person's suffering is unbearable and irreversible or when the burdens of living outweigh the benefits for a person suffering from a terminal or fatal illness, the cessation of life may be considered a relative good ([30], pp. 141-142).

This appeal to "benefits and burdens" is then followed by the concluding paragraph on stewardship:

Christian theological and ethical reflection shows that the obligations to use life-sustaining

treatments cease when the physical, emotional, financial, or social burdens exceed the benefits for
the dying patient and the care givers ([30, p. 142).

It is of some interest that the United Methodist – Roman Catholic report
had been careful to distinguish between benefits and burdens to the dying
patient and to care givers. That statement had concluded that obligations for
life-sustaining treatments cease when the burdens for the dying patient *and* the
care givers exceed the benefits to the *patient*, while recognizing that care givers'
benefits should not outweigh the burdens to the patient.

X. ACTIVE EUTHANASIA AND ASSISTED SUICIDE

It is accurate to say, on the one hand, that no new ethical positions on actively
ending life appeared in the 1990-92 period in the "Methodist tradition". The
theological concern previously voiced by the Christian Methodist Episcopal
Church, that humans not take on a "God-role" ([6]), is unchanged in that
denomination's official statements. The resolution on "Understanding Living
and Dying as Faithful Christians" adopted by United Methodists in 1992 is not
substantially different, in its discussion of active termination of life, from the
United Methodist-Roman Catholic document reported in Volume One.

At the same time, some subtleties in the statement adopted by the General
Conference reflect an uncomfortable ambiguity within Methodism, one
obviously shared in other communities of Christians. The United Methodist –
Roman Catholic joint statement acknowledged that differences emerged about
the status of assisted suicide and active euthanasia as "ethically permissible
action[s] . . . given certain circumstances . . ." ([9], p. 13). The official Roman
Catholic position could not be open to that possibility, and one of the United
Methodist participants in the dialogue, J. Robert Nelson, has acknowledged
that he likewise preferred not to "open that door". The "door" of ambiguity
is found in two segments of the "Understanding Living and Dying" resolution.
The first, discussed in section IX above, recognizes that "the history of
Christian thought" has "generally" found "direct, intentional termination of
human life" to be contradictory to "loving stewardship of life". That sentence
is followed, however, by a recognition of exceptions in cases of martyrdom or
sacrifice for others, and turns to the first portion of what Nelson saw as the
opening of the "United Methodist door": "When a person's suffering is
unbearable and irreversible or when the burdens of living outweigh the benefits
for a person suffering from a terminal or fatal illness, the cessation of life may
be considered a relative good" ([30], p. 142). The second opening comes in
a section on suicide and summarizes the growing experience of persons facing
the clinical, hospice, and home bedside dilemmas:

Some persons, confronted with a terminal illness that promises prolonged suffering and anguish
for themselves and for loved ones, may consider suicide as a means to hasten death. When the
natural process of dying is extended by application of medical technology, the emotional,

economic, and relational consequences for self and others may lead a responsible person seriously to question whether continued living is faithful stewardship of the gift of life. Some may ask caregivers for assistance in taking their lives. Churches need to provide preparation in dealing with these complex issues ([30], p. 144).

Both of these "openings" are somewhat countered by the section on "Pain and Dying". The "belief held by some that euthanasia and suicide" may be acceptable solutions to "excruciating pain experienced by the terminally ill" is tempered by the increasing ability of medical science to manage pain, thus "minimizing the use of [the] options" of euthanasia and suicide ([30], p. 147). The concluding discussion of pain management echoes a major thrust of the section on suicide by emphasizing the importance of "community, family, and competent pastoral care givers" in overcoming or alleviating the "loneliness, fear and anguish, which is often more painful than physical suffering" ([30], p. 147).

This document's acceptance by the General Conference was apparently the stimulus for an initiation of wider debate on the issues in the magazine published for United Methodist clergy. Under the title, "Shall We PULL the Plug?", three points of view were presented by clergy who are professionally involved in clinical settings and/or bioethics research and writing ([48]). Dale Wilson presented a brief history of significant ethical issues in response to the Patient Self-Determination Act of 1990, in "What is Now Legal is Also Moral". J. Robert Nelson rejected suicide, assisted suicide, and euthanasia as a matter of theological principle in "Is it Life's Ending or Ending Life?". Bruce Hilton supported the possibility of "a swifter end to life on this earth" as being a moral act in "Is Active Euthanasia a Moral Option?". In addition to relevant sections from the resolution (discussed above), the article concluded with responses from each writer to the others.

Wilson's discussion focuses primarily on the right of self-determination as expressed through advance directives provided by the patient and/or family that would allow termination of treatment. Nelson and Hilton discuss the active termination of life. Nelson argues strongly, from what he considers both sound theological – biblical tradition and humanistic principle, that the possibilities of active euthanasia or suicide, cannot be given moral credibility. He prefers that United Methodists "shut" the door that was opened "a crack" in the 1992 resolution. Hilton surveys arguments concerning the active "causing of death", including a cautious consideration of the concerns expressed by the Hemlock Society. He responds to Nelson with the assertion, "There is still room – and maybe the need – for ambiguity in theology and ethics" ([48], p. 11). This openness to ambiguity seemed, to several members of the dialogue team and apparently to those who supported the resolution at General Conference, in harmony not only with Methodism's founder, John Wesley, and the "quadrilateral" of Wesleyan tradition (scripture, tradition, experience and reason), but also with a wider range of Christians, including some Roman Catholics who are willing to dissent from Vatican pronouncements. As was pointed out by a Roman Catholic physician who participated in the dialogue (who in his own position held firmly to his church's anti-suicide or active euthanasia line), his experience demanded a recognition that suicide and euthanasia are sometimes considered by very caring and faithful Christians. He insisted that the churches must provide thoughtful and caring assistance to persons in the throes of such dilemmas. As Hilton said in commenting on the option of suicide, "I wish it would never come up, but on rare occasions it does, and the statement leaves room for choices that a compassionate pastor may need to respect" ([48], p. 11). The statement to which he refers, "Understanding Living and Dying . . . ", strongly urges that others become involved in deliberations about ending life, attempting to assure engagement with such issues as:

(a) God's sacred gift of life and the characteristics or boundaries of meaningful life; (b) the rights and responsibilities of the person in relationship to the community; (c) the exercise and limits of human freedom; (d) the burdens and benefits for both the person and the community ([30], p. 144).

Having brought these issues before the General Conference, it is likely that theological and ethical reflection will continue. Methodist scholars are contributing major publications. Especially noteworthy among recent efforts are Bruce Hilton's *First, Do No Harm* and Robert Weir's *Abating Treatment With Critically Ill Patients - Ethical and Legal Limits to the Medical Prolongation of Life*.

XI. DEFINITION OF DEATH

In one sense, there has been no change since Volume One regarding the definition of death in the Methodist tradition. As was the case then, the definition of death, as usually discussed in medical ethics, is not found in any documents adopted by official church bodies. The fact that the United Methodist Church Board of Church and Society, in signing an *amicus curiae* brief in the Nancy Cruzan Supreme Court case ([24]), supported a definition from a Presbyterian source indicates that this standard understanding is satisfactory. In more general terms, the brief cited the loss of capacity for human relationship. In medical terms, the brief listed such criteria as cessation of brain function and cardiovascular activity, flat electroencephalogram, and negative responses to other tests.

In another sense, however, "Understanding Living and Dying as Faithful Christians" has raised theological considerations about the ways that death is understood. The document's section on "Christian Hope" affirms the following:

In the face of the ultimate mystery of why humans suffer and die, our hope rests in the God who brought again Jesus from the dead. God offers us, in the midst of our struggle and pain, the promise of wholeness within the unending community of the Risen Christ. Nothing, neither life nor death, can separate us from the love of God in Jesus Christ ([30], p. 142).

To many, of course, it is not at all clear what a "resurrection faith" actually means in understanding one's own death. The Methodist tradition certainly would not "trivialize" death, in whatever of its many forms such trivialization might take. On the other hand, Methodist traditions have included such common interpretations of death as punishment for sin, as mystical "transition" to other forms or stages of life, or as satisfaction of "God's will". The nature of "wholeness within the unending community of the Risen Christ" is more easily proclaimed than it is described. Thus, the people called Methodist can be as confused as other Christians in the face of death, proclaiming a belief in afterlife on one hand, while uttering questions of what one may have done "wrong" to have brought on death. Coming to terms with, or defining, death remains a major theological challenge and thus an ethical concern in this tradition.

XII. ORGAN DONATION AND TRANSPLANTATION

United Methodists reasserted in 1992 their firm commitment to organ and tissue donation, as voiced in a 1984 statement ([19]). As a life-giving act, as a positive outcome for persons grieving the loss of a loved one, and as an expression of humanitarian ideals, United Methodists are strongly encouraged to join others in actively working to meet the need for organs and tissues. This is also affirmed in a special section of the "Understanding Living and Dying . . ." document:

The gift of life in organ donation allows patients and survivors to experience positive meaning in the midst of their grief. Donation is to be encouraged, assuming appropriate safeguards against hastening death and with determination of death by reliable criteria. Pastoral-care persons should be willing to explore these options as a normal part of conversation with patients and their families ([30], p. 145).

XIII. GENETIC ISSUES

Christians have approached concerns about genetic science and "engineering" cautiously for several years. Bishops of the African Methodist Episcopal Zion Church warned in their 1984 Episcopal address: "The Church must teach that genetic engineering interferes with God's natural order. Genetic engineering is a science which pulls man away from and not towards God" ([1], p. 45). The 1988 General Conference of the United Methodist Church "approved a statement affirming the positive prospects and warning of the potential dangers of genetic technologies" ([39], p. 325). It established a Task Force with an impressive, almost overwhelming, charge to:

review and assess scientific developments in genetics and their implications for all life; take initiatives with industrial, governmental, and educational institutions involved in genetic engineering to discuss further projections and possible impact; convey to industry and government the sense of urgency to protect the environment as well as animal and human life; support a moratorium on animal patenting until the task force has explored the ethical issues involved; cooperate with other churches, faith groups, and ecumenical bodies sharing similar concerns; explore the effects of the concentration of genetic engineering research tasks and applications in a few crops; and recommend to the 1992 General Conference such further responses and actions as may be deemed appropriate ([39], pp.325).

The term "genetic science" was adopted to identify collectively the aforementioned issues, and the task force was thus named the Genetic Science Task Force.

The task force was appointed in March 1989. Task force members included scientists, educators, health professionals, ethicists, theologians, a social worker, a lawyer, and a farmer. Informational hearings in the following areas provided basic data on the issues: Houston and College Station, Texas; Boston, Massachusetts; Washington, D.C.; San Leandro, California; Ames, Iowa; Durham, North Carolina; and Oak Ridge, Tennessee. Testimony was received from geneticists, physicians, theologians, ethicists, social workers, attorneys, officers of biotechnology companies, journalists, insurance executives, governmental regulatory agency representatives, educators, and persons with genetic disorders and the family members of such persons. The hearing process formed the basis of the recommendations contained in this resolution ([39], pp. 325-326).

Although the resolution concludes with a very significant number of recommendations for action, an early section lays out the theological and ethical foundations of the recommendations. Beginning with the declaration that "Creation has its origin, existence, value and destiny in God", the statement upholds traditional doctrinal claims regarding the Creation, and affirms that "The goodness of our genetic diversity is grounded in our creation by God". Human beings are recognized as stewards of Creation, and one sentence in the stewardship section offers strong ethical grounding for subsequent discussion: "Humans are to participate in, manage, nurture, justly distribute, employ, develop, and enhance creation's resources in accordance with their finite discernment of God's purposes". Such stewards are not to exploit or waste, nor are they to refuse to "act creatively with intelligence, skill and foresight". Humans acting in God's image base their power and responsibility in love. "Failure to accept limits by rejecting or ignoring accountability to God and interdependency with the whole of creation is the essence of sin". The question, then, is not "can", but "should" humans "perform prodigious work of research and technology". The document rejects the notion that mere ability should be equated with permission to act; whether or not to do what can be done must be guided by "the principle of accountability to God and to the human community and the sustainability of all creation" ([39], pp. 326-327). The document therefore calls for both ethical and legal oversight in research design and in the application of research to technologies ([39], p. 332).

"Genetic diversity" in humans is to be embraced and respected: "Barriers and prejudices based on biological characteristics fracture the human family and distort God's goal for humanity" ([39], p. 328). Thus, one essential component of understanding more about genetic science is the contribution of doctrines of redemption and salvation to ethical responses to genetic diversity. Those genetic qualities that leave some persons "defenseless", "powerless" and "voiceless" require the response of the Christian community as a matter of both love and justice ([39], p. 328).

How are Christians to gain insight in this "emerging age of genetics", including the alteration of DNA in plants and animals? The coming of God's reign offers hope: "It is both the vision of God's new heaven and new earth and the recognition of our limits which must inform and shape our role as stewards of earth and life . . ." in this age ([39], p. 329). Theological and ethical issues are again brought into focus to explain "why the church is addressing these issues":

God's sovereignty over all creation, our status as stewards of creation's resources, and the Church's nature as a nurturing and prophetic community living toward God's reign over all existence propel us to consider the theological/ethical implications of genetic science. As genetic science probes the very structure of biological life and develops means to alter the nature of life itself, the potential for relief of suffering and the healing of creation is enormous. But the potential for added physical and emotional suffering and social and economic injustice also exists. Developments in genetic science compel our reevaluation of accepted theological/ethical issues, including determinism versus free will, the nature of sin, just distribution of resources, the status of human beings in relation to other forms of life, and the meaning of personhood ([39], p. 329).

Referring to a position taken by the General Conference in 1984, genes are declared to be "a part of the common heritage of all peoples". Thus, serious theological and ethical concerns are raised by claims to exclusive ownership rights of genetic materials for technological purposes. Patenting must be assessed then, for both its negative potential to invade common property and for its positive potential to support new developments.

Medical and health issues are of particular concern in relation to genetic science and technology:

a. We support the right of all persons to health care and health-care resources regardless of their genetic or medical conditions.

b. We support equal access to medical resources including genetic testing and genetic counseling by appropriately educated and trained health-care professionals. We affirm that responsible stewardship of God's gift of human life implies access of all persons to genetic counseling throughout their reproductive life.

c. We support human gene therapies that produce changes that cannot be passed on to offspring (somatic), but believe that they should be limited to the alleviation of suffering caused by disease. We urge that guidelines and government regulations be developed for the use of all gene therapies. We oppose therapy that results in changes that can be passed to offspring (germ-line therapy) until its safety and the certainty of its effects can be demonstrated and until risks to human life can be demonstrated to be minimal.

d. We support the use of recombinant DNA for the purposes of genetic therapy and the prevention of genetic disorders. However, we oppose its use for eugenic purposes or genetic enhancements designed merely for cosmetic purposes or social advantage ([39], p. 335).

Overall, the statement insists that time is short, and the church is encouraged to become involved at all levels in research, debate, discussion, and decision-making on these issues.

XIV. RESOURCE ALLOCATION: LEGITIMATE CONTROL AND STEWARDSHIP

Methodism was born in an era of increasing awareness of inequities in the distribution of life's goods, including health care. John Wesley has been credited with influencing democratization in the England of his time; as Martin Marty puts it, "... some prominent historians have argued that [Wesley] bought off discontent and channeled energies so that England was spared a shooting revolution" ([43], p. xii). Twentieth-century followers of Wesley, in their writings from the 1908 Social Creed through official statements in 1992, have demonstrated increasing awareness of how resources are owned, managed, controlled, distributed, and redistributed. A thorough analysis of the 1992 *Book of Resolutions* from the perspective of how resources are controlled would demonstrate that deepening perceptions of stewardship have led increasingly to calls for more shared and sensitive management of environmental resources. Issues that have been discussed include rural development, the distribution of infant formula in developing countries, industrial expansion, safety in the workplace, the needs of farm workers, world hunger and poverty, Native American issues, and health and bioethics concerns.

One example of such discussion is the 1992 resolution, "Enabling Financial Support For Domestic Programs", which examines both the effects of and opportunities created by reduced military spending. Among programs to which public funds should be redistributed, the resolution lists "adequate health care" and other social programs that would have an effect on health ([49], p. 499). Another example is the lengthy 1992 resolution on genetic science, which encourages public funding of genetic research projects in order that more public accountability of the outcome and direction of such research can be assured ([39], p. 333). A third example is a 1992 resolution, "Drug and Alcohol Concerns", which discusses health issues related to tobacco usage. The resolution recommends targeting domestic advertising and international marketing plans of tobacco companies and urges the Agriculture Department and other government agencies to work toward the orderly transition of the tobacco industry into "other, more benign, lines of production" ([36], p. 235). Finally, the recognition that toxic wastes are much more likely to be disposed of on land inhabited primarily by racial minorities led to an identification of such practice as "environmental racism", and a call to the church at large to participate in gaining control over this major health hazard ([35], pp 67-70).

XV. AIDS AND RELATED ISSUES

The Bishops of The African Methodist Episcopal Zion Church introduced their comments on Acquired Immune Deficiency Syndrome (AIDS) in an especially gripping fashion. After asking what AIDS is, and providing a dictionary definition of it, they continued:

> But AIDS is more than this. It is an enemy that deprives infants and youth of their futures; that deprives the world of contributions of future scientists, teachers, engineers whose lives are snuffed out far too soon; that takes from parents valuable moments which should be shared and remembered with children; that prevents grandparents from expounding words of wisdom to grandchildren; that holds young adults captive, preventing them from seeing the beauty and vastness of the world ([2], p. 23).

This Bishops' address is especially compelling in comparison to their address of 1988. The earlier statement had more to say about the various "sins against God and society" that produce AIDS than it did about the victims of AIDS. Adultery, fornication, homosexuality, lesbianism, and infidelity were twice denounced as "ungodly and unChristian", although the address also emphasized the repentance and forgiveness available to sinners. "Sociological links" were acknowledged between the spread of AIDS and drug abuse, use of contaminated needles, contaminated blood in transfusions, and heterosexual transmission of AIDS. Three brief sentences spoke to serving AIDS victims, concluding with: "Jesus Christ cares, and so should the Church ([2], p. 16). Four years later, however, the Bishops declare AIDS to be "a problem of people, not of classes. As long as the Church is in the business of caring for people, we cannot afford the luxury of condemning people . . ." ([3], p. 23). Instead, they would commit the church to "a wholesome educational approach and . . . scientific and medical controls".

Following the lead of three of its General Boards – Discipleship, Church and Society, and Global Ministries – The United Methodist Church in its 1988 General Conference officially adopted a comprehensive statement on "AIDS and the Healing Ministry of the Church". Placing the issue in the context of the "Gospel of Wholeness", the church resolved to function as a "healing community, empowered by the Holy Spirit, . . . called to confession, celebration and action" ([25], pp. 115-116). The confession was as follows:

> . . .until now our response to AIDS has been tardy and inadequate; . . . we have failed to call political leaders to account for their slowness and lack of compassion; and . . . when challenged

by the assertion that AIDS is God's punishment we have failed to offer a grace-filled alternative, consistent with an understanding of the whole Gospel of Jesus Christ ([25], pp. 116-117).

The "celebration" and thanksgiving was for persons who had developed service and educational ministries and who had provided leadership and guidance at all levels of the church. The intended action was lengthy and comprehensive, touching on: pastoral and medical care; educational efforts involving scientific/medical, and theological/biblical components; collaborative ministries involving community, interfaith, and ecumenical efforts; worship life that provides both pastoral care and education; support to those providing care to a person with AIDS; and use of local church resources for response. The church at all levels was called upon to become involved in a long list of specific actions that, if pursued, would put United Methodists in the forefront of ministry to AIDS victims and those who serve them. The work that was to be done between 1988 and 1992 was focused as follows:

The global AIDS pandemic provides a nearly unparalleled opportunity for witness to the Gospel and service to human need among persons, many of whom would otherwise be alone and alienated from themselves, other people and from God. The Christian gospel of wholeness calls us to a complete and full dedication of our bodies as temples of the Holy Spirit. We are called, also, to a ministry with and among all persons, including those whose lives are touched by AIDS. As members of The United Methodist Church we covenant together to assure ministries and other services to persons with AIDS, based on the reality of meaning and hope in and for their lives, whatever duration they may have. We acknowledge the spiritual and personal growth that can be experienced by persons facing AIDS in their own life or the life of a loved one, and we give thanks for the witness to God's empowering love contained in that growth. We ask for God's guidance that we might respond in ways that bear witness always to Jesus's own compassionate ministry of healing and reconciliation; and that to this end we might love one another and care for one another with the same unmeasured and unconditional love that Jesus embodied ([25], p. 120).

By 1992, United Methodist involvement in all aspects of AIDS ministry resulted in the document adopted by the General Conference, "The Church and the Global HIV/AIDS Epidemic". In relatively brief form, information is provided about the extent of the epidemic world-wide, the ways that it is transmitted, the forms of impact on economic, social, demographic, political and health systems, and the extent to which the Church had responded around the globe since 1988. Local churches are urged to "be places of openness where persons whose lives have been touched by HIV-infection and illness can name their pain and reach out for compassion, understanding, and acceptance in the presence of persons who bear Christ's name" ([40], p. 566). This openness is meant to extend to care and support for the ill and their families, as well as to education and support for refraining from behavior that transmits HIV infection. General program agencies are encouraged to participate in a variety of detailed activity related to treatment, care, research, education and advocacy. The document urges annual conferences (regional groupings) and episcopal leadership to provide necessary stimulation and support for local activities. The extent of the denomination's commitment and its theological context are clear in the concluding portion of the document:

The unconditional love of God, witnessed to and manifested throughout Christ's healing ministry, provides an ever-present sign and call to the church and all persons of faith to be involved in efforts to prevent the spread of HIV infection, to provide care and treatment to those who are already infected and ill, to uphold the preciousness of God's creation through proclamation and affirmation and to be a harbinger of hope, mercy, goodness, forgiveness, and reconciliation within the world.

The United Methodist Church unequivocally condemns the rejection and neglect of persons with HIV-infection and illness and all crimes of hate aimed at persons with HIV infection or who are presumed to be carriers of the virus. The United Methodist Church advocates the full involvement of the church at all levels to be in ministry with and to respond fully to the needs of persons, families, and communities whose lives have been affected by HIV-infection and illness. In keeping with our faith in the risen Christ we confess our belief that God has received those who have died, that the wounds of living loved ones will be healed, and that Christ, through the Holy Spirit, is present among us as we strive to exemplify what it means to be bearers of Christ's name in the midst of the global HIV/AIDS epidemic ([40], p. 568).

XVI. ENVIRONMENTAL ISSUES

"Humankind is destroying the global ecological balance which provides the life-support systems for the planet" ([33], p. 62). With this ominous declaration, United Methodists began their most recent declaration on the environment, continuing a tradition of concern that, in its modern manifestation goes back to the 1908 "Social Creed", but finds its origins in John Wesley's concerns with industrial and sanitation issues of his own day. The Methodist Episcopal Church (the northern portion of the denomination at the time) adopted a Social Creed in 1908 that included a focus on health and environment hazards faced by workers. General Conferences of The Methodist Church, in the 1940's, 50's and 60's, urged active conservation measures in the face of soil erosion and dwindling natural resource reserves. These statements included emphasis on stewardship and the ethical claim that "community rights take precedence over property rights" ([34], p. 72). In 1984, The United Methodist Church adopted a commitment to "Environmental Stewardship" which included a succinct grounding of the moral commitment in biblical and theological tradition. A brief discussion of the Greek terms, *oikos, oikonomos,* and *oikonomia* leads to a "broad" conclusion that "stewardship, economics, and ecology are, and should be, related. Indeed, a 'faithful and wise steward' (Luke 12:42) must relate them". Equally important is the Judaic understanding of *shalom,* which provides the goal of wholeness and harmony for the steward ([34], p. 71).

Ethical affirmations and specific program directions in 1992 are grounded in confession that has considerable moral significance:

Confronted with the massive crisis of the deterioration of God's creation and faced with the question of the ultimate survival of life, we ask God's forgiveness for our participation in this destruction of God's creation. We have misused God's good creation. We have confused God's call for us to be faithful stewards of creation with a license to use all of creation as we see fit. The first humans had to leave the Garden of Eden when they decided they had permission to use all of creation despite warnings to the contrary. We have denied that God's covenant is with all living creatures (Gen. 9:9). We have even denied that all of the human family should enjoy the covenant. We forget that the good news that we are called to proclaim includes the promise that Jesus Christ came to redeem all creation (Col. 1:15-20).

We believe that at the center of the vision of shalom is the integration of environmental, economic, and social justice.

We are called to eliminate over-consumption as a life-style, thus using lower levels of finite natural resources.

We are called to seek a new life-style rooted in justice and peace.

We are called to establish new priorities in a world where 40,000 children die of hunger each day.

Therefore, we are called to a global sense of community, solidarity leading to a new world system of international relationships and economic/environmental order. In this way the misery of one billion poor now living in absolute poverty can be alleviated and the living ecosystem be saved ([33], p. 63).

The vast majority of the program recommendations making up the body of this 1992 resolution have implications for health and medical concerns. Though not couched in the language of much of the "medical ethics" literature of recent years, concerns for acid rain, the "greenhouse effect", depletion of the ozone layer, reforestation, sound agricultural practices, limitations of water quantity and quality, all have profound meanings in regard to individual and group health.

The importance of bringing social ethics to bear on these matters is highlighted in the 1992 resolution on "Environmental Racism". Because "[r]ace is consistently the most statistically significant variable in the location of commercial hazardous waste facilities" ([35], p. 67), documented situations of blatantly unjust damage to health, even lives, of people of color amount to a major form of racism. When "out of sight, out of mind" tends to rule production and disposal of hazardous wastes, the demands of justice require recognition that" ... 'out of sight, out of mind' is most often where the poor and powerless live and work" ([35], p. 68). The clear advocacy for the poor and powerless in the Gospels, as well as the centuries-long tradition in Christian ethics and moral theology about such concepts as justice, stewardship, and diversity in creation, support the elevation of this issue to major prominence in both religious and secular communities.

XVII. THE MEANING OF EMBODIMENT AND IMPLICATIONS FOR BIOETHICS

It is clear in all statements concerning medical or health care ethics that the Methodist tradition is reverential, respectful, and serious in its view of the human body as the creation and gift of God which provides the earthly houses of the spirit that human beings share with their God. Following the lead of John Wesley, in each of the areas discussed in this report, physical and mental well-being are advocated as divine intentions, ways in which human persons share in the wholeness ordained by God.

This commitment is particularly acute with regard to persons with "handicapping conditions", whatever form those handicaps may take. United Methodist actions have increasingly insisted that the inclusiveness of the body of Christ is indeed *all* inclusive. That emphasis requires reexamination of human community norms that have systematically excluded or made more difficult the lives of those persons whose embodiment does not fit the norms. A 1992 resolution, updating language adopted in 1984, required inclusion of both the "gifts" and the "concerns and needs" of all persons, whatever their embodiment ([21].

Another 1992 statement, "Health in Mind and Body", discusses embodiment in straightforward terms: "Mental, physical, social, emotional and spiritual health are intricately interwoven" ([37], p. 280). Just as "health" is an interweaving of these many factors, the form of embodiment taken by any particular individual is that person's representation of God's presence in the human community. Health and wholeness for all, including that individual, depends on the ways that the community responds to God's presence within each embodiment. This recognition, inherent in earliest aspects of Methodist tradition, is reflected in major programmatic commitments for (among others):

- persons with physically or mentally handicapping conditions;
- children and youth throughout the world whose lives are shaped by situations producing fear, anxiety, anger and aggression;
- changing forms of the family;
- sexuality issues and sexual abuse;
- substance and drug abuse and its effects on all parties involved;
- persons victimized by racism, sexism and classism;
- persons infected by HIV and AIDS related illnesses, and those touched by their condition;
- violence in its many forms and effects;
- environmental effects on health.

XVIII. CONCLUSION

It is clear from this admittedly incomplete survey of the most recent developments in the Methodist tradition(s) that awareness, analysis, and reexamination of previous understandings and precepts is growing significantly. The descendants of John and Charles Wesley, Philip Otterbein, Jacob Albright, Richard Allen, Lucius Holsey and Isabella Thoburn retain an attribute shared by all of them, but noted by Martin E. Marty as a marked characteristic of Wesley:

. . . this modern – no enemy of science and a friend of medicine – was not afraid of modernity. While we may chuckle at some of the Wesleyan nostrums and bizarre medical theories, they were not far off the mark of the best scientific efforts of his time. And they did show a passionate regard for humans in their suffering, a warm concern for their bodies, and a sense that he and his workers must care and cure not only in the realm of soul-saving, their chosen sphere, but also in the search for temporal well-being. That tradition has not been exhausted. It is, in fact, only now being recovered widely ([43], p. xi).

This "wide recovery" comports with the directive of the United Methodist Church *Discipline* to be alert to the reality that: "new issues continually arise that summon us to fresh theological inquiry. Daily we are presented with an array of concerns that challenge our proclamation of God's reign over all of human existence" ([27], p. 82).

The University of Kansas
Lawrence, Kansas U.S.A.

BIBLIOGRAPHY

1. Board of Bishops of the African Methodist Episcopal Zion Church: 1984, *The Quadrennial Episcopal Address*, 42nd Session of the General Conference, St. Louis, Mo., July 25 - August 3, 1984, African Methodist Episcopal Zion Church, Charlotte, North Carolina.
2. Board of Bishops of the African Methodist Episcopal Zion Church: 1988, *The Quadrennial Episcopal Address*, 43rd Session of the General Conference, Charlotte, N.C., African Methodist Episcopal Zion Church, Charlotte, North Carolina.
3. "The Response of the Church to the Spread of AIDS", Board of Bishops of the African Methodist Episcopal Zion Church: 1992, *The Quadrennial Episcopal Address*, 44th Session of the General Conference, Atlanta, Ga., July 22-31, 1992, Shaw Temple African Methodist Episcopal Zion Church, Atlanta, Georgia.
4. Board of Social Concerns, Christian Methodist Episcopal Church: (no date), *Denominational Statements on Issues of Social Concern*. Christian Methodist Episcopal Church, Atlanta.
5. General Conference, Christian Methodist Episcopal Church: 1966, "Social Creed", in [4], pp. 3-8.

6. General Conference, Christian Methodist Episcopal Church: 1978, "Euthanasia", in [4], p. 14.
7. General Conference, Christian Methodist Episcopal Church: 1978, "Abortion", in [4], pp. 14-15.
8. "A Position Statement from the College of Bishops on Abortion", from the 1990 Annual Christian Methodist Episcopal Convocation, in *The Christian Index*, Vol. 125, No. 1, January 1, 1992, pp. 4-5.
9. Delaney, J., and Oliphint, B. (eds.): 1989, *Holy Living and Holy Dying - A United Methodist/Roman Catholic Common Statement*, Prepared by the General Commission on Christian Unity and Interreligious Concerns of The United Methodist Church and the Bishops' Committee for Ecumenical and Interfaith Affairs, National Conference of Catholic Bishops, General Board of Global Ministries, Cincinnati.
10. The General Conference of The United Methodist Church: 1988, *The Book of Resolutions of The United Methodist Church - 1988*, The United Methodist Publishing House, Nashville.
11. The General Conference of The United Methodist Church: 1988, "AIDS and the Healing Ministry of the Church", in [25], pp. 115-120.
12. The General Conference of The United Methodist Church: 1988, "Genetic Science", in [10], pp. 213-216.
13. The General Conference of The United Methodist Church: 1984, "Health and Wholeness", in [25], pp. 273-278.
14. The General Conference of The United Methodist Church: 1980, "Health Care Delivery Policy Statement", in [10], pp. 241-247.
15. The General Conference of The United Methodist Church: 1984, "Health For All By the Year 2000", in [25], pp. 278-280.
16. The General Conference of The United Methodist Church: 1980, "Human Rights", in [25], pp. 506-507.
17. The General Conference of The United Methodist Church: 1976, "Medical Rights for Children and Youth", in [25], pp. 308-311.
18. The General Conference of The United Methodist Church: 1988, "Mental Health", in [10], pp. 268-272.
19. The General Conference of The United Methodist Church: 1984, "Organ and Tissue Donation", in [25], p. 123.
20. The General Conference of The United Methodist Church: 1988, "Suicide: A Challenge to Ministry", in [25], pp. 377-382.
21. The General Conference of The United Methodist Church: 1984, 1992, "The Church and Persons With Mentally, Physically and/or Psychologically Handicapping Conditions", (adopted 1984, revised 1992), in [25], pp. 200-204.
22. Lyons, C.: 1989, "Abortion and Responsible Parenthood: The Faithful Witness of a Church to Complex and Critical Issues", Health and Welfare Ministries Department, General Board of Global Ministries, The United Methodist Church, New York.

23. Lyons, C.: 1989, "On Not Misrepresenting The Faithful Witness of The Church", Health and Welfare Ministries Department, General Board of Global Ministries, The United Methodist Church, New York.

24. Martin, T., Verelli, D., and Lopez, M.: 1989, "Brief of the General Board of Church and Society of The United Methodist Church As Amicus Curiae in Support of Petitioners, Nancy Beth Cruzan, by Her Parents and Co-Guardians, Lester L. and Joyce Cruzan, in the Supreme Court of the United States, October, 1989.

25. The General Conference of The United Methodist Church: 1992, *The Book of Resolutions of The United Methodist Church - 1992*, The United Methodist Publishing House, Nashville, Tennessee.

26. The General Conference of The United Methodist Church: 1992, "The Social Principles", in [25], pp. 31-52. This important formulation of social statements is also published in the denomination's official book of law and procedures, *The Book of Discipline of the United Methodist Church - 1992* ([27], pp. 87 -106).

27. *The Book of Discipline of the United Methodist Church –1992*, The United Methodist Publishing House, Nashville, Tennessee.

28. The General Conference of The United Methodist Church: 1992, "Universal Access to Health Care in the United States and Related Territories", in [25], pp. 395- 398.

29. The General Conference of The United Methodist Church: 1976, "Responsible Parenthood", in [25], pp. 125 - 128.

30. The General Conference of The United Methodist Church; 1992, "Understanding Living and Dying as Faithful Christians", in [25], pp. 140-150.

31. The General Conference of The United Methodist Church: 1992, "Care-Giving Teams for Persons with AIDS", in [25], pp. 120-121.

32. The General Conference of The United Methodist Church: 1992, "Circumcision", in [25], p. 121.

33. The General Conference of The United Methodist Church: 1992, "Environmental Justice for a Sustainable Future", in [25], pp. 62-67.

34. The General Conference of The United Methodist Church: 1992, "Environmental Stewardship" (1984), in [25], pp. 70-76.

35. The General Conference of The United Methodist Church: 1992, "Environmental Racism", in [25], pp. 67-70.

36. The General Conference of The United Methodist Church: 1992, "Drug and Alcohol Concerns", in [25], pp. 229-241.

37. The General Conference of The United Methodist Church: 1992, "Health in Mind and Body", in [25], pp. 280-284.

38. The General Conference of The United Methodist Church: 1992, "Ministries on Mental Illness", in [25] pp. 313-317.

39. The General Conference of The United Methodist Church: 1992, "New Developments in Genetic Science", in [25], pp. 325 - 338.

40. The General Conference of The United Methodist Church: 1992, "The Church and the Global HIV/AIDS Epidemic", in [25], pp. 564 -568.
41. The General Conference of The United Methodist Church: 1992, "Infant Formula Abuse", in [25], pp. 584 - 588.
42. The General Conference of The United Methodist Church: 1988, "Supportive Policies for Families With Children", in [25], pp. 135 - 140.
43. Holifield, E. Brooks: 1986, *Health and Medicine in the Methodist Tradition*. New York: Crossroad.
44. The General Conference of The United Methodist Church: 1992, "United States-Mexico Border", in [25], pp. 644-647.
45. The General Conference of The United Methodist Church: 1992, "Oppose Food and Medicine Blockade or Embargoes", in [25], pp. 605-606.
46. Interreligious Health Care Access Campaign: 1992, *Working Principles for Assessing National Health Care Legislation* (a consensus document created by religious leaders through five national consultations over a period of two years) Washington, D.C.
47. The General Conference of The United Methodist Church: 1988, "Aging in the United States of America", in [25], pp. 165 - 176.
48. Wilson, D., Nelson, J.R., and Hilton, B.: 1992 (October), "Should We PULL the Plug?" *Circuit Rider*, pp. 4-11. Dale Wilson, "What is Now Legal is Also Moral" (pp. 4-5); J. Robert Nelson, "Is it Life's Ending or Ending Life?" (pp. 6-8); Bruce Hilton, "Is Active Euthanasia as Moral Option?" (pp. 8-9). In addition to relevant sections from the resolution (discussed above), the article concluded with responses from each writer to the others.
49. The General Conference of The United Methodist Church: 1992, "Enabling Financial Support for Domestic Programs", in [25], pp. 498-499.
50. Short, M.K.S.: 1992 (December), "Health Care, A Matter of Justice", *Response*, December, 1992, pp. 28-31.

PAUL D. SIMMONS

BAPTIST-EVANGELICAL MEDICAL ETHICS

I. INTRODUCTION

The purpose of this essay is to outline and analyze developments in various
areas of bioethics among Baptists and Evangelicals since 1990. It will examine
both perspectives and activities. There are important caveats to be made,
however, in dealing with perspectives in medical ethics among Baptists and
evangelicals.

First, it is both problematic and necessary to treat evangelical and Baptist
opinion in the same article. Differences between evangelicals and Baptists are
increasingly difficult to discern, at least at the level of denominational
affiliation. However, it is arguable on scholarly and historical grounds that
important distinctions between the two can and should be made ([16], p. 28).

Shifts in emphases in recent years make public perceptions and the realities
of power within and among the various groups more determinative than
scholarly distinctions. Evangelicals are the theological siblings of fundamentalism. Both hold to the five fundamental doctrines. Biblical inerrancy and
infallibility, the virgin birth, penal substitutionary atonement, the bodily
resurrection, and the literal, bodily return of Christ are all necessary and
irreducible foundations of belief and therefore non-negotiable bases for
Christian faith. These particular doctrines function virtually as dogma for
defining orthodox belief (or eliminating the unorthodox "unbeliever"). Those
who hold strongly to these notions will often refuse to have "fellowship with"
those who reject the doctrinal formulation (i.e., belong to the same church).

Baptists hold generally to these doctrines without insisting on these
particular ways of stating them. The authority of Scripture in all matters of
faith and practice, the incarnation of God in Christ, the atoning life and death
of Jesus, the resurrection of Christ from the dead, and a belief in his return in
glory are important doctrines to Baptists. They define themselves as "born
again believers", as do evangelicals. But Baptists also hold strongly to beliefs
in religious liberty, the separation of church and state, and "the direct,
unmediated, undelegated lordship of Jesus Christ" ([16], p. 29). The lordship
of Christ and the competency of the individual soul before God are the
doctrinal bases for rejecting any imposition of priestly, ecclesiastical, or
governmental authority between the believer and God. It becomes a non-
negotiable belief to assert that no group or religious leader may impose creeds,

B. Andrew Lustig (Sr. Ed.), Bioethics Yearbook: Volume 3, 243-270.
©1993 Kluwer Academic Publishers.

doctrines, or prescribed practices upon individual believers.

The distinctive or foundational issue for Baptists is "the priority of voluntary and uncoerced faith or response to the Word and Act of God" ([16], p. 173). Faith must be free and uncoerced in order to be authentic; voluntarism is the *sine qua non* of genuine religion and morality. Their emphasis on the liberty of conscience is rooted in their experience of persecution for being dissenters. And their revision of the Westminster Confession underscores and clarifies their distinction from evangelicals. Baptists believe strongly that coercion does not and cannot produce conversion. Further, their revision of Article 3 shows their belief that Christians sin when thinking themselves to be the ultimate judges of their fellow human beings ([16], p. 176). It was their deletion of Article 4, however, that shows the Baptist abhorrence of attempting to legislate solutions to moral and doctrinal beliefs.

A Baptist's approach to bioethical issues will likely be far more tolerant of differing perspectives/solutions than will those of an evangelical/fundamentalist, therefore. Baptists will support the legal protections of religious liberty, while evangelicals will move more easily from morality to legal prohibitions in good theocratic/Puritan fashion. Baptists will likely see no threat to faith in God as Creator in theories of evolution, while evangelicals resist evolution as contradictory to their notion of creation as miracle.

For reasons like these, distinguishing between Baptists and evangelicals will require more than determining denominational or church affiliation. Many "Baptists" in name are evangelical-fundamentalists in spirit and practice. Pat Robertson and Jerry Falwell are typical examples; both are called Baptists, but both are more fundamentalist-evangelical than "Baptist".

Ron Hamel points out that there are over thirty Baptist denominations in the United States. They are noted for their diversity of opinion, he says, representing as they do a tradition of independence and theological diversity, and a history marked by controversy and division. He calls them "one of the most democratic religious bodies in America" because of the emphasis on complete autonomy of the local congregation as well as individual freedom of thought and expression. There is no central religious authority vested in a church hierarchy, and thus no "official" position of the various churches on particular issues in biomedical ethics ([19], p. 63).

What is true formally is often a different matter functionally. There are strong levers of power and influence available to those in positions of leadership and/or authority, including the directors of agencies, boards of trustees, and seminary administrations. Among Southern Baptists, for instance, there has been a claim to "authoritative positions" on various issues from abortion to women in ministry that various agencies have been pressured to adopt by their boards of trustees. In turn, administrators are pressured to impose them upon their employees. Extensive intrusions into seminary educational processes by trustees and administrators have made the notion of academic freedom meaningless. Resolutions from the annual meeting of messengers are represented as reflecting the beliefs of "the vast majority" of Southern Baptists and thus normative for all employees of the agencies, commissions, and seminaries. Resolutions are now treated as if they were the formulations of dogma by ancient Councils – an approach one would more typically identify with Evangelicalism.

The Preamble to the 1963 Baptist Statement of Faith and Message allowed for differences of interpretation and gave room for diversity of opinion among Southern Baptists. That toleration for diversity is now largely a thing of the past. The Cooperative Baptist Fellowship and the Alliance of Baptists are splinter groups attempting to correct the rapid shift toward doctrinaire and authoritarian fundamentalism. They represent the democratic ecclesiology of which Hamel speaks. The corrective effort has been largely unsuccessful and certainly comes too late to rescue the agencies of the convention from the new ecclesiasticism. It is doubtful that the openness of traditional Baptist democratic polity will ever return to the Southern Convention. The forces of authoritarianism are well positioned to maintain control for the foreseeable future. It is now far more evangelical than Baptist, but the name remains.

A further characterization of Baptist-evangelical medical ethics is a moral seriousness that takes the form of conservative attitudes toward politics and political solutions to ethical issues. The "social conscience" of evangelicals tends toward an extension of what are regarded as personal sins. The avoidance of "worldliness" is both a matter of personal piety and social salvation. Prohibition was an experiment at social reform rooted in a moral revulsion against "demon rum" and a personal piety of total abstinence from alcoholic beverages. Censorship of artistic or written materials that might be considered obscene or pornographic extends the concern for personal purity to the protection due the innocent and the harm done to society at large. That moral fervor might be a virtue can be granted; that it is often misguided in the social context is also arguable.

Further distinctions among fundamentalist/evangelicals are also necessary. The type fundamentalism of associated with Bob Jones University is typically more cultic, with minimal involvement in the larger social context. This type advocates personal piety but eschews social action. Ironically, one of Bob Jones' most controversial graduates is Randall Terry, founder and inspiration for Operation Rescue, one of the most radical and reactionary social movements ever among evangelical Christians.

The left wing of evangelicalism is represented by Evangelicals for Social Action (ESA) and *Sojourners* magazine, and includes leaders such as Jim Wallis, Ronald Sider, and Tony Campolo. ESA leaders are deeply involved in efforts to influence policy on social justice issues, including economics and race. They are known for a strong emphasis on human rights and peacemaking as basic to justice. Conservative religion is wed to "liberal" politics.

Militant fundamentalist/evangelicals, on the other hand, are thoroughly politicized on the side of right-wing issues. They are ideological, intransigent, authoritarian, and belligerent in their approach, and often in coalition with right-wing political action groups. The heavy involvement of militant evangelicals in the political scene for the past two decades is hardly an aberration. Their Puritan forebears attempted to develop a type of covenantal political theology whereby laws would be molded by the piety of Christian believers. That theocratic posture was seen in the alliance of fundamentalists like Carl McIntyre with the political conservatism of Barry Goldwater, and the wedding of Moral Majority concerns with the politics of Ronald Reagan and, to some extent, of George Bush. In such cases, religious zeal is linked with conservative political and economic ideology. A type of civil religion that combines fervent nationalism with religious zealotry has been the result.

The most extreme of all such groups is what is called Christian Reconstructionism. Rousas John Rushdoony, Gary North, and Greg Bahnsen are prominent names in this movement and promote its ideas in journals like *The Counsel of Chalcedon* and *The Journal of Christian Reconstructionism* and in numerous books. These leaders propose to reform society and establish a theonomy under the laws of the Old Testament. The public school system would be abolished as would all entitlement programs. A tithe would replace the income tax system, and an unregulated, laissez-faire capitalist economy would be instituted backed by a gold standard. Capital punishment would be imposed for eighteen crimes, including juvenile delinquency, blasphemy, homosexuality, and abortion. Pluralism would be denied; America would be declared Constitutionally a Christian nation.

While most evangelicals give little support to such extremism, the movement is active at grassroots levels, running for school boards and local government posts. Low-key campaigns have shown a remarkable degree of success in places like California.

Evangelicals and Baptists are thus a diverse lot, and distinctions among them are as important as the emphases that unite them. Careful attention to every nuance or detail of difference is impossible and unnecessary for present purposes. But this brief survey might provide some points of reference for discerning the primary variables at work as approaches to biomedical ethics are explored.

II. NEW REPRODUCTIVE TECHNIQUES

Reproductive techniques that involve technical intervention to bypass infertility are hardly addressed in the resolutions of the various groups under discussion. Such topics are discussed in the writings of ethicists within the various groups, however. These writings reflect the views not only of the writer but of large numbers of people within the traditions. Little consensus can be found on these exotic techniques, making Hamel's comments about a lack of an authoritative position certainly apropos in this area [19].

There are at least seven means of assisting pregnancy that involve biotechnical assistance or intervention. These include various techniques of In-Vitro Fertilization (IVF), Artificial Insemination (AI) by Donor (AID) or by husband (AIH), and surrogate parenting. Opinions differ widely on the moral acceptability of various procedures, but strong reservations are found against surrogate parenting. Some writers worry about the personal dimensions of maternal bonding and the confusion of roles and relationships, though they do not condemn surrogate parenting as such ([35], p. 169-170). John Davis, for example, calls surrogacy a type of prostitution, says it is often done to atone for an abortion, and that it is clearly immoral ([11], p. 77).

AIH is typically accepted since it furthers God's purpose and blessings on marriage. In contrast, Davis says AID is immoral, since it involves the intrusion of a third party into the marriage relationship. He fears that the marriage bond might be harmed, and that the child may feel deceived as to its true origins ([11], p. 73).

Genetic studies are progressing rapidly, as are the techniques for assisting pregnancy for an infertile couple. The cryopreservation of the pre-embryo has made it possible for couples actually to achieve pregnancy using the genetic materials of total strangers (it is thus sometimes called pre-adoption). Examining the pre-embryo for genetic anomalies prior to implantation has enabled couples with lethal genetic factors that are afflicting their offspring to know in advance that the child will be healthy. Sometimes called BABI (Blastomere Analysis Before Implantation), the procedure identifies such lethal genes as Fragile X syndrome, hemophilia, Lesch Nyhan, and cystic fibrosis.

A great advantage of this technique is that sex selection need not determine whether to maintain the pregnancy. Healthy males can be brought to term since those that would be afflicted with hemophilia, for instance, can be isolated ([33]). The procedure promises to be a blessing to large numbers of couples since it is simple, inexpensive and extremely accurate. Unfortunately. it runs into the abortion debate since not all pre-embryos are selected for implantation.

The issue of birth control or the use of contraceptives was the subject of a *Christianity Today* Institute prompted by the claim of some prolife evangelicals that birth control is immoral ([28]). Randall Terry of Operation Rescue, for instance, says that birth control is selfish and sinful. He thus links his opposition to abortion to an anti-contraceptive morality in a way similar to that of traditional Roman Catholicism. But he stands virtually alone among evangelicals and Baptists in opposing family planning and the use of contraceptives.

Stanley Grenz approaches the issue in a way more typical among evangelicals. Theologically, he says, the question and its answer are rooted in God's ultimate purposes in history. God ordains marriage, but raising children is not the highest goal or outcome of marriage. One's spiritual family has precedence over one's biological family, as Jesus clearly showed (Matt. 12:50; John 3:31-59). Under certain circumstances, he says, a couple might in good conscience remain childless. However, both selfishness and sterilization should be avoided ([28], p. 38).

Similarly, Raymond C. Van Leeuwen, challenges home-schooling advocate Mary Pride's contention that the Bible forbids birth control based on Genesis 1:28. Van Leeuwen argues the "be fruitful" passage is not a command but a blessing. Those who argue for a categorical prohibition of birth control have fallen prey to legalism, imposing a burden on couples never intended by God. Birth control, he says, is a matter of Christian freedom ([28], p. 37).

Debra Evans cautions against separating sex and procreation. Her own experience leads her to believe that the availability of the pill has encouraged premarital promiscuity and a devaluation of childbearing by women. Evans claims that maternity and motherhood helped her to rediscover her own femininity, although she affirms the celibacy of Mother Teresa. She stops barely short of saying family planning is wrong, and expresses fear of the social pressures that embody eroticism but are disgusted by pregnancy and mother-hood ([28], p. 40).

George Brusaber argues that the Bible does not categorically prohibit birth control, but does require morally appropriate methods. However, some forms of birth control, such as abortion, are morally reprehensible; others are morally neutral, such as those that block conception or prevent fertilization ([28], p. 45). Typically, if an ovum has been fertilized, any act to interrupt or destroy the tissue is condemned ([28], p. 41). Thus, the issue of abortion seems inextrica-bly tied to evangelical perspectives on reproductive techniques, as these comments by Brusaber and Grenz indicate.

Both the intra-uterine device (IUD) and RU-486 are condemned as abortifacients. The running battle with Planned Parenthood seems unending and inevitable, because of that organization's support for abortion, abortion counseling, and the distribution of contraceptives to teens. Those Baptists and evangelicals who are strongly anti-abortion, will place careful restrictions on the types of "birth control" to which they subscribe. Not even concerns about population growth justify what they see as tantamount to "mass execution" ([5], p. 113).

Others give positive and unqualified support to any form of contraceptive, including RU-486. The American Baptist Convention for instance, acknowl-edged the linkage between widespread abortion and the unavailability of reliable and safe contraceptives. It implicitly admitted that the moral objections to contraception by certain religious or faith communities complicate the provision of contraceptives in programs to control population growth.

American Baptists encouraged government, industries, and foundations to support the research and development of safe, reliable, affordable and culturally appropriate methods of contraception for both men and women worldwide ([6], p. 3).

The government ban on RU-486 was criticized by a Southern Baptist theologian as an unwarranted intrusion into medical and scientific ventures by political ideology ([33], p. 32). Unless and until it can be shown on scientific grounds that a fertilized ovum is a person, a government ban is unjustified. Citing John Rawls, this theologian argued that laws or government regulations should "be supported by ordinary observation and modes of thought . . . which are generally recognized as correct". The notion that a zygote is a person and thus should be protected by law is based on abstract metaphysical speculation, not ordinary logic.

III. ABORTION

Abortion continues to be *the* bioethical issue at the top of the evangelical-Baptist list of moral/social priorities. No topic generates either the passion for social reform nor the deep divisions within the ranks of conservative Christians. It is probably "the largest social and political issue to divide the nation since slavery", as C. Everett Koop notes ([20], p. 19). Koop also embodies the evangelical perspective on the issue in many ways.

Koop rejects the idea that abortion is a medical issue, preferring to see it as a thoroughly moral matter, since so few women terminate pregnancies for medical reasons ([20], p. 18). He views the procedure as one of killing babies, adopting a genetic definition ([20], p. 80) of fetal personhood and believing that conception is the logical point at which "to draw the line", both morally and legally ([20], p.27). He is committed to a "reverence for the sanctity of human life" and believes that view is supported by such biblical passages as Jeremiah 1:5 and Psalms 139 ([20], p. 29). Unlike many evangelicals who are adamantly anti-abortion, Koop believes there are great inequities in the availability of abortion services for the poor and that the real answer to abortion is contraception ([20], p. 31). He is also unwilling to use just *any* argument against legalized abortion. As Surgeon General, he refused to manipulate the data so as to condemn abortion on grounds of the supposed negative psychological or emotional consequences to the woman who has an abortion. He is thus one of the more moderate of those evangelicals who are nonetheless adamantly opposed to abortion. His view amounts to a condemnation of the procedure on *moral* grounds without attempting to resolve the thornier legal or personal dilemmas that often attend the decision.

Many evangelicals/Baptists are far more radical in seeking a political or legal prohibition of what they perceive as a great social evil. The 1992 political campaign witnessed the extensive involvement of evangelicals in anti-abortion politics, most of it in opposition to Bill Clinton. *USA Today* carried a full page advertisement against Clinton on Friday, October 30, paid for by Pierce Creek Church, Binghampton, New York. The advertisement claimed that to vote for Clinton would be a sin, a charge repeated in a brochure apparently mailed to all evangelical and Southern Baptist pastors. The advertisement reflected the strong opposition to abortion of Operation Rescue leader Randall Terry, who believed it incredible that any Christian could advocate a public policy that would make or keep abortion legal. The Internal Revenue Service seems ready to investigate the church's action, since the ad solicited tax deductible contributions ([48]).

The Republican National Convention featured speakers such as Pat Robertson, Southern Baptist televangelist, who championed a "family values" agenda that is strongly anti-abortion. The argument of Pat Buchanan that America is in need of a religious war, captured the sentiment of many evangelicals and Southern Baptists. The argument reflects their Puritan past and its theocratic approach to church-state issues. They not only move easily from absolutistic moral beliefs to legislative solutions, but also seek to break down the traditional wall of separation by seeking public revenues to finance private schools and court approval for prayers in the public school system.

The Clinton victory prompted a threat from Jerry Falwell that he might resurrect Moral Majority, the now-defunct political action agency that had been so influential with the Reagan administration. What had been supportive of the political agenda and two successive national administrations will now become a reactionary movement, opposing and seeking to block many items on the agenda of the Clinton administration. The disruptive social activism of Operation Rescue is itself a divisive issue among evangelicals and Baptists and will be given additional attention below.

Abortion is also the primary issue driving the politicization of Southern Baptists. Their annual conventions continue to support efforts to bring an end to legalized abortion. Southern Baptists like Pat Robertson have become major players in the Republican Party. His Christian Coalition claims 550 chapters throughout the fifty states with a $12 million budget in 1992, and is active in the politics of the Republican Party. Such issues as the use of fetal tissue, blocking the distribution of RU 486, and support for the "gag rule" on health care providers in clinics that receive federal funds are obvious and focused targets of such political activity.

There is great irony in the fact that the three most prominent Southern Baptists in America are pro-choice. They are President Bill Clinton, Vice President Al Gore, and former President Jimmy Carter. Their perspective is moderate by any measure. They are not *for* abortion, but do believe it should be legally available. The position reflects that of millions of Southern Baptists, though it is not widely perceived to be representative of that denomination. Polls indicate that the Clinton-Gore ticket did not enjoy the support of a majority of their Southern Baptist constituency, and that is largely related to the abortion stance of the democratic ticket. Clinton has promised to sign the Freedom of Choice bill into law and has declared that he will move against the anti-abortion extremists who block abortion clinics.

The current leadership of the Convention is strongly anti-abortion; it believes that a legislative prohibition is a simple solution to what is regarded as a moral tragedy and a major social evil. The executive director of the Christian Life Commission wrote an "Open Letter" to President-Elect Bill

Clinton expressing an unalterable commitment to the protection of unborn human life. "The vast majority of Southern Baptists", he said, "believe that a pre-born baby is a distinct human life, according to both science and the Bible. The euphemisms of 'choice' or 'reproductive freedom' cannot disguise or justify killing a baby" ([21]).

All curriculum materials from the Baptist Sunday School Board advocate a strict "sanctity of life" approach. The concept was applied originally only to abortion; issues relating to elective death have been added since 1991. But such issues as war, capital punishment, or animal rights are not included as sanctity of life topics.

A special Sunday School lesson by Jimmy Draper, a former pastor who served as Convention President and is now head of the Baptist Sunday School Board, argued that the Bible teaches a strict anti-abortion ethic, and that Christians are to support laws to restrict or prohibit its availability. No attention is given to the merits or even the arguments of a pro-choice position ([12], pp. 36 ff.).

Michael Whitehead, the general counsel of the Christian Life Commission of the SBC, resigned from the American Bar Association to protest its resolution supporting abortion rights. He felt his membership constituted paying "dues to help fund its advocacy in public policy against values which we hold most dear". He also called on other Southern Baptist attorneys to follow his lead. Many Southern Baptists observe "Sanctity of Life Sunday" the third Sunday of January, commemorating what they regard as the infamous *Roe v. Wade* decision. Various activities have included: (1) planting crosses in a "cemetery of the innocents" in the front lawn of the church, each cross symbolizing a "child" aborted each day in the county or state; (2) organizing "life chains", which involve adults and children lining major thoroughfares while holding signs saying "Abortion kills Children" and "Jesus Forgives and Heals"; (3) the Christian Life Commission video, "The Sanctity of Human Life", offering sermon outlines, and literature for local churches; (4) the Baptist Sunday School Board anti-abortion curriculum for youth through adults; and (5) the Home Mission Board provides resources and training for establishing crisis pregnancy centers under the rubric of evangelism through its Alternatives to Abortion Ministries.

Southern Baptists who support choice regarding abortion believe that the decision is morally ambiguous, and is best left to the discretion of the woman facing a problem pregnancy. Strong arguments are made on logical, moral, biblical, and theological grounds. The notion that a fertilized ovum should be regarded as a person is rejected as radically reductionistic and non-biblical. No prohibitions are found against elective abortion in the Bible, which portrays human life made in the *imago dei* as having birth and breath (Gen.2:7), and human free moral agency as the zenith of the divine creative activity. The silence of the Scripture regarding abortion "is eloquent testimony to the sacredness of this choice for women and their families and the privacy in which it is to be considered* ([37], p. 28).

The curriculum materials distributed by Smyth & Helwys, a publication group identified with the moderate wing of the Southern Convention, takes a similar approach. The sanctity of life is seen in terms of the union of the sacred and secular. Life in all its dimensions is sacred, for it is a gift of God who blesses us with joy and sustains us with grace. Using the story of the wedding at Cana, the writer argued that all of life is sacred when the believer can discern the presence and power of God in nature, ordinary events, social occasions, and individual people [9].

A statement by the General Board of the American Baptist Convention disavowed any intention to speak on behalf of all constituents. Rather than proposing a uniform or national policy, the board insisted *that ministry to persons in situations of crisis pregnancy and abortion is a concern that primarily affects the local churches*. It affirmed *life as a sacred and gracious gift of God*, but admitted genuine diversity of opinion among its membership regarding the morality and legal acceptability of abortion.

The Board acknowledged agreement at several points. Abortion is opposed as a means of avoiding responsibility for conception, as a primary means of birth control, and when used without regard for the far-reaching consequences of the act. Acts of sexual violence that contribute to abortion are denounced, as is violence and harassment against abortion clinics. The membership is urged to work to prevent the causes of unplanned and unwanted pregnancies that lead to the widespread resort to abortion.

The Board statement expresses support and sympathy to all who struggle with the abortion decision. Individual moral responsibility is affirmed as the arena of personal struggle with abortion, while those considering abortion are encouraged to seek spiritual counsel and to engage in conscientious prayer. Concerning legislation to regulate the availability of abortion, the General Board affirmed the right of every American Baptists *to advocate for a public policy on abortion that reflects his or her beliefs* ([6]).

Strong divisions among evangelicals and Baptists will continue to exist, creating dissension in the ranks and different patterns in social goals. The primary variables determining those differences will be opinions about the nature of personhood, the place of women in church and society, pluralism as a corollary of religious liberty, the relation of God to natural processes, and attitudes toward birth control and population growth.

IV. EXPERIMENTATION, INFORMED CONSENT

Experimentation on human subjects continues to generate moral concerns among bioethicists. The debate focuses on such issues as informed consent, risks versus benefits to the patient, social costs, and the politicization of medicine. The principles of autonomy, beneficence, and justice are clearly at issue. During the past two years, concerns about experimental devices such as the artificial heart have hardly surfaced. The more recent introduction of a more sophisticated model than the Jarvik heart will undoubtedly bring debates about totally implantable artificial hearts to the attention of the evangelical public. Experimental transplantation of vital organs such as livers and hearts from baboons to persons will also attract attention, if not comment. The issue that has generated the most emotion has clearly been the use of fetal tissue.

Southern Baptists are profoundly divided over the issue of experimentation with human fetal tissue. Attitudes toward the topic generally parallel those concerning abortion. Those who are avidly anti-abortion typically oppose the use of fetal tissue transplants, believing it will encourage women to opt for abortion, despite the fact that using such tissue shows great promise in treating Parkinson's disease, Huntington's chorea, and perhaps even Alzheimer's.

Ben Mitchell of The Christian Life Commission (SBC) regards the use of human fetal tissue as a "technology" that cannot be supported biblically or ethically. His objection is directly related to his concern that such tissue will be used from elective abortions, and that it will be a further inducement to elective abortion. He thus supports the federal moratorium on the use of fetal tissue, despite its promise in treating neural disorders and genetic diseases ([26], p. 8). He argues that the focus must remain on "the baby who is being brutally murdered *in utero*" ([26], p. 10).

Guy Walden, former pastor of Broadway Baptist Church, Houston, TX is an outspoken advocate of fetal tissue transplants. He and his wife are adamant in their opposition to abortion, especially for reasons of fetal deformity. However, their experience with children born with Hurler's Syndrome leads to their equally strong insistence on the moral rightness of fetal tissue transplants. They have had two children to die of the disease, but a third treated *in utero* with fetal tissue was born without many of the presenting symptoms of this dread genetic disease ([17]). Other arguments supporting the use of fetal tissue transplants can be found among Baptists. Dorothy Vawter argues that the ban "is based on false and groundless assumptions about women's intellectual and moral capacities, the reasons they have abortions, as well as on ignorance of fetal tissue procurement practices". The notion that women would be encouraged to abort to donate tissue to anonymous recipients is without empirical evidence. The idea that women abort for frivolous reasons or without assessing risk and consequences is insulting and degrading. In short, Vawter says, a myth about women has been constructed that is disrespectful and harmful to them ([47], p. 10).

Others argue that the basis for the ban is ideological and thus violates sound procedure for the development of regulations governing experimental medical procedures. Public policy should not be premised on metaphysical speculation in a pluralistic society. Empirical data, scientific findings, and other types of evidence which is available to all people is basic to democratic processes. Appeals to special knowledge or basing claims in abstract metaphysics is a type of gnosticism ([25], p. 546) that is often found in religious circles but is extremely problematic as the basis for public policy.

V. EUTHANASIA AND SUICIDE

The issue of assisted suicide gained extensive public attention in 1992. Dr. Timothy Quill's admission that he had prescribed sleeping pills to a leukemia patient, knowing of her intention to commit suicide, and Dr. Jack Kevorkian's openly assisting persons to commit suicide, were items that gained national attention and generated heated debate.

The dilemma of people facing a slow and ugly death and a rapid decline into total debility has created a climate of desperation for remedies. *Final Exit*, a "how to" manual for potential suicides written by Derek Humphry of the Hemlock Society, was at the top of the best-seller list during the Fall of 1991. "Initiative 119", a ballot measure to approve physician-assisted suicide, was barely defeated by voters in the state of Washington in November 1992.

The evangelical community apparently played a major role in the 54% to 46% defeat of the measure. A Christian Action Council anti-119 video was widely distributed among churches and other organizations. Prayer rallies, radio programs, and a telethon all were part of an intensive statewide campaign. The Christian Medical and Dental Society also issued a statement opposing euthanasia and physician-assisted suicide.

Even so, a survey by *Christianity Today* of people who said that they would vote for the Washington initiative indicated that 49% described themselves as "born again believers", while 57% called themselves Protestants. Fifty-two percent would consider some option to end their own life if they had an incurable illness with a great deal of physical pain. The motives and actions contemplated varied widely: nearly half did not want to be a burden; one in five did not want to live in pain or be dependent on a machine; nearly two-thirds would consider asking a doctor to withhold life-sustaining treatment; over one-half the respondents would consider asking a doctor to prescribe a lethal drug dosage or asking a physician to assist in suicide ([23]).

Such findings are not treated sympathetically by evangelical commentators. Nor are the moral demands of mercy in the medical context ever considered beyond that of "keeping the patient alive". Helping a patient die who is *in extremis* and has requested assistance as merciful relief from suffering is hardly viewed as a "countervailing requirement of agape". The typical attitude portrays such a physician as an "executioner" unworthy of moral support ([23]).

Evangelicals recognize the pressures to commit suicide created by depression and by certain social factors, including soaring medical costs. Joni Tada deals helpfully with those feelings as one who has "been there". She is a quadriplegic who served on the National Council on Disability and thus also speaks from the role of advocacy for the disabled. She fears the trend toward devaluing the life of the handicapped and the pressures placed upon them to commit suicide. She encourages those in despair to have hope and to recognize the sacredness of life as gift; she also implies that suicide is an unforgivable sin that will consign one to hell ([44], p. 105). Further, she believes that the final outcome of a socially approved policy of euthanasia will be the elimination of the disabled and others of limited utilitarian value ([44], p. 76).

C. Everett Koop argues that there are no legitimate circumstances in which a physician should assist the suicide of a patient for that would be to cross the line from being healer to being a killer. Koop is also concerned about the "slippery slope": society tends to expand the number of conditions and groups targeted for this "final solution" or "special treatment" ([20], p. 56). Even so, Koop acknowledges that there is an appropriate time to withdraw or withhold treatment and allow death to come. He also accepts the moral argument of "indirect effect". Drugs can be given to alleviate pain even if death comes more quickly as a result. The motive makes the moral difference: if one intends to shorten the patient's life, that is euthanasia and thus immoral.

Southern Baptists addressed the issue in a 1992 Convention resolution strongly opposing euthanasia or assisted suicide, based on the biblical prohibition of taking innocent human life, including one's own. They affirmed the need for more effective pain management, companionship, and appropriate ministries to the dying. No action intended to cause a person's death was deemed morally appropriate. They recommended that any physician or other person who practices euthanasia or assists patients with suicide should be prosecuted to the full extent of the law ([1], p. 92), an apparent though indirect reference to the widely publicized actions of Dr. Jack Kevorkian.

VI. CARE OF SEVERELY HANDICAPPED NEWBORNS

Strong family values and the mystique of innocent and vulnerable infants predispose evangelicals to support medical care for severely handicapped infants. The moral rule against killing is stringently applied to "innocent" newborns. Any such action is considered infanticide, a term used both to reflect and evoke moral revulsion against assisting the death even of those born dying. Beckwith and Geisler draw a connection between arguments that support abortion and those that support infanticide: "if it is right to kill (by abortion) babies who might be deformed, then why not kill children who are handicapped?" ([5], p. 134; [20], p. 55). They oppose any action that crosses the moral line between allowing an infant to die and actually killing a newborn. Nonetheless, they accept the rightness of withholding or withdrawing treatment to infants when it is futile ([5], p. 135), with the same standard for decision making applying to children as to adults. Beckwith and Geisler do fear the abuse of this principle, citing the "Infant Doe" case in Indiana in which interventionist surgery to correct a life-threatening abdominal condition was refused by the parents.

The moral rule against killing is so focused that evangelicals seldom struggle with the morality of leaving infants to a slow and ugly death by starvation. A theology that relates God to the dying process and an ethic that prohibits "killing the innocent" combine to foreclose the possibility of merciful assistance. Typically, "Christian hope" takes the form of praying for a quick death and taking comfort in a belief in the afterlife.

The issue of authority in decision making regarding treatment of handicapped newborns was insightfully examined by Earl Shelp, but few evangelicals or Baptists have thoughtfully considered the issue or responded to his challenge. Shelp challenges the passivity of parents who typically leave such decisions to the physician or acquiesce to government regulations. He also attacks the imperialism of the medical establishment and government agencies who impose treatments in the name of beneficence. He says parents are the proper focus of authority for decisions regarding medical care. Both historical precedent and familial burden underscore the priority of parental authority in such matters. Proper constraints are required, of course, against those who would make unreasonable decisions, as in cases of Phenylketonuria that would require only dietary care or infants needing blood transfusions. What is medically sound and reasonable is balanced against parental authority in deciding what is morally acceptable and thus to be permitted or rejected. Nonetheless Shelp argues that the court of final appeal regarding "the patient's best interest" should be parents, not doctors, hospitals, or federal regulators.

Shelp also questions the morality of "allowing to die" versus that of "assisted dying" in the neonatal intensive care unit (NICU). He argues that the morality of "always sustaining life" is morally untenable and often inhumane. Providing a merciful and quick death for the most severely impaired is not only morally tenable but perhaps ethically mandated ([30], p. 174).

Shelp has the advantage of analyzing and responding to crises in the NICU from a clinical perspective. Most evangelicals deal with such issues in the abstract, as problems to be resolved by appeals to moral absolutes. That moralistic approach takes little if any account of the rapid advances in medical technology that present a vast array of treatment options but cannot offer any reasonable hope for cure.

VII. WITHHOLDING, WITHDRAWING TREATMENT

Withholding or withdrawing treatment from the dying patient is morally acceptable to evangelicals ([20], p. 55), since death is to be accepted as inevitable and a strong belief in the afterlife provides an overriding hope. Some distinctions are made between the two actions, of course, because "withdrawal" often includes nutrition and hydration, which are more difficult to integrate into an ethic of "not killing". Withdrawing a ventilator from a patient who will die shortly afterward is different than withdrawing a gastronomic tube from a patient in a persistent vegetative state (PVS) and may otherwise live for years.

A 1992 resolution by the Southern Baptist Convention insisted that nutrition and hydration be viewed as part of compassionate medical care, in opposition to a portion of the Supreme Court's *Cruzan* decision. A copy of that resolution was included in an *amicus curiae* brief filed against the petition of Martha Elston on behalf of her daughter, Sue DeGrella. Sue had been in a PVS in a nursing home in Louisville, Kentucky, for nine years following a severe beating. She was maintained by nutrition and hydration through a gastronomic tube. Her mother, Mrs. Elston, had lovingly cared for Sue but was now dying of pancreatic cancer. She desired to see closure on her daughter's dying before her own death removed her from the scene. A district court judge ruled in favor of Mrs. Elston, based on the often-expressed wishes of the patient, the unanimous support of the family, and the *Cruzan* case. An appeal by the *guardian ad litem* delayed implementing the decision until well after the death of Mrs. Elston.

The Elston family were active members of a large Baptist church in Louisville. Two Southern Baptist neurosurgeons and a Southern Baptist seminary professor and bioethicist had given supportive testimony at the trial in favor of the Elston petition. Mrs. Elston felt personally insulted that her own denomination would show such insensitivity to her daughter's plight and her own by filing the *amicus* brief against her petition.

The 1992 resolution by the Executive Committee is indicative of the shift toward authoritarianism in moral matters toward members of the Convention. In the past, it would have been unthinkable for Baptists to call for court intervention concerning family decisions about dying loved ones. The twin emphases on compassion for families and individualism in decision-making would have combined with a suspicion of government authority as intrusive. The past decade, however has seen the emergence of leadership that is inclined toward control of decisions by those in "authority" – whether governmental or religious.

Contrary to Hamel's description of Baptists as democratic, the Southern Convention is rapidly moving toward a type of hierarchical ecclesiology. The bylaws of the Convention speak of democracy, while the actions of the elected leadership speak of centralized authority. All Baptist agencies and their employees, including seminary professors, are expected to follow the "dic-tates" of convention resolutions which are regarded as "official" statements of belief or policy. Resolutions like that condemning euthanasia and suicide would become normative for orthodox belief and action. Professors would have no latitude for questioning the ethical or theological justifiability of such statements. Those who would do so on grounds of logic, biblical interpretation, or conscience grounded in experience would be subject to investigation and/or removal. It is hardly a fruitful environment for the development of scholarly opinion on bioethical issues.

VIII. HEALTH CARE

The 1992 Presidential campaign was marked by a clear consensus on the part of American voters that health care reform is long overdue. Bill Clinton regards reform as mandatory and has placed it high on the list of priorities for his administration. He intends to propose legislation within 100 days of taking office to guarantee insurance to all Americans. States like Kentucky, Oregon, Florida, and Minnesota have been attempting health care reform that takes account of both affordability and accessibility. Morally, we can neither deny Americans access to health care, nor break the bank in doing so.

In the industrialized world, only the United States and South Africa have no national health care system. In 1991, 37 million Americans had no health insurance coverage; 81 million (25% of the population) were at risk for costs for catastrophic or long-term medical needs. Health care costs in America reached 14% of the gross national product in 1992; it was 13.2% in 1991, according to the Commerce Department. The Department estimates that health spending will increase 12% in 1993, for a total expenditure of $939.9 billion, and that annual increases between 12% and 15% will continue unless significant changes in America's health care system take place. In 1994 costs will likely exceed $1 trillion.

The debate often turns on whether health care is a right or a privilege. If it is a right, as the 1948 United Nations Declaration of Human Rights declared, then access should not be limited by ability to pay. The basic premise of current practice in America is that health care is a privilege, thus care is premised on fee-for-service. Accessibility is determined by affordability.

C. Everett Koop once said that the American system of health care is "broken". He now calls not only for radical reform of the way that we pay for care, but for a new type of physician ([20], p. 92). The reforms he suggests include subsidizing training for physicians ([20], p. 91), changes in malpractice laws ([20], p. 95), and a lowering of expectations on the part of consumers ([20], p. 133). He admits that not everything can be provided to patients at public expense, and that some type of rationing is inevitable and necessary.

American Baptists support the notion of health care as a human right. Their 1991 policy statement affirms support for programs, legislation, and research toward "a new comprehensive health care delivery system" and advocates "the availability of, access to and funding for quality health care for all persons". The statement supports universal coverage based on human need, rather than any calculus of economic, geographic, or racial factors. It acknowledges the lack of consensus on how to fund universal coverage, and discusses a number of complex issues that must be addressed, including quality of care, cost of technology and research, reimbursement of providers, and accessibility for the working poor and indigent ([15], p. 5). But the *moral* mandate to provide universal health care should not be ignored because of technical questions, most of which can be worked out by people of good sense and compassion.

Southern Baptists have made only modest calls for reform. The Annuity Board, which provides health care insurance for numerous employees of churches and agencies, has admitted the need for change but not dealt with specifics. Change is addressed more as a matter of economics than of ethics or human rights since soaring costs are eroding the financial security of many Baptists insured through the Board ([49]).

The extensive involvement of Southern Baptists and other evangelicals in the politics of the Reagan era makes it difficult for them to support national health care insurance, various types of single payer approaches, or federal funding. The great specter is that of "socialized medicine", which is seen as a direct challenge to laissez-faire capitalism, the economic ideology wed to Christian rhetoric by groups like Falwell's Moral Majority, Bill Bright's Campus Crusade, and reconstructionists like Greg Bahnsen. Socialism in any form is a favorite target of this right-wing religious coalition.

Even so, there are persons in positions of power that will influence the direction of health care reform more than all the resolutions that might be passed. Both Bill Clinton and Al Gore, like former President Carter, are Baptists who are firmly committed to extensive revisions in U.S. delivery and funding of health care. The fact they were reared and nurtured in a tradition that emphasized human rights and the morality of compassionate care for others speaks volumes about the orientation of Baptists and other evangelicals to person-centered values. These, in the end, will win out over the morally problematic arguments of economic ideology.

IX. AIDS (ACQUIRED-IMMUNE DEFICIENCY SYNDROME)

More than 260,000 Americans have now died of AIDS and it is estimated that over one million are infected with the HIV virus. An effective response to AIDS has been limited by medical, political, and religious factors. Scientists were slow to respond to the crisis because of its sudden appearance in 1981. Ignorance about its nature and origin contributed to the hysteria that followed the awareness of its devastating impact on health. Religious sensibilities about open discussion of sexual matters and moral attitudes about homosexuality complicated the scientific response. Euphemisms such as "exchange of bodily fluids" were used to warn people about the way that the disease was spread by sexual contact. Anal intercourse was the first positive evidence of a manner of transmitting the HIV virus, but public rhetoric was governed by the rules of polite society, thus limiting the public understanding of AIDS.

Politically, the revolution for gay rights of the 1970s collided with the Reagan revolution of the 1980s and its heavy involvement with the religious right ([20], p.62). A politically sensitive issue was religiously explosive, since traditional Christian approaches to homosexual behavior are highly negative and repressive.

Evangelical opinion typically regards those who are homosexual as morally perverse and religiously degenerate. The Bible is thought to teach that homosexual behavior is an abomination to God deserving of the death penalty, based on such passages as Genesis 19:1-14, Leviticus 18:22, and Leviticus 20:13, which calls for capital punishment.

Resolutions passed by the Southern Baptist Convention in 1987 and 1988 reflected these assumptions ([1]). The 1988 resolution regarded homosexuality as the cause of AIDS, related suffering to God's wrath, and called on those who are homosexual to seek forgiveness for their "abomination". The resolution has not been rescinded and a more informed and compassionate statement is not likely.

A 1992 resolution by the Executive Committee of the Southern Baptist Convention (SBC) condemned two North Carolina Churches for "accommodating homosexuality", one by licensing a gay man to preach, the other by blessing a gay union. The churches were removed from membership in their local associations and state conventions, and their messengers were rejected for the annual convention. The resolution expresses "abhorrence of homosexuality", argues that "God regards homosexuality as a gross perversion and unquestioned sin", and states that "unrepentant homosexuality is repeatedly condemned in Scripture". The convention will vote in 1993 on an amendment to its bylaws that would ban any church open to homosexuals from membership in the convention ([1], p. 118).

Linking AIDS and homosexuality is extremely problematic, since AIDS is a human health issue, not one of sexual orientation. Even so, the linkage is strong in conservative Christian circles and will not easily be displaced by more informed perspectives. The 1987 SBC resolution on AIDS rightly called it "a major health threat" but lapsed into a moralistic posture by blaming it on a rejection of "biblical standards of decency and morality" and by opposing the distribution of condoms and any talk of "safe sex". The resolution's most positive note was a call for "Christlike compassion" for the "victims of AIDS and their families". Despite publicity surrounding AIDS, and its appearance in local church families, the resolutions are not likely to be rescinded or revised toward more compassionate and common-sense understandings. Even so, many Baptists are aware of the inadequacy and moral intolerance of such statements and are engaged in supportive and healing ministries. Numerous conferences at local and state levels have included testimonies by persons either infected with the AIDS virus or family members of persons who have died with AIDS.

Earl Shelp, an ordained Baptist minister and director of Interfaith Research and Ministry in Houston, Texas, was a recipient of the America's Award in 1992 because of his work with AIDS patients and his efforts to organize ministries to them.   The recognition is given to "unsung heroes" by The Positive Thinking Foundation, which praised Shelp for "mobiliz[ing] volunteers and organiz[ing] training seminars for clergy, in a campaign of education, persuasion, and judicious arm-twisting" [2].

The national publicity given to the experience of a third-generation Baptist minister and his family infected with AIDS on NBC's "Dateline" has set AIDS firmly on the theological-ethical agenda of the largest Protestant denomination in America. Scot Allen has received little comfort from churches and has been rejected when attempting to find comfort from a local congregation. His story is a case study in how biblical-theological beliefs and traditional approaches to the moral issue of homosexuality influence if not determine attitudes toward victims of AIDS. Scot Allen's wife, Lydia, received HIV-tainted blood in a transfusion in 1982. Scot's son, Brian was born three and one-half years later with AIDS. Both have subsequently died. Scot's son Matt, now 10, was also infected through a transfusion.

Removed from his position as associate minister in Colorado when he admitted the HIV infection of his child, Scot moved his family to his native Texas. Two Baptist churches offered neither support nor acceptance, aside from the usual verbal assurances of concern and prayers. Even the church where his father was a member rejected Matt for child care. When Brian died, the church again was rejecting and distant.

A complicating factor in family dynamics was that Scot's brother is homosexual, a fact that their father has been unable to accept. At one time, Scot's rage about AIDS caused him in anger to turn against gays, including his brother. He worked through the issue by recognizing that sexual orientation is not a choice, but is rooted in formative factors related to psycho-sexual development. Scot's work to find a place of acceptance for his son, Matt, has had some positive outcomes. First Baptist Church in Arlington, Texas, has since instituted guidelines for accepting HIV-infected children. The minister now says insightfully that churches must move beyond the ignorance and fear that clouds the issue and provide acceptance and support to such families. Scot has served on the President's Commission on AIDS for three years, and works with the Dallas AIDS Interfaith Network to find churches for those who are HIV positive.

At the heart of the ethics debate about AIDS are important theological variables. The condemning, rejecting, punitive approach builds upon beliefs about God as stern judge – the giver and enforcer of rigid moral standards for sexual conduct. This theology is dominated by images of divine power and wrath. Such notions pervade fundamentalist and evangelical thought. In spite of an emphasis on salvation by grace through faith, preachments are often harshly legalistic, resulting in a type of works righteousness. When combined with the fervency and heat of profound conviction, evangelicals generate intense feelings of opposition against those they perceive as acting contrary to God's stern rule. That angry intolerance has pervaded the political activities of evangelicals associated with the New Political Right, generally grouped together under the heading of the "Moral Majority" made famous by Jerry Falwell.

Former Surgeon General of the U.S., C. Everett Koop, who is one of the most prominent evangelicals in America, expressed his sense of betrayal by those on the religious right who criticized him so vehemently for his report on AIDS. His own position, he said, was dictated by scientific integrity and Christian compassion. He felt strongly, however, that his Christian opponents had lost any commitment to compassion or integrity ([20], p.63-64).

Those evangelicals who accept and minister to the victims of AIDS do so by suspending moral judgment. The ethics of compassion builds upon the biblical themes of hospitality and love of neighbor. As Earl Shelp puts it, "we are called to care", not to engage in harsh judgmentalism ([2]).

The most important theological variable in the debate about AIDS is belief about the nature of God ([36]). Is God engaged in efforts to kill those who are gay by creating and inflicting them with the AIDS virus as so many evangelicals claim? Central to the teachings of Jesus is the image of God as loving and caring Father/Parent. The Christian conception of God stresses love, not power or wrath, as the essence of the divine nature (I John 4:8). God's action flows from the divine being. Jesus rejected emphatically the idea that God does evil things to people, when responding to those who wanted harsh explanations for a man born blind (John 9). He also provided a simple test for knowing whether God would do evil things to a person. The test is that of the caring and beneficent parent. Would a decent and loving parent trick a child who is hungry by giving a rock instead of bread or a poisonous viper instead of fish? The answer is an emphatic No! Jesus then drove home the moral: "if you who are sinful" would not do such an evil thing to a vulnerable child, "how much more will your Father who is in heaven give good things to those who ask?" (Matt. 7:9-11; Lk. 11:11-13).

At issue in the AIDS debate is the Christian conception of God and the moral imperative of love for needy neighbors. Evangelicals find themselves in the awkward, confusing and often contradictory position of clinging to strong moral convictions that appear shaped more by sexual fears and social mores than by the revelation of God in Christ. The concern for good morals often overwhelms a concern for good theology and ethics.

A consistent *Christian* ethic will also require a re-examination of absolutistic and moralistic approaches to homosexuality. The question is not so much the authority of Scripture as it is the accuracy with which Scripture has been interpreted, and the moral justifiability of the way that it has been used to reject and condemn those who are gay. That compassion is normative is frequently confirmed; that its limits are tested severely by the AIDS crisis is equally obvious.

X. ANIMAL RIGHTS

The issue of animal rights has not caught the attention of nor generated passion among evangelicals or Baptists. The topic has been broached ([38], p. 18) but little systematic religious reflection has been devoted to it. The reasons for this neglect are both theological and practical in nature.

Baptists and evangelicals in many ways are products of a rural past in which animal husbandry and the necessities of farm life provide the central images or models for dealing with animals. The language of "rights" for non-human creatures is a difficult concept to accept. Hunting and the preparation of meat for dietary needs hardly lend themselves to protectionist attitudes toward animals.

Theologically, the emphasis on personal salvation and the uniqueness of being human in the *imago dei* tend toward anthropocentrism. An ethic of exploitation has been the result; animals are creatures of God but exist for the good of humanity. They are not included in God's redemptive purpose for eternity, and thus are not part of the umbrella of protection provided by a "sanctity of life" ethic. One can be "completely pro-life" without placing animal rights on a list of moral priorities.

Theological anthropocentricity and ecological exploitation are inextricably related. The result is not only a ravaging of the environment "to meet human needs", but an exclusion of animals from the realm of redemption. But a biblically based and rightly informed Christianity cannot long ignore the facts concerning animal species. One scientist has estimated that 100 species of plants and animals will be driven into extinction each day within the next two decades, a rate 1000 times that of natural evolution. Many of these species are never catalogued. On the endangered list are such animals as the panda, the Spanish lynx, the black rhinoceros, the Asiatic lion, the elephant, the snow leopard, the wild yak, the Drill monkey, the golden tamarin, and the humpback whale.

The human population explosion is probably the greatest factor threatening animal existence. In pressing for new frontiers to an ever-expanding system of human needs, the habitat of animals is inevitably threatened. Tropical rain forests and their plant and animal denizens are being rapidly depleted in order to accommodate the burgeoning growth of the human population. It is not that frontier settlers are evil and their intentions toward animals malicious; it is that people have inadequate conceptual models for granting status rights to animals that protect their existence on earth as a gift from God.

There is hope that the biblically-oriented theology of evangelicalism will develop a critical consciousness regarding the place of animals in God's scheme of creation and redemption. Most sympathetic treatments now emphasize Christian responsibility to *care for* animals. The image is one of the stewardship of superior powers toward subordinate and less worthy creatures ([22], [50]). Such approaches are not without merit, they may prove inadequate to alter present trends toward the extinction of animal species.

A dissertation is in progress under my supervision that raises the issue in terms of the dilemma between the conservation of non-human creation and what is perceived as meeting human needs. The case is drawn from the medical arena. An extract from the Yew tree is useful in treating human breast cancer. Since each treatment requires sacrificing five trees, the impact on this scarce species of tree is enormous. Animal species are also threatened as their habitat is removed. Other cases from medical experimentation could also be used, such as the transplantation of baboon livers and hearts to human subjects. The Baby Fae case was simply one in a series of efforts to exploit the healthy vital organs of animals to replace diseased human organs. Animal rights activists pose the substantive moral question by asking whether a healthy animal should be sacrificed for the sake of experimental treatments on people that have little likelihood of success.

The theocentric ethics of James Gustafson is also beginning to influence evangelical/Baptist thought ([18]). A theologian of the reformed tradition, his project profoundly questions the theological justifiability of an ethic that revolves around an assumption of the absolute moral value of people. He argues rightly that, in Christian theology, it is God who is the center of value and who establishes the norms for moral truth. What is needed is a *theo*centric ethic to replace the present *anthropo*centric ethic.

In both biblical and scientific perspectives, the uniqueness of being human consists in the ability of people to know that they are part of a larger whole. Their glory and dignity are found in their ability to relate responsibly to their place in the universe. But to order human priorities and actions in such fashion as to diminish or denigrate the existence of other creatures is arrogance by any measure.

The claim to absolute value symbolized both in notions of human immortality and the sanctity of human life is partially the result of such thinking. Could it be that a major factor in human *hubris* – original sin – is the notion that *only* people are somehow reflective of the *imago dei*? When people are regarded as of supreme and absolute value, all other creatures have only a secondary or utilitarian value and are available to be exploited as people decide. Might it be that the moral crisis with regard to the treatment of animals is rooted in bad theology and an unjustifiable ethic that claims too much for people and too little for the rest of God's good creatures?

XI. OTHER ISSUES

Predictions about the future are always problematic. But they are also necessary if trends are to be taken seriously and the future is to be sought and not simply awaited. The particular issue confronting evangelicals and Baptists during the 1990's concerns the connection between politics and the bioethical matters they pursue with such vigor. This involves not only the politicization of religious beliefs and goals, but also their pursuit through various channels of social action.

1. *Politics and Religious Pursuits.* Especially troubling for thoughtful evangelicals and Baptists is the way in which religion has become so intertwined with politics. Conservative religion in America has not only traditionally supported strong opinions regarding the separation of church and state, but has regarded political processes themselves as degrading and unworthy. That the importance of politics and of Christian involvement in public discourse have been acknowledged should be welcome to any person interested in the moral shaping of public policy. But the open identification of particular religious values with political parties or programs poses fundamental problems for both theology and politics.

The narrow "pro-family" agenda of conservative politics is clearly difficult if not impossible to reconcile with a concern for justice in the social order. The voting patterns of self-proclaimed pro-life evangelicals has often been shaped almost exclusively by the abortion issue, which determines everything from family leave bills to scientific research involving fetal tissue. Clearly the use of power in pursuit of such narrow interests is obstructive to scientific progress, blind to larger issues of justice for women and minorities, and a denial of a pluralistic Christian witness.

The election of Bill Clinton and Al Gore in 1992 seems to indicate a widespread rejection of the politics of the new right which has attracted so many evangelicals and Baptists in recent years. Not only has the rationale been non-persuasive to large numbers of people, the tactics and strategies employed have given the movement very negative marks.

The question for evangelicals and Baptists is whether they will continue the quest for political power at the price of sacrificing the integrity of the Christian vision. Cal Thomas, syndicated columnist and evangelical Christian who once worked for the Moral Majority, has rightly and insightfully called for a revision of strategy. He has appealed to Jerry Falwell not to resurrect the Moral Majority. He believes it is time for evangelicals/Baptists to get out of politics and return to doing what they do best, namely, build the foundations of moral society by shaping the character of religious people ([46]).

The new right coalition of religion and politics has done injury to both the evangelical witness and the political process. Unless evangelicals recapture their own ethic of personal piety that transcends and judges the many moral compromises necessary to the pursuit of political power, they will be regarded as simply another political party and the country will continue to suffer from a reactionary religious zealotry.

2. *Social Activism: The Question of Civil Disobedience.* The second major issue is related to the first. It is one posed by Operation Rescue (OR) and the religious mentality that supports its particular brand of civil disobedience. OR is the civil action arm of the coalition against abortion rights. It intends to engage in clinic disruptions until abortion is either banned or severely curtailed

([24]).

Evangelicals and Baptists are deeply divided over OR, though they are in general agreement that there are circumstances under which Christians should engage in civil disobedience. Beckwith and Geisler helpfully distinguish between the anti-promulgation view and the anti-compulsion approach ([5], p. 166 *ff.*). OR argues that government should be disobeyed if it promulgates laws and thus allows actions that are contrary to God's law. Thus, its actions are only indirectly related to permissive abortion laws. It trespasses against clinics, but is not able to engage in direct disobedience since no one is compelled to have an abortion.

The anti-compulsionists argue that only those laws that compel a person to break God's law should be broken. Beckwith and Geisler, using this approach argue strongly against OR and are more representative of evangelical/Baptist thought. When OR strategies of civil disobedience were used to block clinics in Atlanta, it was opposed by Charles Stanley, the pastor of First Baptist Church and probably the most influential evangelical in the city. For Stanley, the basic biblical command is to obey the governing authorities (Rom. 13:1-7; Titus 3:1). The only exceptions are those cases in which a civil law either requires an act that is contrary to God's law or prohibits an act that is consistent with God's word ([42]).

There are even stronger arguments against OR. These are rooted in concerns for religious liberty. The basic premise of the movement is that the fetus is a person from the moment of conception, thus the claim of protesting "the brutal murder of babies". OR uses images of the Holocaust and claims that it is adopting the rationale and tactics of Martin Luther King, Jr's civil rights campaign. If OR is right in the basic premise, it is right in the campaign of civil disobedience, as Tim Stafford says ([39], p. 18).

It is precisely this ground-of-meaning belief that is the Achilles heel of the movement. The claim that the Bible teaches that fetuses are human beings and that abortion is murder is especially problematic. Scholars equally committed to biblical authority find neither a prohibition of elective abortion in Scripture nor any support for the notion that zygotes are persons. To the contrary, the biblical portrait of personhood focuses on birth and breath (Genesis 2:7) and attributes such as self awareness, moral reasoning, spiritual gifts, social relationships, and capacities of introspection and imagination. The woman clearly and undeniably fits the biblical portrait as one who bears the *imago dei*, but a conceptus clearly does not. The very Bible to which anti-abortionist evangelicals claim such allegiance seems to refute their argument at every significant point ([37].

The OR contention that a fetus is a person amounts to a claim to special knowledge. The dogmatic way in which the belief is argued reveals an intolerance for differing opinion, even if the latter is also rooted in religious tradition and theology. OR thus denies religious pluralism. Somehow OR members are able to discern what others find untenable on logical, moral or scientific grounds. Failing to produce an adequate argument for banning abortion, OR has resorted to heavy-handed tactics designed to coerce the nation to conform to their version of laws based on metaphysical speculation.

That is one of the major differences separating King's civil disobedience campaign from that of OR. African-Americans are indisputably persons by any ordinary definition of the term. It takes no special revelation to know that King was seeking to enlarge the scope of those whose civil rights should rightly be protected by law. The OR campaign reveals an ideological posture in seeking to protect a fetus "from the moment of conception". The most problematic of all definitions of personhood (a genetic code is a person) is proposed as a legal solution to what OR perceives as a moral issue.

Another major problem with Operation Rescue is that it sacrifices civility in pursuing a distinctively religious goal. The vehemence of rhetoric and the disruptive and coercive nature of its tactics reveal strategies Roland Bainton associated with a crusade ethic ([3], p. 148). Whether the war is against foreign enemies of state, or against domestic "enemies" of morality, four characteristics appear: (1) the cause is holy; (2) God fights for the crusaders and against their opposition; (3) the crusaders are godly, the enemy ungodly; and (4) the campaign is prosecuted unsparingly; as a battle to the finish. OR strategists make all these claims in justifying their tactics and goals ([45]).

The sincerity of their belief is not at issue. They are true believers who accept without question the profound beliefs that promote their actions. In a pluralistic society, however, such narrow claims to truth and heavy-handed approaches to public policy seem prima facie violations of the religious liberties to which all Americans are entitled. The social disruptions also threaten the loss of civility between various religious groups necessary for social cohesion and stability. OR strategies conjure up images of the Inquisition and the religious wars of the middle ages. Such recognitions seem to be a part of the modest criticisms against OR by fellow evangelicals and Baptists.

The proper forum for criticizing and finally undermining support for such civil disruptions is in the religious arena. Those theologians and ethicists among evangelicals and Baptists who see the errors of OR's ways need to say so strongly. The courts have only limited powers to control or punish their actions, since they are basically protected by First Amendment guarantees. But OR has pushed the laws to their absolute limits and government patience is wearing thin. Laws that might be passed to punish or control OR may well have a chilling effect on other types of actions that will have a more supportable moral base. Whether evangelical leaders will rise to this challenge will be a major issue to watch in the coming years.

Southern Baptist Theological Seminary
Louisville, Kentucky, U.S.A.

BIBLIOGRAPHY

1. *Annual of the Southern Baptist Convention*.
2. *America's Awards*: 1992, Positive Thinking Foundation, New York.
3. Bainton, R.: 1960, *Christian Attitudes Towards War and Peace*. Abingdon, Nashville.
4. Barron, S.: 1991, "Searching for Life's Beginning", *Christianity Today*, November 11.
5. Beckwith, F. and N. Geisler: 1991, *Matters of Life and Death: Abortion and Euthanasia*, Baker Book House, Grand Rapids.
6. Board of Social Ministries: 1987, "Abortion and Ministry in the Local Church", American Baptist Convention, Valley Forge.
7. Boston, B.: 1988, "Thy Kingdom Come: Christian Reconstructionists Want to Take Dominion Over America", *Church and State*, September, pp. 6-12.
8. Campolo, T.: 1988, *Twenty Hot Potatoes Christians are Afraid to Touch*, Word Publishers, Dallas.
9. Christopher, P.: 1992, "A Concern is Expressed", *Formations*, January 19. Smyth & Helwys, Greenville, SC.
10. Cromartie, M.: 1992, "Fixing the World: The Saga of Evangelicals and Social Action", *Christianity Today*, April 27, 23-25.
11. Davis, J.: 1985, *Evangelical Ethics: Issues Facing the Church Today*, Presbyterian and Reformed Publishing Co., Phillipsburg, NJ.
12. Draper, J.: 1991, "Respect for Human Life", *The Adult Teacher*, January-March, 36-47, Baptist Sunday School Board, SBC, Nashville, Tn.
13. Falwell, J.: 1987, "An Agenda for the 1980's", in J. Neuhaus and M. Cromartie (eds.), *Piety and Politics*. Ethics and Public Policy Center, Washington.
14. Falwell, J.: 1987, "AIDS: the Judgment of God", *Liberty Report*, April, Lynchburg, Virginia.
15. Franklin, C.: 1991-92, "Health Care Captures Attention–Finally", *Advocate*, Winter.
16. Garrett, J., E.G.Hinson and J.E.Tull: 1983, *Are Southern Baptists "Evangelicals"*? Mercer University Press, Macon, GA.
17. Goldberg, J.: 1992, "Who Gets to Play God"? *Life*, February 15:2, 50-56.
18. Gustafson, J.: 1984, *Ethics from a Theocentric Perspective*, 2 vols., University of Chicago, Chicago.
19. Hamel, P. (ed.): 1991, *Choosing Death: Active Euthanasia, Religion and the Public Debate*, Trinity Press, Philadelphia.
20. Koop, C. and T. Johnson: 1992, *Let's Talk: An Honest Conversation on Abortion, Euthanasia, AIDS, Health Care*, Zondervan, Grand Rapids.
21. Land, R.: 1992, "Open Letter to President-Elect Bill Clinton", *Salt*, November 12, p. 3.

22. Land, R. and L. Moore: 1992, *The Earth is the Lord's*, Broadman, Nashville.
23. Lawton, K.: 1991, "The Doctor as Executioner", *Christianity Today*, December 16, 50-52.
24. Leber, G.: 1989, "We Must Rescue Them", *Hastings Center Report*, November/December, 26-27.
25. Marty, M.: 1992, "All Gnostics Here", *The Christian Century*, May 20-27, pp. .
26. Mitchell, C.: 1992, "Keep Ban on use of aborted Babies", *Light*, January-February, Christian Life Commission, Nashville.
27. National Ministries: 1991, *Christian Action*, American Baptist Convention, Valley Forge, PA.
28. Neff, D. (ed.): 1991, "Is Birth Control Christian?" *Christianity Today*, Nov. 11, pp. 34-45.
29. Neff, D.: 1992, "Politics, Polemics, and RU-486", *Christianity Today*, September 14, p. 19.
30. Shelp, E.: 1986, *Born to Die? Deciding the Fate of Critically   Ill Newborns*, Free Press, New York.
31. Shelp, E.: 1992, *AIDS and the Church: The Second Decade*. Westminster/John Knox, Louisville.
32. Sider, R.: 1987, *Completely Pro-Life*, Inter-Varsity Press, Downer's Grove, IL.
33. Simmons, P.: 1992, "Preimplantation Genetic Screening: Theological and Ethical Issues", Second National Conference on Genetics, Religion and Ethics, March 13-15, The Institute of Religion and Baylor College of Medicine, Texas Medical Center, Houston.
34. Simmons, P.: 1990, "Religious Liberty and the Abortion Debate", *Journal of Church and State*, Summer, Baylor University, Waco, TX.
35. Simmons, P.: 1983, *Birth and Death: Bioethical Decision Making*, Westminster, Philadelphia.
36. Simmons, P.: 1991, "AIDS: God's Curse or Divine Challenge?" *Clergy in Crisis*, Spring, 2:1, Memorial Medical Center, Savannah.
37. Simmons, P.: 1990, "The Fetus as Person: a Biblical Perspective", in E. Doerr & J. Prescott, eds. *Abortion Rights and Fetal 'Personhood'*, 2nd ed., Centerline, Long Beach.
38. Stafford, T.: 1990, "Animal Lib", *Christianity Today*, June 18, p. 18.
39. Stafford, T.: 1992, "In Reluctant Praise of Extremism", *Christianity Today*, October 26, 18-22.
40. Stafford, T.: 1992, "Ron Sider's Unsettling Crusade", *Christianity Today*, April 27, 18-22.
41. Stafford, T.: 1992, "Inside Crisis Pregnancy Centers", *Christianity Today*, August 17, pp. 20-24.
42. Stanley, C., *et al*: 1988, "A Biblical Perspective on Civil Disobedience", August 28, First Baptist Church, Atlanta.

43. Strode, T.: 1992, "Clinton Plans to Move Against Operation Rescue", *Baptist Press Release*, October 26.
44. Tada, J.: 1992, *When is it Right to Die?* Zondervan, Grand Rapids.
45. Terry, R.: 1990, *Accessory to Murder: the Enemies, Allies, and Accomplices to the Death of Our Culture*, Wolgemuth & Wyatt, Brentwood, TN.
46. Thomas, C.: 1992, "The GOP Ruins", *The Courier Journal*, Thursday, November 5, Forum.
47. Vawter, D.: 1992, "Ban Unjustified, Should be Removed", *Light*, January-February. Christian Life Commission, Nashville.
48. Wall, J.: 1992, *The Christian Century*, Dec. 23-30, p.1183.
49. Warnock, K.: 1992, "Baptists Share Nation's Concern about Health-Care System's Ills", *The Years Ahead*, Summer, The Annuity Board, SBC, Dallas.
50. Yancey, P.: 1991, "A Voice Crying in the Rain Forest", *Christianity Today*, July 22, 26-28.

AVRAHAM STEINBERG

JEWISH MEDICAL ETHICS

Two years are a rather short period for reporting on significant developments
in theological thinking and ruling. The following is, therefore, merely a
supplement to the material discussed in Volume One of the *Bioethics Yearbook*,
pp. 179-199. Part I of the current report corresponds to the lettering of
subtitles in the first volume, and is intended only to add to the material that
was covered in the previous volume. Part II discusses developments on other
issues.

I. ADDITIONS TO VOLUME ONE

A. *In Vitro Fertilization (IVF)*

Surrogate motherhood via a donor ovum is generally characterized by
contemporary halakhic scholars as offensive to moral sensitivities and is
prohibited a priori. One of the leading halakhic authorities expresses the
opinion that such a procedure might be biblically prohibited [16].

Nevertheless, if a donor ovum or a donor womb is utilized, a fundamental
issue arises: Who is the legal mother of the born child? The dilemma and
dispute among a number of rabbis concerning this question was discussed in
the first volume (p. 184). Recently, three of the most prominent current
halakhic authorities have publicized their opinions: Rabbi E. Y. Waldenberg
considers the nurturing woman to be the legal mother; Rabbi Y. S. Eliashiv
tends to concur with that view, but with reservations; Rabbi S. Z. Auerbach
concludes that there is no clear halakhic evidence in the sources to support one
approach or the other, and, therefore, that both the ovum-donor and the
surrogate mother should be considered as legal mothers [2].

If one obtains several ova from a woman's ovary and fertilizes all of them,
is one permitted to destroy those that will not be reimplanted? The Sephardi
Chief Rabbi of Israel, Rabbi Mordechai Eliahu ruled the following: It is
prohibited to destroy fertilized ova that were intended to be implanted, but ova
not chosen for implantation may be discarded [8]. (For other opinions see
Volume 1, p. 185).

Finally, it is prohibited to desecrate the Sabbath in order to salvage
fertilized ova that have not been implanted ([8]; [11], p. 141).

B. Andrew Lustig (Sr. Ed.), Bioethics Yearbook: Volume 3, 271-279.
©1993 Kluwer Academic Publishers.

D. *Newborns with Anomalies*

The general halakhic approach to newborns with anomalies was summarized in the first volume of the *Bioethics Yearbook* (p. 187). Several specific conditions, including meningomyelocele and Down's syndrome with duodenal atresia, were also discussed.

If the baby has a reasonable chance of survival, it is imperative to apply all available aggressive resuscitative measures to prematurely born infants, even though such procedures may cause untoward severe side effects. Hence, if a high concentration of oxygen is required, it should be provided with due care, even though it may cause blindness because of retinopathy. Similarly, aggressive resuscitation should be applied whenever needed, even though it may result in intracerebral hemorrhage with significant brain damage ([151; [12], pp. 127-128).

Parents who refuse to treat their defective newborn can be forced to do so, and should be forced to bear all the expenses of the necessary treatments and operations. That judgment, however, pertains only to life-saving procedures. If treatment is intended only to improve the quality of life, the parents cannot be coerced to bear the costs ([12], pp. 129, 130).

It is immoral for parents to abandon any newborn, whether for medical, social or economic reasons ([12], p. 129).

It is forbidden to kill an anencephalic newborn, even for purposes of transplantation. However, such an infant should not be resuscitated in the event of arrest [8].

I. *Definition of the Moment of Death*

The most highly debated and controversial medico-halakhic issue in the past few years concerns the definition of the moment of death. Many articles, reviews and discussions have recently been published attempting to define the moment of death according to Jewish law (see volume 1, pp. 192-193). In addition to the two classic definitions of death, namely cardiac death and brain death, some important variations have been advocated.

A variation of classic cardiac death, which places the ultimate significance upon the cessation of the function of the heart, was proposed by one prominent rabbi. In his opinion the definition of death depends on the cessation of blood circulation. This theory is based on the importance of the blood as the soul (Deuteronomy 12:23), and the prominence attributed by the ancients to the heart, brain and liver as the organs upon which the soul is dependent. Hence, on this view, the cessation of blood circulation to any one of these organs, or to all three of them, constitutes death [14].

Brain death criteria were accepted by the Chief Rabbinate of Israel, as reported in the first volume (p. 193). However, according to that opinion, it is not brain death per se that defines life or death; rather, respiration is the function that indicates life or death. If absolute and irreversible cessation of respiration can be reliably proven, the person is defined as dead. Irreversible cessation of respiratory activity can be assumed if one can demonstrate unequivocal medical criteria of brain death, which must of necessity involve the respiratory center in the brainstem. An important and significant variation of this opinion was articulated by Rabbi S. Z. Auerbach, a leading contemporary halakhic authority. In his opinion, the whole brain as an organ-defines life or death, and the destruction of the entire brain therefore constitutes death. However, because of halakhic and scientific restrictions, Rabbi Auerbach ruled that there is currently no reliable way to prove beyond any doubt that a person's brain is entirely destroyed, unless the heart has stopped functioning.

Nonetheless, organismal death may occur despite the fact that the heart is functioning normally, and in fact a fetus can continue to live in the uterus of an indisputably dead animal! To demonstrate that principle the following experiment was performed in Israel. In a large hospital with appropriate facilities, a pregnant sheep was anesthetized, intubated and ventilated. Subsequently, decapitation above the point of tracheal intubation was performed. Fatal bleeding was prevented by tying the large cervical blood vessels and replacing blood loss by intravenous fluids. The decapitated pregnant sheep was kept in this condition for 25 minutes, during which her heart functioned normally and fetal monitoring showed normal fetal heart beats. After 25 minutes a live, normal lamb was delivered by cesarean section [13].

By all criteria, including strict halakhic criteria, a decapitated sheep is dead. Nevertheless, this sheep's in-vivo heart function was normal. Moreover, the fetus continued to live in her womb and was delivered alive and well. Only two criteria of death were fulfilled here – absolute and irreversible cessation of spontaneous respiration, and absolute destruction of the entire brain. The heart and the blood circulation continued to function normally, indicating that they cannot serve as independent criteria of life or death.

J. *Organ Transplantation*

With regard to live donation of bone marrow by a living donor, it is preferable to convince the prospective donor to consent to the donation. If he refuses because he fears that the procedure might endanger him, no pressure should be applied to him. If, however, he is afraid only of the pain and discomfort that might result from the procedure, if he is the only matching donor, and if the donation is required for a lifesaving treatment, society then has the power to insist upon the donation in order to save life [11]. If the prospective bone marrow donor is a minor and is of an age that he can express his wishes, he should be asked to consent. If he is incapable of expressing an opinion his parents' consent may be sufficient to permit the donation [5].

According to one scholar, a live donor is permitted to accept monetary compensation for organ donation [13]. A more cautious approach is adopted by others ([11]. pp. 218-219). However, family members are prohibited from demanding payment for their consent to harvest organs from the deceased, because deriving benefit from the dead is prohibited. If, however, the money is needed for the life-saving treatment of a relative, it is permissible [12].

II. OTHER ISSUES

Disclosure of Information

The decision whether or not to disclose the truth to the patient depends on factual, ethical, and halakhic considerations. It must also be determined who is best qualified to decide whether or not the patient is to be told the truth, and what approach is appropriate in implementing that decision.

There is no doubt that the truth is an exceptionally valuable principle in Judaism (see, for instance, Exodus 34:6: Zechariah 8:16; Maimonides' Mishneh Torah, De'ot 2:6). However, according to halakhah, truth-telling is not an absolute ethical imperative. Therefore, in certain specific and well-defined circumstances of conflict between the truth and other values (e.g., situations where a human life or peace are at stake), it is permissible to deviate from the truth.

In the patient-physician relationship, the fundamental and primary obligation of a medical practitioner is to avoid harming the patient and to act in the patient's best interests. These considerations outweigh the purely philosophical principle of autonomy (see my introduction in volume 1, p. 181). Hence, the most important factor in deciding whether or not to disclose information is the factual assessment of harm versus benefit.

There are several opinions among rabbinic legislators and thinkers concerning the disclosure of the truth to the patient. Some rabbis argue that one should not disclose a fatal disease to a patient, so as not to destroy his spirit and make treatment more difficult. The rabbis maintain this opinion despite the fact that most patients react favorably to the disclosure. They argue that because an occasional patient may react negatively and his death hastened, it is prohibited to disclose the full truth in all cases. Other rabbis have ruled that in general it is preferable to remain silent and withhold the truth, unless one is absolutely certain that disclosure will not harm the patient.

Some writers distinguish between different categories of patients. In cases where there is hope for cure and revealing the truth may help by allowing the patient to actively participate in the medical treatment program, it is proper to disclose the truth. For patients with a terminal condition for which there is no medical treatment other than pain relief, the condition should not be disclosed to the patient but only to the closest relatives [1].

Other Jewish scholars opine that the question of revelation or concealment of the truth, from a halakhic viewpoint, depends on what is best for the patient.

One cannot make a general, definitive rule: Each case must be individually assessed on its own merits and a decision made as to what is best for that patient [9]. Since the general atmosphere in many Western societies today favors the disclosure of information to patients, and since studies have proven that the benefit of disclosure in many instances significantly outweighs the withholding of information, these scholars generally favor disclosure.

However, the more important issue is not "whether" to disclose to the patient the truth about his illness, but "how" to do so. Practical answers to questions about the timing and setting of disclosure are more important than the principle itself. The answers to such questions are intended to benefit and/or minimize the harm to each individual patient ([10], p. 139).

Suicide

In most instances suicidal acts are prohibited by Jewish law. There are certain circumstances, however, where the act is prohibited but the person is not judged to have committed a willful suicide.

According to Jewish law, suicide is regarded as murder. Moreover, some authorities opined that a person who commits suicide is worse than a killer, because all transgressions are purged at the time of death, but a person who commits suicide transgresses by his very death. In the act of suicide, death, which should be an atonement for the individual, instead becomes a major sin.

Several reasons are given for the prohibition of suicide. The value of life is paramount; therefore, one is obligated to preserve one's life. Moreover, a person is not the master of his body and thus is not allowed to take his own life or to harm himself. In accordance with the Scriptures and ethical principles, a person's body is entrusted to him as a deposit by God to fulfill God's wishes. One does not have the right to damage this deposit in any manner whatsoever. A person who commits suicide denies fundamental Judaic beliefs in reward and punishment and the world to come. A person who commits suicide cannot repent and his death does not atone for him.

The act of suicide is punishable. According to Jewish law, most acts of respect that are usually accorded to the deceased, are denied to the person who commits suicide. There is also a requirement to bury that person more than eight cubits away from other graves. However, to actually carry out punishment, a variety of strict conditions and specific circumstances are required, and thus, the imposition of punishment is very rare in practice.

Because of the strong opposition to the act of suicide in Jewish law, it is obligatory to save one who survives a suicide attempt.

The Elderly

The general Jewish approach to the elderly is to accommodate them in the family environment. In the Bible and Talmud, the elderly are not included in groups of underprivileged people (such as the poor, the proselytes, the orphans, and the widows) who require special considerations of charity and compassion because of their underprivileged status. Similarly, there is no mention ln the Bible and Talmud about institutions or organizations specifically designated to help the elderly. By contrast, organizations are described that care for the ill, the poor, and the dead. Thus, the integration of the elderly into family life, and care of the elderly by the family, have been normal and accepted practice.

For this reason, old age homes among the Jews were only recently established in contrast to the establishment of old age homes by other groups at much earlier historical periods ([11], 338).

Judaism essentially views old age in a positive light because it is the stage of life associated with a richness of experience, accumulated knowledge, decrease in libido, and free time to study Torah and fulfill commandments. There are also negative aspects to old age because of physical and mental deterioration. Thus, the Rabbis speak of both the good and bad features of old age ([11], p. 352).

There are a myriad of biblical and rabbinical laws and customs pertaining to respect and honor toward the elderly. The most notable example is the biblical commandment: "Thou shalt rise up before the hoary head, and honor the face of the old man" (Leviticus 19:32). The requirement to respect the elderly applies to all old people, even an elderly sinner, an elderly wicked person, or an elderly ignoramus (Tractate Kiddushin 32a; Maimonides' Mishneh Torah, Talmud Torah 6:9; Karo's Shulchan Aruch, Yoreh De'ah 244:7).

Acquired Immune Deficiency Syndrome (AIDS)

At the moment, AIDS is, unfortunately, a lethal, contagious disease with no available cure or immunization. Therefore, preventive measures are the only available means of fighting this pandemic.

There is a clear obligation incumbent on each individual and on society at large to do everything possible to prevent the spread of such a lethal disease. In general, society has both the right and the duty to implement any measure that is helpful in saving its members from contracting the disease, provided that the suggested measure is efficacious. This is true even when the measures undertaken by society deny individuals rights such as liberty, confidentiality, and autonomy. In other words, the need to protect innocent third parties and society at large takes precedence over the rights and liberties of the individual, provided that the actions taken by society are effective, and there is no other available solution to protect both society and its individuals.

In the first decade of the outbreak of AIDS, the only preventive measure recommended by health-care policy-makers was "safe sex", namely the utilization of a condom during sexual engagement with unknown partners. This recommendation is halakhically difficult to accept for two major reasons: a) the use of a condom is generally strictly forbidden because it violates the biblical prohibition of improper emission of seed; b) morally and educationally, the lesson of that campaign is that homosexuality, prostitution, or adultery are acceptable lifestyles, so long as technical precautions are taken to avoid contracting the disease! From the Jewish standpoint, that is a fallacious message.

Moreover, because of politically influential high-risk groups (such as homosexuals) in the USA, the AIDS epidemic was handled by using an exceptional epidemiologic approach. In order to protect the individual rights and liberties of homosexuals, it was forbidden to perform HIV screening tests even on hospitalized AIDS patients, unless they specifically consented to this test; it was forbidden to inform sexual partners of AIDS patients; it was forbidden to report HIV carriers to public health authorities; and it was forbidden to disclose the carrier state of health-care providers to their patients. This approach has undergone some changes in recent years, and a more reasonable, epidemiologic approach is gaining support.

One of the most significant AIDS risk groups are homosexuals. Judaism regards homosexual conduct as a serious transgression of divine law, as is clearly stated in the Bible: "And with a man thou shalt not lie as one lies with a woman: it is an abomination" (Leviticus 18:22). Countenancing a homosexual lifestyle as morally or socially acceptable constitutes deviation from divinely dictated norms. The validity or non-validity of the claim that homosexuality is natural rather than aberrant, or a normal state rather than an illness, is irrelevant to Jewish teaching. Not everything that is normal and natural is also licit and morally acceptable. Divine commandments, by their very nature, are designed to curb and to channel human desires. They are not necessarily reflective of that which comes naturally to man. Homosexuality is one aspect of human nature in which natural tendencies must be confronted and subdued, and represents an additional (and perhaps more difficult) trial. For some, the challenge is undoubtedly greater than for others, but the standard is enunciated for all with utmost clarity [20].

Judaism makes a clear and sharp distinction between sinners and sins, as stated in the Talmud: "Let sins cease out of the earth but not the sinners" (Tractate Berachot 10a). In our association with patients who are afflicted with AIDS, we must react with compassion and love to those persons. We must treat them and alleviate their suffering to the best of our ability. However, that acceptance need not, and dare not, encompass any form of illicit conduct that may lie at the source of the affliction – whether homosexuality, prostitution, or drug addiction. The question of punishment should not arise in our relationship to individuals who are engaged in deviant sexual or social behavior. Although the act must be deplored, the person who commits such an act remains a Jew to whom our hearts and arms are open. No human being can declare with certainty that there is a direct cause and effect relationship between a Specific misdeed and any particular misfortune. Hence, it remains our obligation to relate positively and to be helpful to any fellow man afflicted with any disease, including AIDS, whether or not his previous immoral or illicit behavior has led to his suffering. Society is duty-bound to treat victims of AIDS as it treats the victims of any other infectious disease.

From the Jewish standpoint, the preventive campaign would emphasize educational efforts to eliminate deviant behavior, including homosexuality, prostitution and drug addiction. It would thereby aim at preventing the major sources of contracting and spreading of the disease, rather than permitting or even encouraging such deviant behavior by merely recommending (often inadequate) technical measures to reduce the chance of infection.

With regard to the moral dilemma of screening for HIV carriers, the most significant problem concern how to design and implement testing programs that will effectively protect the lives and health of members of the society at large. If scientists and epidemiologists determine that compulsory screening can effectively reduce the number of AIDS victims and arrest the spread of this lethal disease, it would be appropriate from the Jewish standpoint to implement such actions, despite the fact that compulsory testing is certainly a gross violation of individual liberty and autonomy ([12], p. 598: [20]).

Similarly, despite the well established commitment of physicians to keeping patients' medical information confidential, if it is clearly judged that withholding the information may harm a third party, e.g., the medical team, or a sexual partner, it is imperative to convince the patient to disclose the fact that he is suffering from AIDS to those that may be infected by him. If he refuses, it is the duty of the health-care provider to warn those that might be endangered by the patient [7].

A final issue posed by AIDS is the question of the physician's obligations to his patients and to himself. Since the risk of contracting AIDS from a patient when established and necessary precautions are strictly adhered to is minimal, it is the obligation of health-care providers to treat AIDS patients, and the basic commandment incumbent upon everyone to visit the sick is applicable to AIDS patients ([12]. pp. 599-600).

Hadassah Medical School
Hebrew University
Jerusalem, Israel

BIBLIOGRAPHY

1. Abraham, S.A.: 1985, *Nishmat Avraham, Yore De'ah* 338:3, Jerusalem (Hebrew).
2. Abraham, S.A.: 1991, *Nishmat Avraham*, Vol. 4, Even Ha'ezer 5:2, Jerusalem (Hebrew).
3. Auerbach, S.Z. cited in: Abraham, S.A.: 1991, *Nishmat Avraham*, Vol. 4, *Orach Chaim* 330:5, Jerusalem (Hebrew).

4. Auerbach, S.Z. cited in: Abraham, S.A.: 1991, *Nishmat Avraham*, Vol. 4, *Even Ha'ezer* 80:1, Jerusalem (Hebrew).
5. Auerbach, S.Z. cited in: Abraham, S.A.: 1991, *Nishmat Avraham*, Vol. 4, *Choshen Mishpat* 243:1, Jerusalem (Hebrew).
6. Auerbach, S.Z. cited in: Abraham, S.A.: 1991, *Nishmat Avraham*, Vol. 4, *Choshen Mishpat* 420:1-2, Jerusalem (Hebrew).
7. Bleich, J.D.: 1992, "AIDS: A Jewish perspective", Tradition 26(3), 49-80.
8. Eliahu, M.: 1990, "Destruction of Eggs", *Techumin* 11, 272-274 (Hebrew).
9. Shafran, Y.: 1987, "Telling the Truth to the Patient", *Assia* 42-43, 16-23 (Hebrew).
10. Steinberg, A.: 1988, *Encyclopedia Hilchatit Refuit*, Vol. 1, The Dr. Falk Schlesinger Institute for Medical Halakhic Research at Shaare Zedek Medical Center, Jerusalem (Hebrew).
11. Steinberg, A.: 1991, *Encyclopedia Hilchatit Refuit*, Vol. 2, The Dr.Falk Schlesinger Institute for Medical Halakhic Research at Shaare Zedek Medical Center, Jerusalem (Hebrew).
12. Steinberg. A.: 1992, *Encyclopedia Hilchatit Refuit*, Vol. 3, The Dr.Falk Schlesinger Institute for Medical Halakhic Research at Shaare Zedek Medical Center, Jerusalem (Hebrew).
13. Steinberg, A.: Personal communication.
14. Schachter, H.: 1990, "Concerning the Laws of the Dead and the Dying", *Assia* 49-50, 119-137 (Hebrew).
15. Waldenberg, E. Y.: 1990, *Responsa Tzitz Eliezer*, Vol. 18, No. 19, sec.1, Jerusalem (Hebrew).
16. Wasner, S.: 1981, *Responsa Shevet Halevi*, Vol. 3, No. 175. Sec. 2, Bnei Brag (Hebrew).

KENNETH VAUX

BIOETHICS IN THE REFORMED TRADITION

INTRODUCTION

As 1992 drew to a close, a new liberal spirit was felt throughout the world, especially in the West where the ideal of freedom first took cultural form. Bioethical developments both contributed to this exhilarating ethos and were in turn influenced by it. This essay reviews bioethics developments over the last biennium in the Reformed tradition. I will first discuss that new cultural ethos and its peculiar relation to the Reformed tradition. I will then explore three illustrative bioethical issues: abortion, aid-in-dying, and gay and lesbian rights to ordination. Finally, I will return again to socio-cultural analysis, trying to assess the significance of these developments.

I. LIBERTY AND THE REFORMED ETHOS

One of the important books of recent years is Francis Fukuyama's *The End of History and The Last Man*. The study chronicles the success of freedom in the modern world. Focusing on economic and political history and the flourishing of free-enterprise social systems, the study also alludes to an underlying individual and collective consciousness of spiritual freedom. The book takes this fundamental turn by virtue of its grounding in Hegelian philosophy. Liberty is a virtue with deep roots in the history of civilization, but it takes on a pervasive force in the Calvinistic Reformation in western Europe beginning in the sixteenth century [1]. The libertarian revolution, enlivened through the English Revolution of the 1640's and the American and French revolutions of the next century, was very much the product of Calvinist convictions about conscience, toleration, non-interference, and autonomy. The Reformed Tradition has been a potent bearer of liberty into world civilization, with all the awesome ambiguities that such freedom inspires.

The liberal and secular spirit has made a deep imprint on contemporary medical decision-making. In late 1992 the American electorate selected Bill Clinton President of the United States. It soon became clear that this Southern Baptist Calvinist, steeped in the human rights heritage of Anglo-American thought through philosophers such as his Oxford compatriot John Locke, would make a series of biomedical policy discussions that would accent personal "free choice". Abortion would be available in publicly funded facilities such as

B. Andrew Lustig (Sr. Ed.), Bioethics Yearbook: Volume 3, 281-289.
©1993 Kluwer Academic Publishers.

military hospitals. Research on RU 486, the abortifacient drug, would be approved. Fetal tissue research and therapeutic development would be resumed.

At the same time, the ambiguities of freedom were also evident in a number of decisions in late 1992. With a sense, perhaps, that freedom had gotten out of hand, the New York City School Board dismissed Chancellor Joseph A. Fernandez, in part for his policy of distributing condoms in the public schools. The Board was also critical of his programs commending sympathy for and understanding of the homosexual life style. By contrast, the Baltimore School Board authorized Norplant sterilization in its magnet school. Similarly, in an Illinois case, a judge offered a child-abusing mother a reduced sentence if she would accept Norplant. To date, these developments have been hailed by some as offering greater freedom and condemned by others as endorsing sexual promiscuity.

In overview, then, the early 1990s were witnessing a shift in our understanding of bioethics. Freedom was moving to complement earlier authorities and solidarities. Increasingly, responsibility was being emphasized as the correlative of autonomy. A decade of resurgent conservatism and fundamentalism in worldview and morals was giving way to an affirmation of personal liberty and societal tolerance.

II. ABORTION

Abortion is an interim tragedy in an otherwise purposive and prolific creation. It is a human arrogation that must be diminished as we ameliorate the circumstances that make it necessary. In ethics, freedom calls for allowance.

The Reformed tradition and its member communions have a long history of discussing the religious and ethical aspects of abortion. For centuries, Reformed Church bodies, including American Presbyterian denominations, condemned abortion. This condemnation was expressed as silent concurrence with the prevailing ecclesial and social ethic. Then, beginning several decades ago with the strong advocacy of women's rights, ethical policy shifted toward freedom of choice. In 1984, this author chaired the denomination's Task Force on Science, Medicine, and Human Values. In its conclusions, the Task Force unanimously concurred on matters such as health care access and social justice, care for the dying, and genetic engineering. Although opinions were divided on the issue of abortion, a strong pro-choice position was eventually adopted based on freedom of conscience. The Task Force affirmed the *responsibility of women, guided by Scripture and the Holy Spirit, to make good moral decisions regarding problem pregnancies*.

In the late 1980s, the Presbyterian Church grew less comfortable with the *pro choice* position. A desire emerged among pastors and congregations to formulate a more nuanced view. Initiatives and overtures were submitted to the General Assembly each year and, although "pro-life" appeals were always voted down, convictions in that direction mounted. From 1989-1992, the General Assembly Special Committee on Problem Pregnancies and Abortion worked to forge a new synthesis between "pro-life" and "pro-choice" positions. By early 1992, it was clear that a decidedly moderate majority position would emerge. A minority position generally discouraged abortion except in cases of rape, incest, fetal deformity, and threat to the mother's life. In its report, the Special Committee affirmed that "all life is precious to God", that "we are to preserve and protect life", and that abortion "should be an option of last resort".

In novel initiatives, the Church was asked to establish centers for alternatives to abortion. The issue was also raised as to whether churches were required to support the domination's health insurance plan, which funds abortions, or whether, in "free choice", churches could dissent from this plan. As is the case for health care facilities, judicatories have also supported such conscientious objection for churches. The 1992 General Assembly voted a more moderate "freedom of choice" policy with a strong emphasis on family covenant and care of children.

Passages from majority and minority spokespersons portray the rich colors of the debate. Howard Rice, a Professor of Ministry at San Francisco Seminary and a handicapped person, and Elizabeth Achtemeier, a biblical scholar at Union Seminary in Richmond, Virginia, respectively express those views:

One track (of the report) emphasizes the biblical theme of the preciousness of life as a gift from God and the special tenderness which we are called by God to have for the weakest and most vulnerable in our world. The other track emphasizes another biblical theme, that of our God-given responsibilities to make difficult decisions in a fallen world

...all life, born and unborn, belongs to the God who has made it, and to destroy that life is to "rob God" (Malachi 3:8) of what belongs to Him. To destroy that life is further to deny that we are not our own, but rather bought with the price of God's only begotten Son (I Corinthians 6:19-20)[2].

Expressed here is the tension or dialectic between liberty and solidarity. The world is fallen and is being redeemed. Abortion will continue to be a tragic necessity. We need seek to ameliorate its agony and diminish its incidence. Biotechnology, perhaps in the form of abortifacients such as RU 486, may cast the problem in a new moral light. Just as it is becoming more unconscionable to knowingly give birth to a severely genetically or congenitally injured baby, it may become conscionable to unknowingly thwart the implantation of an unwanted embryo. Cell analysis (e.g., amniocentesis and ultrasound) now discloses information about the physical condition of a nascent human being. Just as we would not morally prolong the agonal dying of an old and sick person with an infinite array of death-defying devices, we should not condemn one born-to-die to a living death. In the same spirit, it may be morally acceptable to contravene the initial or continued implantation of an embryo when one lacks the human strength or divine summons to receive a new life.

In a strange twist of logic, it maybe the case that selective allowance of abortion is the only way to limit its occurrence. Abortion is wrong as a contraceptive, a population control policy, for sex selection, or as a mere convenience. Abortion is right in situations of teen-age rape, incest, danger to a mother's life, severe genetic or congenital anomalies, or when pregnancy poses a life-threatening burden to the woman or couple. Reason and religiously informed conscience affirms something like this morally nuanced tableau. How to effect such a moral policy in personal decision-making and public policy is an enormously complex task, one calling for great measures of understanding, forgiveness, and support.

III. AID IN DYING

Late in 1992, Dr. Jack Kevorkian continued to make headlines by assisting in a number of suicides in southern Michigan, the American homeland of Dutch Reformed faith. Using either a thanatron (a Rube Goldberg device whereby a patient would self-inject a barbiturate and a killing cardioactive drug) or a mask delivering a lethal dose of carbon dioxide, Kevorkian helped several severely ill patients to commit suicide before the 1993 law against assisted suicide took effect in Michigan. Kevorkian mused at the frantic political machinations of the horrified Michigan legislators:

I feel pleasure that they're making fools of themselves, disgust, even contempt, that they would even think of perpetuating human misery by law . . . I don't call it a law. It is the arbitrary codification of an edict, for the sole benefit of a barbaric religious clique [3].

Again, the debate about aid in dying centers on issues of freedom of personal and professional action versus the traditional moral proscription of such action. The Michigan law outlawing assisted suicide and physician-assisted suicide is being challenged by the American Civil Liberties Union, which argues that the law will infringe on the privacy rights of patients, families, and doctors. The law is also being challenged by a coalition of physicians, pharmacists, and nurses serving the elderly, who argue that it will limit the range of their care. Finally, the Wayne County Medical Society objects to the law, asserting that it will *impair medical practice in the relief of pain and suffering*[3].

It is no coincidence that Kevorkian's work takes place in the seed-bed of the Reformed tradition in America. It is also no coincidence that the world's most liberal euthanasia practice is found in another culture deeply shaped by the Calvinist heritage, i.e., the Netherlands. Calvinism has generated individuals and cultures deeply committed to autonomous and theonomous conscience, values often defined in resistance to civil and ecclesial authority. The tradition has stimulated laissez-faire entrepreneurialism, economic independence, the Protestant work ethic, and the Puritan sex-ethic. The "aging and dying ethic" of this tradition is captured in the words of Joe Harotunian, another Armenian Calvinist. Toward the end of his life, Harotunian, a Chicago theologian, is said to have remarked, "No right is so fundamental as that of a person to give his life back to God".

But renegade ethics are discomforting. The ethics of freedom are risky, adventurous, and often bizarre. The Kevorkian protest clearly reminds us that the dominant ways our culture deals with the dying are deficient, verging on the atrocious. Cancer physicians today are beginning to understand that honesty and humanity with patients require a candid sharing about cost, side-effects, life-expectancy and quality of life, as well as about projected benefits of beginning another round of surgery, chemotherapy, or radiation therapy. This sobering candor, it is argued, is an appropriate requirement of truly informed consent as one enters what is now being called the "last illness". We tend to spend our last days in hospitals, our last hours in intensive care units, our last dollars in medical expenses. Kevorkian's provocative gestures challenge this "American way of death".

An editorial in the New York Times, entitled "Why Dr. Kevorkian was Called In", reads as follows:

Last Wednesday a man named Jack Miller dropped his hand, thereby pulling a clip off the plastic tubing that connected a canister of carbon monoxide to a mast over his face. The gadget was yet another of the egregious Dr. Jack Kevorkian's suicide devices, and Mr. Miller was the ninth person to take advantage of his ingenuity. Eighteen minutes later, Mr. Miller was dead. Jack Miller wanted to end his life because the pain from metastatic bone cancer had made it unbearable. In pulling that clip he put himself in the driver's seat - which is precisely where most people want to be as they approach the end of their life. If they aren't, it's not because of a lack of directives defining what is legally and ethically appropriate in the care of the dying. It's because of the gap between the intellectual constructs and the realities of the respirator, the IV tube and the oxygen hose [4].

Responding to the death-denying excesses of modern medicine, social policy has already moved to allow passive euthanasia and, in limited circumstances and jurisdictions, active euthanasia. The right to refuse life-prolonging care is well-established, and information about advance directives is now required of institutions by the Patient Self-Determination Act. Unfortunately, technological and economic imperatives often take ascendancy and, like Oppenheimer's fearful aphorism regarding the bomb, we find that "what is technically sweet becomes irresistible".

Reformed church bodies have responded in two ways to the challenge posed by the discussion of aid-in-dying. In California and Washington state, Presbyterian voters were more inclined to support initiatives allowing physician-assisted suicide than were conservative Baptists. Kevorkian's own clients were more apt to come from liberal Protestant or Unitarian denominations than from fundamentalist Christian groups. Mainline Presbyterians, we might assume, would be somewhat sympathetic, although not as free-thinking as

Unitarians, nor as involved in groups like the Hemlock Society. On the other hand, much of the conservative reaction against Kevorkian comes from Christian Reformed churches. In an informal poll of ministers in this tradition taken by the author, it is clear that they are generally opposed to euthanasia on biblical grounds.

Presbyterian documents on death and dying continue to emphasize the right of persons to refuse treatment, to accept death without resorting to frantic measures to prolong life, to protect the poor from coercion on these matters, and to balance the imperatives of social and community justice with individual demands for longevity.

IV. GAY AND LESBIAN RIGHTS

As the decade turned, the issue of civil and ecclesial rights for homosexual persons again become prominent. Central to that discussion were issues concerning the status of sexual preference and the morality of overtly homosexual behavior.

In the United Presbyterian Church (USA), a moderate Reformed body bracketed by more conservative communions like the Christian Reformed Church and Orthodox Presbyterian Church on the right and the more liberal United Church of Christ on the left, the controversy on these issues was acute. In 1991, the General Assembly's Special Commission on Human Sexuality issued a report that extolled free expression, toleration of different sexual styles and patterns of relationships (e.g. pre-marital sexual practice) and a reaffirmation of the moral legitimacy of homosexual being and behavior. Although not a matter within its specific purview, the Commission also counselled broad acceptance of homosexuals in the church, and even their inclusion in the ordained ministries. The report, however, was resoundingly rejected by the General Assembly.

In late 1991 and 1992, a single case arose to focus the ethical reflection of United Presbyterian Church (USA). Jane Adams Spahr, a Presbyterian minister ordained in the 1970's before gay persons sought to be publicly acknowledged, sought to become co-pastor in the Downtown Presbyterian Church in Rochester, New York. The local church wished to call her and the Presbytery and Synod affirmed the call in response to an appeal by disgruntled minorities in both bodies who questioned the legitimacy of her call. Presbyter and Synod cited a "grandfather clause" to justify the appointment. The "grandfather clause" refers to an element in the 1978 denominational policy that offered "definitive guidance" to the church on the matter of authorizing the ministry of "avowed practicing homosexual" person. That report counselled that there be no retroactive exclusion.

Spahr, who had written her Doctor of Ministry thesis at San Francisco Theological Seminary on "Lesbian Spirituality", was held in abeyance by a "stay of enforcement" while the judicial process worked its way to the denomination's permanent Judicial Commission. On November 3, 1992, the Permanent Judicial Council "set aside the call".

The gay and lesbian community within the church was outraged. As the biennium closed, numerous overtures to the General Assembly dealing with the judgment of the Permanent Judicial Council were being formulated in the Presbyteries. For example, the New Brunswick Presbyter decided to " ... allow Presbyter or session to ordain anyone they want without regard to the 'definitive guidance' of the General Assembly". The New Brunswick judgment affirmed parochial autonomy and rightful jurisdiction: "a person's fitness can best be judged by the governing body that has direct knowledge of that person".

The ethics of religious bodies on this issue provide a fascinating glimpse of the sociology of moral sentiment in contemporary religion. In affirming, however tentatively, the right to ordain anyone by a given Presbytery, the New Brunswick and Chicago Presbyteries move the church away from the depth and breadth of its own moral heritage toward the more libertarian emphasis of progressive Protestantism found, for example, in the Minneapolis Jurisdiction of the United Church of Christ or in the Unitarian Church. In seeking the right to acknowledge ordain practicing homosexuals to ministry, those Presbyteries also depart from the millennia-long condemnations of homoerotic practice. They also part company with the broad body of communions in the biblical tradition: Judaism, Roman, Catholicism, Eastern Orthodoxy and most forms of evangelical Protestantism.

How shall this agonizing issue be interpreted? What are the theological and ethical themes that cast light on the subject? If the issue is one of purity and fidelity, we may wish to discountenance homosexual practice and the implied approval of the practice that ordination implies. At the same time, we should acknowledge that heterosexual persons can also violate standards of purity and fidelity, as well as the requirements of compassion and care.

A. *Liberation/Stigmatization*

The holiness strand of ethics in the Hebrew Bible and the virtue compendium of Stoicism have posed the problem of how to typify homosexuality? Is it disorder, sin, misbehavior, a flaw of character, or an alternative life style? The Levitical litany and Pauline profile are often invoked too facilely and flippantly. First, in Leviticus and Paul, behavior rather than being is at issue. Both scriptures are ignorant of genetic or ontologic aspects of homosexuality. Leviticus catalogues behaviors that are offensive to a jealous and holy God: incest, adultery, child-sacrifice, homosexuality, bestiality, spiritism, and cursing one's parents. These actions, which were pervasive in Egyptian and Canaanite cultures, were unconscionable to followers of Jehovah.

Nonetheless, the present-day question is this: can and should homosexual relationships be dissociated from this tableau of culpable and abominable

behaviors?   One the one hand, one is inclined to say yes.   Consensual
homosexual relations do not appear to entail the stigmata of violence,
degradation, and harm of the other practices listed.   On the other hand, later
Greeks and Romans would not only strip homosexual behavior of harm, but
would also claim that homoeroticism, even pedophilia, were natural phases of
human development and fulfillment.   Against this new counterpart of ancient
paganism, primitive Christianity would again speak the word of separation,
chastity, and the exemplary life.   Against a cultural backdrop of infanticide,
abortion, and all varieties of homoeroticism, the intensely ascetic and
apocalyptic followers of the Nazarene, both Hebraic and Hellenistic, would
employ the behavioral canons of the Pythagorean and pious Stoics and
formulate ethical teachings like Paul's moral instruction to the Romans and the
Didache.   In Romans (1:18-32), Paul couples homosexuality with idolatry as
consuming and compulsive passions that draw energy away from the proper
center of devotion and service.   Paul, we should recall, had a similar, though
muted sentiment toward marriage itself, seeing it as a disorienting distraction
from the urgency of Kingdom come (I Corinthians 7:9).

These comments are offered to support the contention that the end of the
matter is ambivalence and arbitration.   Sexual being, what our consumer age
irreverently calls sexual preference, is neither blameworthy or praiseworthy, but
simply is.   It belongs in the moral category that Calvin calls *adiaphoria* –
something morally neutral.   Homosexual behavior does not belong to the order
of edification or damnation.   It is, "for the time being", an inscrutable mystery
of the fallen world.   Its conjunction with the HIV pandemic in the late
twentieth century is surely further reason for cautious reappraisal.

As the 1978 Presbyterian instruction and guidance on homosexually stated:
"Civil discrimination, expulsion of gays and lesbians from the military, is
unconscionable".   Ecclesial discrimination, e.g. restricting ordination, is
conscionable. A calling body is the ultimate authority on this matter. To order
its own life, any jurisdiction of the church; congregation, Presbyter, Synod or
General Assembly should be free to ordain or not ordain the self-avowed
practicing homosexual person. Authority cannot be escaped or avoided. If (as
in the New York City Presbyter case in 1976) "definitive guidance" is sought
from the General Assembly, it must be heeded. If the church is not willing to
accept guidance, it should not ask for it.

We are left, of course, with the frustrating political reality of plebiscite
decision-making and democracy, the political form that Calvinism anchored into
world history. How should we deal with the ecclesial-legal phenomenon of an
individual or minority asking for appeal to a superior court? Only one answer
is appropriate: there must be the opportunity for a counter-appeal on behalf
of the majority. For all its theological moorings and sacramental trappings,
ordination is an ordinary, pragmatic ordering of the churches to activate
mission and achieve unity and peace.

V. SUMMARY

This essay has sought to capture the convictions of one stream of modern religious tradition on bioethical matters. I stand in the Reformed tradition in the moderate center of that pathway. I have singled out several recurrent themes that are relevant to a number of issues. The Calvinist and Reformed heritage is biased toward freedom, asceticism, and unity. It has fostered these ideals not only in the secular history of Western civilization, but also in Eastern cultures, such as the Armenian and Korean, which it has helped to shape.

University of Illinois Medical Center
Chicago, Illinois, U.S.A.

BIBLIOGRAPHY

1.   Fukuyama, Francis: 1992, *The End of History and the Last Man*. New York. Free Press.
2.   "Abortion: Top Issue of Assembly ...": 1992. *The News of the Presbyterian Church (U.S.A.)* (May), pp. 4-5.
3.   "Lull for Kevorkian May Presage New Furor Over Suicides He Aids." *New York Times*, February 22, 1992, C8.
4.   "Why Dr. Kevorkian Was Called In." *New York Times*, January 25, 1993, A10.

NOTES ON CONTRIBUTORS

Theo A. Boer, Ph.D., is Research Fellow at the Centre for BioEthics and Medical Law at Utrecht University, The Netherlands.

Joseph Boyle, Ph.D.,is Professor of Philosophy, St. Michael's College, University of Toronto, Toronto, Ontario, Canada.

Courtney S. Campbell, Ph.D., is Assistant Professor of Philosophy, Oregon State University, Corvallis, Oregon, U.S.A.

Prakash N. Desai, M.D., is Professor of Clinical Psychiatry, Department of Psychiatry, University of Illinois Medical Center, Chicago, and Chief of the Psychiatry Service, Veterans Administration West Side Medical Center, Chicago, Illinois, U.S.A.

Judith A. Granbois, M.A., is Program Associate, Poynter Center for the Study of Ethics and American Institutions, Indiana University, Bloomington, Indiana, U.S.A.

Stanley S. Harakas, Th.D., is Professor of Christian Ethics at Holy Cross Greek Orthodox School of Theology in Brookline, Massachusetts, U.S.A.

Hassan H. Hathout, M.D., Ph.D., is Advisor, Islamic Center of Southern California, Los Angeles, California, U.S.A.

B. Andrew Lustig, Ph.D., is Research Fellow in Theological Ethics at the Institute of Religion and a Member of the Center for Ethics, Medicine, and Public Issues at Baylor College of Medicine, Houston, Texas, U.S.A.

Paul T. Nelson, Ph.D., is Associate Professor, Chair, and Director of the Honors Program, Department of Religion, Wittenberg University, Springfield, Ohio, U.S.A.

Kathleen Nolan, M.D., M.S.L., is Visiting Associate for Medicine at the Hastings Center, Briarcliff Manor, New York, and a Zen student in full-time residential training at Zen Mountain Monastery, Mount Tremper, New York, U.S.A.

Egbert Schroten, Ph.D., is Professor of Christian Ethics on the Theological Faculty and Director of the Centre for Bio-Ethics and Medical Law, Utrecht University, The Netherlands.

Robert L. Shelton, Ph.D., is Associate Professor and Chairman, Department of Religious Studies, University of Kansas, Lawrence, Kansas, U.S.A.

Paul D. Simmons, Ph.D., has recently retired as Professor of Christian Ethics and Director of the Clarence Jordan Center for Christian Ethical Concerns, Southern Baptist Theological Seminary, Louisville, Kentucky, U.S.A.

David H. Smith, Ph.D., is Professor of Religious Studies and Director of the Poynter Center for the Study of Ethics and American Institutions, Indiana University, Bloomington, Indiana, U.S.A.

Avraham Steinberg, M.D., is Director, Center for Medical Ethics, Hadassah Medical School, Hebrew University, and Pediatric Neurologist, Department of Pediatrics, Shaare Zedek Medical Center, Jerusalem, Israel.

NOTES ON CONTRIBUTORS

Kenneth L. Vaux, Ph.D., is Professor of Theological Ethics and Director of the Center for Ethics in Public Life, Garrett Evangelical Theological Seminary, Evanston, Illinois, U.S.A.

There are numerous errors in the references for "Bioethics in Scandinavia: 1989-1991", by Reidar K. Lie and Jens Erik Paulsen, pp. 279-307 in Volume 2 of the *Bioethics Yearbook*. The corrections are as follows.

On page 279: note [47] corresponds to bibliographical reference 49.
On page 282: notes [59,60] correspond to references 61,62.
On Page 283: note [53] corresponds to reference 55;
               note [5] corresponds to reference 6.
On page 285: note [23] corresponds to reference 24.
On page 286: note [52] corresponds to reference 54;
               note [23] corresponds to reference 24;
               note [57] corresponds to reference 60.
On page 287: note [61] corresponds to reference 64;
               note [6] corresponds to reference 7;
               note [8] corresponds to reference 9;
               note [20] corresponds to reference 21.
On page 288: note [54] corresponds to the following missing reference:
               Socialstyrelsen: 1990, "Socialstyrelsens allmänna råd
               omhändertagande av foster after abort", <u>Socialstyrelsens</u>
               <u>författningssamling</u>, SOSFS 1990:8, Stockholm;
               notes [38,39] correspond to references 39,40;
               note [35] corresponds to reference 36;
On page 289: note [34] corresponds to reference 35.
On page 290: note [10] corresponds to reference 11;
               note [50] corresponds to reference 52.
On page 291: note [47] corresponds to reference 48;
               notes [24,30] correspond to references 25,31.
On page 292: notes [31,32] correspond to references 32,33;
               notes [9,21] correspond to references 10,22;
               notes [43,44] correspond to references 44,45;
               note [64] corresponds to reference 65;
               note [17] corresponds to reference 18;
               note [52] corresponds to reference 53;
               note [16] corresponds to reference 17.
On page 294: notes [42,69] correspond to references 42,70;
               note [19] corresponds to reference 20;
               note [60] corresponds to reference 63.
On page 296: note [58] corresponds to reference 59;
               note [27] corresponds to reference 28;
               note [49] corresponds to reference 50;
               note [18] corresponds to reference 19.
On page 297: note [45] corresponds to reference 46.
On page 304: note [[57] corresponds to reference 5.

INDEX OF AUTHORS AND DOCUMENTS DISCUSSED

The manufacturer's authorised representative in the EU is Springer
Nature Customer Service Centre GmbH, Europaplatz 3, 69115 Heidelberg,
Germany. If you have any concerns regarding our products, please
contact ProductSafety@springernature.com

Printed and bound by CPI Group (UK) Ltd, Croydon, CR0 4YY
23/04/2026
02095625-0004